EMERGENCY MEDICINE
CAQ Review
for Physician Assistants

Editor-in-Chief

Jessica J. Britnell, MS, PA-C
Emergency Medicine Physician
Assistant Director
Department of Emergency Medicine
Brigham and Women's Hospital
Boston, Massachusetts

Senior Editor
Hannah S. Dodd, MS, PA-C
Chief Physician Assistant
Department of Emergency Medicine
Brigham and Women's Hospital
Boston, Massachusetts

Content Editors

Matthew Brochu, MPH, MS, PA-C
Physician Assistant
Department of Emergency Medicine
Brigham and Women's Hospital
Boston, Massachusetts

Kristen Vella Gray, MS, PA-C
Physician Assistant
Department of Emergency Medicine
Brigham and Women's Hospital
Boston, Massachusetts

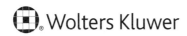 Wolters Kluwer

Philadelphia • Baltimore • New York • London
Buenos Aires • Hong Kong • Sydney • Tokyo

Acquisitions Editor: Jamie E. Elfrank
Product Development Editor: Ashley Fischer
Editorial Assistant: Brian Convery
Marketing Manager: Stephanie Kindlick
Production Project Manager: Marian Bellus
Design Coordinator: Joan Wendt
Manufacturing Coordinator: Beth Welsh
Prepress Vendor: S4Carlisle Publishing Services

Printed in China

Library of Congress Cataloging-in-Publication Data
ISBN-13   978-1-4963-1428-4
ISBN-10   1-4963-1428-X
Available on request from the Publisher

Care has been taken to confirm the accuracy of the information presented and to describe generally accepted practices. However, the authors, editors, and publisher are not responsible for errors or omissions or for any consequences from application of the information in this book and make no warranty, expressed or implied, with respect to the currency, completeness, or accuracy of the contents of the publication. Application of the information in a particular situation remains the professional responsibility of the practitioner.

The authors, editors, and publisher have exerted every effort to ensure that drug selection and dosage set forth in this text are in accordance with current recommendations and practice at the time of publication. However, in view of ongoing research, changes in government regulations, and the constant flow of information relating to drug therapy and drug reactions, the reader is urged to check the package insert for each drug for any change in indications and dosage and for added warnings and precautions. This is particularly important when the recommended agent is a new or infrequently employed drug.

Some drugs and medical devices presented in the publication have Food and Drug Administration (FDA) clearance for limited use in restricted research settings. It is the responsibility of the health care provider to ascertain the FDA status of each drug or device planned for use in their clinical practice.

To purchase additional copies of this book, call our customer service department at (800) 638-3030 or fax orders to (301) 223-2320. International customers should call (301) 223-2300.

Visit Lippincott Williams & Wilkins on the Internet: at LWW.com. Lippincott Williams & Wilkins customer service representatives are available from 8:30 am to 6 pm, EST.

10 9 8 7 6 5 4 3 2 1

Dedication

To Dr. J. Stephen Bohan

Every PA team has a physician champion. You have been that and more: an irreplaceable mentor, professional guide, and an unconditional advocate.

Thank you for opening the doors of Brigham and Women's Emergency Department to the PA profession and teaching us that our career potential is limitless.

With gratitude,

Your EM PA Team

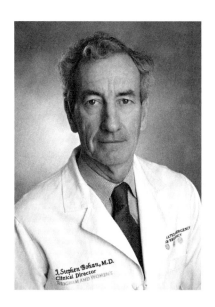

Contributors

Noah Askman, MS, PA-C
Physician Assistant
Department of Emergency Medicine
Brigham and Women's Hospital
Boston, Massachusetts

Heather R. Becker, MS, PA-C
Physician Assistant
Department of Emergency Medicine
Brigham and Women's Hospital
Boston, Massachusetts

MacKenzie Bohlen, MS, PA-C
Physician Assistant
Department of Emergency Medicine
Brigham and Women's Hospital
Boston, Massachusetts

Erin Bradley, MS, PA-C
Physician Assistant
Boston, Massachusetts

Jessica J. Britnell, MS, PA-C
Emergency Medicine Physician Assistant
  Director
Department of Emergency Medicine
Brigham and Women's Hospital
Boston, Massachusetts

Matthew Brochu, MPH, MS, PA-C
Physician Assistant
Department of Emergency Medicine
Brigham and Women's Hospital
Boston, Massachusetts

Michael Cobill, MS, PA-C
Physician Assistant
Department of Emergency Medicine
Brigham and Women's Faulkner
  Hospital
Jamaica Plain, Massachusetts

Donna Collins, MS, PA-C
Physician Assistant
Department of Emergency Medicine
Brigham and Women's Hospital
Boston, Massachusetts

Kelly Devine, MS, PA-C
Physician Assistant
Department of Emergency Medicine
Brigham and Women's Hospital
Boston, Massachusetts

Hannah S. Dodd, MS, PA-C
Chief Physician Assistant
Department of Emergency Medicine
Brigham and Women's Hospital
Boston, Massachusetts

Hana Dubsky, MS, PA-C
Physician Assistant
Department of Emergency Medicine
Brigham and Women's Hospital
Boston, Massachusetts

Nicole Dwyer, PA-C, BS
Physician Assistant
Department of Emergency Medicine
Brigham and Women's Faulkner Hospital
Jamaica Plain, Massachusetts

Rachel Frances, MS, PA-C
Physician Assistant
Department of Emergency Medicine
Brigham and Women's Hospital
Boston, Massachusetts

Patricia Gatcomb, MPH, MS, PA-C
Physician Assistant
Department of Emergency Medicine
Brigham and Women's Hospital
Boston, Massachusetts

Kristen Vella Gray, MS, PA-C
Physician Assistant
Department of Emergency Medicine
Brigham and Women's Hospital
Boston, Massachusetts

Michelle Higgins, MS, PA-C
Physician Assistant
Department of Emergency Medicine
Brigham and Women's Hospital
Boston, Massachusetts

Steven Van Hooser, MS, PA-C
Physician Assistant
Department of Emergency Medicine
Brigham and Women's Faulkner Hospital
Jamaica Plain, Massachusetts

Greg Howarth, MS, PA-C
Physician Assistant
Department of Emergency Medicine
Brigham and Women's Hospital
Boston, Massachusetts

Ashley A. Hughes, MS, PA-C
Physician Assistant
Department of Emergency Medicine
Brigham and Women's Hospital
Boston, Massachusetts

Alaina Iannazzi, MS, PA-C
Physician Assistant
Department of Emergency Medicine
Brigham and Women's Hospital
Boston, Massachusetts

Tara Itrich, MS, PA-C
Physician Assistant
Department of Emergency Medicine
Brigham and Women's Hospital
Boston, Massachusetts

Cathy Jones, MS, PA-C
Physician Assistant
Department of Emergency Medicine
Brigham and Women's Hospital
Boston, Massachusetts

Nicole Kostarellas, MS, PA-C
Physician Assistant
Department of Emergency Medicine
Brigham and Women's Hospital
Boston, Massachusetts

Noelia Kvaternik, MS, PA-C
Physician Assistant
Department of Emergency Medicine
Brigham and Women's Hospital
Boston, Massachusetts

Cathy Llamas, MS, PA-C
Physician Assistant
Department of Emergency Medicine
Brigham and Women's Faulkner Hospital
Jamaica Plain, Massachusetts

Christie Lucente, MS, PA-C
Physician Assistant
Department of Emergency Medicine
Brigham and Women's Hospital
Boston, Massachusetts

AJ Maselli, MS, PA-C
Physician Assistant
Department of Emergency Medicine
Brigham and Women's Hospital
Boston, Massachusetts

Benjamin L Miller, MS, PA-C
Physician Assistant
Department of Emergency Medicine
Signature Healthcare/Brockton Hospital
Brockton, Massachusetts

Carla Novaleski, MS, PA-C
Physician Assistant
Department of Emergency Medicine
Brigham and Women's Hospital
Boston, Massachusetts

Audrey Ranieri, MS, PA-C
Physician Assistant
Department of Emergency Medicine
Brigham and Women's Hospital
Boston, Massachusetts

Mary Beth Samborski, PA-C, MHS
Physician Assistant
Department of Emergency Medicine
Brigham and Women's Hospital
Boston, Massachusetts

Sabrina E. Serino, MS, PA-C
Physician Assistant
Department of Emergency Medicine
Brigham and Women's Hospital
Boston, Massachusetts

Fred Won, MS, PA-C
Physician Assistant
Department of Emergency Medicine
Brigham and Women's Hospital
Boston, Massachusetts

Foreword

Emergency medicine has gone through a number of great evolutionary milestones since its beginnings in a few, scattered centers almost five decades ago. The first of these was the simple recognition that consistent care was required for the most seriously ill and injured patients in society, and that relegating care to a rotating group of interns and residents in medicine and surgery in the academic centers, and rotational or moonlighting physicians in community hospitals, was simply not right. The second milestone was marked by the initiation of residency training programs in emergency medicine in the 1970s, and then energized by the inspirational effort and leadership of those few brave souls who chose to enter these programs, knowing that there was not even the potential for board certification. The third came in 1979, with the first board certification examinations in emergency medicine, and the fourth less than 10 years later, with the formal recognition of emergency medicine as a primary board specialty in the United States. Since then, the specialty has exploded, reaching top three or four status among graduating medical students choosing a specialty and developing broad domain across emergency medical services, disaster preparedness, toxicology, pediatric emergency medicine, emergency ultrasound, resuscitation, and many other related fields.

So, which of these latter developments would I identify as the next great milestone in emergency medicine? Is it the tremendous pace of adoption of emergency ultrasound, the revolution in emergency airway management, the development of board certified sub specialties? Well, no. Although each of these advances, and many others, heralded new directions and scope for emergency care, further enhancing clinical practice, research, and training, none of them, in my opinion, matches the emergence of the physician assistant in a new role as an exceptionally skilled, dedicated, and respected partner in the provision of emergency care.

We have observed the development of the physician assistant in many areas of medicine, but nowhere is the physician assistant as essential and as respected as a clinical colleague as in the emergency departments of hospitals across the nation, ranging from high-volume, tertiary-quaternary level I trauma centers, like my hospital, through busy community hospitals, to smaller centers, challenged by both location and resources. In our department, physician assistants are an essential part of our care team, delivering remarkably proficient and evidence-based care, undertaking procedures, and making incisive diagnoses, all the while demonstrating remarkable professionalism, pride, and leadership that is truly inspiring. In the development of our own department, I count the introduction of physician assistants, over a decade ago, as one of the most influential and positive innovations in our care delivery system. Physician assistants have done something truly exceptional—they have defined a new mode of care delivery, greatly enhancing emergency capability, and have done so in such a way as to make themselves truly indispensible.

This book serves as its own milestone in the climb to specialized care delivery in emergency departments by highly trained physician assistants. Written entirely by physician assistants, for physician assistants, the book is a treasure trove of clinical information, carefully formulated with a question-based format designed to optimally prepare candidates for their emergency medicine examinations. I am indebted to my colleagues, the energetic and visionary physician assistants who have worked tirelessly to produce this valuable work, and to those who will study it, learn from it, and master the core content of emergency medicine, thus taking this next vital step in delivering superior care to those who need it most, that same population of critically ill and injured patients whose precarious conditions spawned an entirely new specialty.

Ron M. Walls, MD
Chair, Department of Emergency Medicine
Brigham and Women's Hospital
Neskey Family Professor of Emergency Medicine
Harvard Medical School

Introduction

About the Certificate of Added Qualifications

National Commission on Certification of Physician Assistants (NCCPA) developed the Certificate of Added Qualifications (CAQ) in 2011 for physician assistants (PAs) to demonstrate a proficiency and expertise in multiple areas of medicine. They offer specialty CAQs in cardiovascular and thoracic surgery, hospital medicine, nephrology, orthopedic surgery, pediatric, psychiatry, and emergency medicine (EM) and continue to add to this list every year. Successful completion of the CAQ provides the PAs with the recognition that they have met certain standards of achievement in their specialty area.

Current CAQ Process for EM

- Documentation of a minimum of 150 hours of Category I CME specific to EM
- ACLS certification
- Certifying EM clinical experience with a minimum experience is 3,000 hours or 18 months of full-time experience working in emergency medicine
- Written certification of your patient management and procedural skills by an EM physician with consideration to a number of specific areas and procedures
- Taking the CAQ examination:
  - The exam contains 120 EM specific questions based on a content blueprint developed by the NCCPA following their 2009 to 2010 PA practice analysis
- After completing all of these requirements and passing the examination, the NCCPA awards the PA the CAQ in EM, which is valid for 10 years as long as the PA-C is maintained and certain specialty-specific CME requirements are maintained.

How to Use This Review Book

This book was written by the Brigham and Women's Health Care Emergency Medicine Physician Assistant team and is currently the first printed and electronic review book for EM PAs looking to achieve the CAQ. The majority of the writers have taken and passed the CAQ exam, and in studying for this, we, ourselves, felt anxious about how to prepare. We understand the importance of passing and wrote this book in order to help our EM PA colleagues feel confident. We enjoyed writing this book and hope that you find it useful as we geared it to EM PAs with 2 years experience. As this book is not all encompassing, we assume that you have a general knowledge and certification of the following:

- Advanced cardiovascular life support
- Pediatric advanced life support
- Advanced trauma life support
- Airway course
- Diagnostic and x-ray interpretation skills

- Lab interpretation
- Pharmacology
- Procedural skills
- HIPPA guidelines

You will notice that the book is organized using the *Content Blueprint* from the NCCPA website by order of the disease and disorder. We have provided the percentage of content on the exam by each chapter title so that you can optimize your study strategy. Our goal was to provide EM PAs across the country an opportunity to have an organized and EM-focused guide to use while studying for this specific examination. It is important to remember that the majority of this content is what you practice in your every day job. We assure you that you need only this review book, your experience, and common sense to pass. You will be prepared!

Tips for Taking the Exam

Given our clinical experience, many of us no longer take written exams frequently and must remember the basics of exam taking. This includes reading the complete test question and thinking about what the answer would be before seeing the actual answers. It is always imperative to look at the exact wording used in the question in order to select the correct answer, such as *most common, gold standard*, etc. It is a timed exam so if you are spending more than 30 seconds on one question, be sure to make an educated guess, flag the question so that you can come back to it, and not dwell on it. Never leave an answer blank in case you don't have time to return to it. A guessed answer is better than no answer at all. Trust your initial instinct and don't change your answers. Studies show your first choice is most often the correct choice. Another strategy is to eliminate the two answers that are clearly wrong, which leaves you with a 50/50 shot. When in doubt—pick C! We recommend, as with all tests, a good night sleep, staying hydrated, a few days off from clinical work prior to exam, and a good breakfast.

Facts About SEMPA

There are currently about 10,000 practicing EM PAs in the United States. This number is only growing as the need for PAs in EM is also increasing. The role of us supporting our professional affiliation, The Society of Emergency Medicine Physician Assistants (SEMPA), as an organized PA voice and representation is imperative in our growth and success as a profession. SEMPA's mission *is to promote and support the professional, clinical, and personal development of PAs involved with emergency medicine and to advance the practice of emergency medicine.* The following is an excerpt taken from SEMPA's website about their own endorsement of the CAQ:

> *The Society of Emergency Medicine Physician Assistants (SEMPA) endorses the National Commission on Certification of Physician Assistants (NCCPA) Certificate of Added Qualifications (CAQ) in emergency medicine as an appropriate measure of knowledge of emergency medical content for physician assistants practicing in emergency medicine. SEMPA further encourages appropriately qualified physician assistants and qualified members to obtain the CAQ in emergency medicine as is deemed necessary for the practice environment, career advancement and objectives of the emergency medicine physician assistant and the attestation of the supervising physician.*

About the Authors and Editors

The authors are the Brigham and Women's Health Care Emergency Medicine PA team, which includes Brigham and Women's Hospital, Brigham and Women's Faulkner Hospital and Foxborough Urgent Care Center.

The editors bring over 25 years of clinical and academic EM experience to the content and knowledge of this book. We are very open and interested in feedback and ideas you may have for future editions as we look to improve. We are very proud of this book and hope you enjoy it. Good luck!

Sincerely,

Editor in Chief: Jessica J. Britnell, MS, PA-C, EM PA Director
Senior Editor: Hannah S. Dodd, MS, PA-C, Chief PA
Content Editors: Matthew Brochu, MPH, MS, PA-C *and*
    Kristen Vella Gray, MS, PA-C

Acknowledgments

Thank you to my family, Ben and Levi; I cannot wait to live by the lake and make happy memories with you.

The PA profession feels like being in a well-kept secret society. . . . we simply have the best jobs in the world. Please stop telling everyone and convince them to go to medical school instead.

Jessica J. Britnell, MS, EM CAQ, PA-C
Editor in Chief

To all the PAs who paved the way, thank you. And to my husband, Eric, who makes me a better person, thanks for making life so fun.

Hannah S. Dodd, MS, EM CAQ, PA-C
Senior Editor

Table of Contents

11 Obstetrics and Gynecology—5% *131*

Heather R. Becker, MacKenzie Bohlen, Hannah S. Dodd, and Noelia Kvaternik

12 Psychobehavioral Disorders—3% *141*

Rachel Frances, Carla Novaleski, and Audrey Ranieri

13 Pulmonary Disorders—9% *153*

Erin Bradley, Kelly Devine, Hannah S. Dodd, Christie Lucente, and Kristen Vella Gray

Abbreviations

AAA abdominal aortic aneurysm
ABC airway, breathing, circulation
ABG arterial blood gas
ACE angiotensin-converting enzyme
ADH antidiuretic hormone
A-fib atrial fibrillation
AIDS acquired immunodeficiency syndrome
AMI acute myocardial infarction syndrome
AMS altered mental status
ARDS acute respiratory distress syndrome
AST aspirate aminotransferase
AV atrioventricular (block)
BP blood pressure
BNP B-type natriuretic peptide
bpm beats per minute
BUN blood urea nitrogen
CA cancer
CBC complete blood count
CHF congestive heart failure
CK creatine kinase
CN cranial nerve
CNS central nervous system
CO cardiac output
COPD chronic obstructive pulmonary disease
CPAP continuous positive airway pressure
Cr creatinine
CSF cerebrospinal fluid
CT computed tomography
CVA costovertebral angle
CXR chest x-ray
DBP diastolic blood pressure
DIC disseminated intravascular coagulation
DKA diabetic ketoacidosis
DRE digital rectal exam
DVT deep venous thrombosis
ECG electrocardiogram
ED emergency department
EDH epidural hematoma

EEG electroencephalogram
EKG electrocardiogram
ENT ear, nose, and throat (specialist)
ESR erythrocyte sedimentation rate
FAST focused assessment with sonography for trauma
FEV1 forced expiratory volume in 1 second
FFP fresh frozen plasma
Fr French (catheter size)
GABA γ-aminobutyric acid
GCS Glasgow coma scale
GI gastrointestinal (specialist)
GIB gastrointestinal bleed
H$_2$ histamine 2
HA headache
HbCO carboxyhemoglobin
hCG human chorionic gonadotropin
HCT hematocrit
HELLP hemolysis, elevated liver enzymes, and low platelets (syndrome)
HIB Haemophilus influenzae type B
HIV human immunodeficiency virus
HOB head of bead
HR heart rate
HRIG human rabies immune globulin
HSV-1 herpes simplex virus type 1
ICH intracranial hemorrhage
ICP intracranial pressure
ICU intensive care unit
IE infective endocarditis
IV intravenous (catheter)
IVF intravenous fluids
IVP intravenous pyelogram
JVD jugular venous distention
JVP jugular venous pressure
KUB kidney, ureter, and bladder
LBO large bowel obstruction
LDH lactate dehydrogenase
LGIB lower gastrointestinal bleed

LP lumbar puncture
LSD lysergic acid diethylamide
LV left ventricular
LVH left ventricular hypertrophy
MI myocardial infarction
mm Hg millimeter of mercury
MRI magnetic resonance imaging
MVC motor vehicle crash
MRSA Methicillin-resistant Staphylococcus aureus
NAC N-acetylcysteine
NGT Nasogastric tube
NIH National Institutes of Health
NOS Not otherwise specified
NPO nothing per os (mouth)
NS normal saline
NSAID nonsteroidal anti-inflammatory drug
NSTEMI non-ST elevation myocardial infarction
O$_2$ oxygen
OB/GYN obstetric/gynecologic
OR operating room
PCI percutaneous coronary intervention
PCN penicillin
PCP phencyclidine
PCR polymerase chain reaction
PE pulmonary embolism
PEP postexposure prophylaxis
PID pelvic inflammatory disease
PNA pneumonia
po per os (by mouth)
POCs products of conception
PPD purified protein derivative
PPI protein pump inhibitor
PT prothrombin time or physical therapist
PTH parathyroid hormone
PTT partial thromboplastin time

PTX pneumothorax
PUD peptic ulcer disease
PZA pyrazinamide
RR respiratory rate
RSV respiratory syncytial virus
RUQ right upper quadrant
SA sinoatrial
SBO small-bowel obstruction
SBP systolic blood pressure
SDH subdural hematoma
SIADH syndrome of inappropriate secretion of ADH
SIRS systemic inflammatory response syndrome
SJS Stevens–Johnson syndrome
SOB shortness of breath
STD sexually transmitted disease
STEMI ST elevation myocardial infarction
STM Streptomycin
T$_3$ triiodothyronine
T$_4$ thyroxine
TB tuberculosis
TBSA total body surface area
TCA tricyclic antidepressant
TEE transesophageal echocardiogram
TIA transient ischemic attack
TM tympanic membrane
TSH thyroid-stimulating hormone
TTP tenderness to palpation
UGIB upper gastrointestinal bleed
US ultrasound
UTI urinary tract infection
VATS video-assisted thoracoscopic surgery
VT ventricular tachycardia
WBC white blood cell
WPW Wolff–Parkinson–White (syndrome)

Abdominal and Gastrointestinal Disorders—10%

1

Heather R. Becker, Jessica J. Britnell,
Hannah S. Dodd, Michelle Higgins,
Nicole Kostarellas, and Kristen Vella Gray

● ANORECTAL DISORDERS

Hemorrhoids

BASICS
- Dilated or bulging veins of hemorrhoidal plexus
- **Internal: above the dentate line**, from the superior cushion (left lateral, right anterior, and right posterior)
- **External: below the dentate line**, from the inferior plexus

ETIOLOGY
- Caused by an increase in pressure in the lower rectum:
  - Straining during bowel movements
  - Sitting for long periods of time on the toilet
  - Chronic diarrhea or constipation
  - Obesity
  - Age
  - Pregnancy

SIGNS AND SYMPTOMS
- Bright red blood per rectum, anal pruritus, prolapse
- Internal are painless; external are painful
- If severe pain, consider thrombosed hemorrhoid

DIAGNOSTICS
- Exam, anoscopy, colonoscopy

TREATMENT
- Pain control, stool softeners, sitz baths, hydrocortisone, banding/surgery
- Incision and removal of clot if thrombosed

Anal Fissure

BASICS
- Tear in the anoderm, distal to the dentate line

ETIOLOGY
- Increased risk with hard stools, chronic diarrhea, anal sex, and vaginal delivery
- Most occur in posterior and anterior line

SIGNS AND SYMPTOMS
- Rectal pain with bowel movements, anal pruritus, minimal bright red blood per rectum
- Many patients will not tolerate digital rectal exam (DRE)
- Most common cause of anorectal pain

DIAGNOSTICS
- History
- Physical exam
- Anoscopy

TREATMENT
- Usually heals within 6 weeks with conservative treatment, stool softeners, pain control, sitz bath, topical nitroglycerin, high-fiber diet

Anorectal Abscess

BASICS
- An abscess in the perianal and perirectal region
- Perianal is the most common anorectal abscess

ETIOLOGY
- Most are result of obstruction of anal gland, which leads to infection and abscess formation

SIGNS AND SYMPTOMS
- Pain and swelling in rectal area
- Tender mass or induration on exam

DIAGNOSTICS
- Physical exam
- CT scan if concern for deeper infection

TREATMENT
- Incision and drainage
- Antibiotics if deeper infection

Pilonidal Cyst

BASICS
- Occur in the upper midline buttock cleft
- High rates of reoccurrence

ETIOLOGY
- Caused by ingrown hair

SIGNS AND SYMPTOMS
- Pain, swelling, redness, fluctuance in gluteal cleft

DIAGNOSTICS
- Physical exam

TREATMENT
- Incision and drainage
- Routine antibiotics are not indicated

APPENDICITIS

BASICS
- Inflammation of appendix
- Most common surgical emergency
- Males > females
- Most common between 10 and 30 years old
  - Perforation rate as high as 80% if <3 years old and >60 years old
- Three percent mortality when perforated

ETIOLOGY
- Due to luminal obstruction
  - Most common cause is fecalith
  - Other causes: tumors, adhesions, dietary matter, hyperplasia of lymphoid tissue
- Organisms usually anaerobic and gram negative
  - Most common: *Bacteroides fragilis* and *E. coli*

SIGNS AND SYMPTOMS
- Diffuse, poorly localized (visceral) pain → right lower quadrant pain between 12 and 24 hours
- ±Fever, anorexia, nausea and vomiting, and urge to defecate, with diarrhea being uncommon
  - Caution: variations in children, elderly, and pregnancy
- Location of appendix determines clinical findings and risk for perforation
  - Retrocecal appendix may localize to right flank; retroileal in men may localize to testicles; pelvic may irritate bladder/rectum with dysuria, suprapubic pain, and urge to defecate; low lying may cause rectal pain
- In pregnancy, patients may have pain in right upper quadrant (RUQ)
- Exam findings: guarding, rebound, and the following special signs:
  - **McBurney**: tender one-third distance from anterior superior iliac crest to umbilicus
    - Only 50% with appendix located within 5 cm of McBurney
  - **Psoas sign:** pain elicited when patient flexes right hip against resistance
  - **Obturator sign**: pain elicited with passive flexion and internal rotation of right hip
  - **Rovsing sign:** manual pressure in left lower quadrant causes pain in right lower quadrant

DIAGNOSTICS
- Elevations of white blood cell (WBC) and C-reactive protein associated with increased likelihood
- Ultrasound: enlarged tender appendix >6 mm with hyperechoic surrounding fat, inability to compress appendix, periappendiceal fluid, and hypervascularity
  - Large variations in sensitivity, increased in thin patients and children
- CT: appendix >7 to 10 mm diameter, wall enhancement, wall thickening >3 mm, and fat stranding
  - Ninety percent sensitive
- MRI in patients where radiation exposure is contraindicated and ultrasound is nondiagnostic (i.e., pregnancy)

TREATMENT
- Surgical removal
- Prophylactic antibiotics to reduce infection
- Complications include perforation and abscess
  - Requires prompt antibiotics with gram-negative and anaerobic coverage

● CHOLECYSTITIS, BILIARY TRACT DISEASE, AND PANCREATITIS

Cholelithiasis

BASICS
- Stones in gallbladder (GB)

ETIOLOGY
- Most common gallstone composition contains cholesterol
- Risk factors: five Fs.
  - Female
  - Fat
  - Fertile
  - Forty
  - Fair

SIGNS AND SYMPTOMS
- Pain in RUQ with radiation to epigastrium or right scapular associated with nausea and vomiting, diaphoresis, often after fatty meal
- Symptoms from 30 minutes to several hours with days or months between episodes
- Exam usually normal because pain is visceral as GB is not inflamed

DIAGNOSTICS
- Ultrasound: presence of stones
- Labs including liver function tests (LFTs), lipase, complete blood count

TREATMENT
- Pain control, dietary changes
- Surgical referral

Cholecystitis

BASICS
- Inflammation of gall bladder

ETIOLOGY
- Inflammation of GB due to obstruction of cystic duct with superimposed infection
  - Common pathogens: *E. coli*, *Klebsiella*, enterococci, and anaerobes

SIGNS AND SYMPTOMS
- Pain is severe, constant, lasting longer than 6 hours worse with movement and deep breaths
- Ill appearing, vomiting, and fever should raise suspicion
- **Murphy's sign**: cessation of inspiration upon palpation in RUQ

DIAGNOSTICS
- Elevations in WBC and LFTs, but may be normal
- Ultrasound: **sonographic Murphy sign**, pericholecystic fluid, GB wall thickening >4 to 5 mm or edema (double wall sign), common bile duct (CBD) dilation >6 mm, intrahepatic, and extra hepatic biliary ductal dilation
  - Ultrasound findings have a 90% positive predictive value
- If ultrasound unclear, hepatic iminodiacetic acid scan (hepatoiminodiacetic acid) is more sensitive and study of choice

TREATMENT
- NPO (nothing per os [mouth]), intravenous fluids (IVF), antiemetics, and analgesics

- Empiric antibiotics: third- or fourth-generation cephalosporin such as ceftazidime and Flagyl
  - Alternatively: combo of β-lactam and β-lactam inhibitor such as Unasyn or Zosyn
- Cholecystectomy for acute cholecystitis within a few days of initial evaluation to decrease morbidity and morality
- Percutaneous cholecystostomy for drainage may be necessary in those who are critically ill or have contraindications to surgery
  - Most common post-op complication: bile leakage
    - ○ Treatment is endoscopic retrograde cholangiopancreatography (ERCP) and stent placement

Acalculous Cholecystitis

- Clinically identical but not associated with gallstone
- Suspect in patients with traumatic injuries, burns, critical illness, total parenteral nutrition (TPN)
- Mortality twice as high as calculus cholecystitis

Choledocholithiasis

BASICS

- The presence of at least one gallstone in the CBD

SIGNS AND SYMPTOMS

- Similar manifestations to biliary colic, ± jaundice, but pain usually more prolonged than with typical colic

DIAGNOSTICS

- Greater than 90% will have elevations in LFTs
- Obstruction of CBD will lead to elevations of bilirubin but usually <15 mg per dL because obstruction is usually intermittent
- Ultrasound: initial imaging modality of choice, but 20% to 90% sensitivity for CBD stones
- ERCP, magnetic resonance cholangiopancreatography, CT with IV contrast may also be used

TREATMENT

- ERCP with sphincterotomy
- Surgery is needed for removal of stones that do not spontaneously pass

Cholangitis

BASICS

- Infection of CBD
- Associated with 5% mortality

ETIOLOGY

- Eighty percent of cases due to obstructing gallstones
  - Most common inciting pathogens: *E. coli*, *Streptococcus*, *Clostridium*, and *Bacteroides*

SIGNS AND SYMPTOMS

- **Charcot triad**: fever, jaundice, RUQ pain
- Reynold pentad: Charcot triad plus shock and altered mental status
- *Caution*: elderly may not complain of RUQ pain

DIAGNOSTICS

- Transaminase levels may be elevated
- Ultrasound and CT low sensitivity
- Magnetic resonance cholangiopancreatography and ERCP detect stones

TREATMENT

- Admit for biliary drainage, surgery consult, gastrointestinal (GI) consult

- Antibiotics
  - Combination treatment with extended spectrum cephalosporin, Flagyl, and ampicillin
    - OR single agent or combination fluoroquinolone
- ERCP with sphincterotomy associated with lowest mortality

Tumors of Biliary Tree and GB

BASICS
- Relatively rare ranging from papillomas and adenomas, which are benign, to carcinoma and cholangiocarcinoma
  - Carcinoma uncommon, associated with chronic cholecystitis and porcelain GB, most commonly arising from fundus or neck
  - Cholangiocarcinoma refers to tumor anywhere from intrahepatic ducts to CBD, spreads through duct wall, extending to lymph nodes, peritoneum, GB, and often liver

SIGNS AND SYMPTOMS
- Painless jaundice and pruritus (suggest obstructing mass distal to biliary tree), malaise, weight loss
- RUQ pain, hepatomegaly, abdominal mass may be palpable

DIAGNOSTICS
- Ultrasound and CT have 60% to 70% sensitivity for detecting carcinoma of GB
- Metastasis present in 50% at diagnosis, 1 year survival rate is 14%

TREATMENT
- ERCP, biopsy, oncology referral

Pancreatitis

BASICS
- Inflammation and self-destruction of pancreas by digestive enzymes
- Males > females; 40 to 60 years old
- Risk factors for severe disease or necrotizing pancreatitis: >55 years old, obesity, pleural effusions, or infiltrates
- Most common complication is pseudocyst

ETIOLOGY
- Most common causes:
  - Alcohol (direct toxin to pancreas)
  - Gallstones (obstruction of pancreatic or CBD)
- Less common: hyperlipidemia, hypercalcemia, medications, infection (mumps), toxins, trauma, surgery, iatrogenic, hereditary, 20% idiopathic
- Usually self-limited but small percentage will lead to multisystem organ failure, systemic inflammatory response syndrome, and death

SIGNS AND SYMPTOMS
- Rapid, severe, constant epigastric pain that may radiate to back
- Pain often worse supine, often associated with nausea and vomiting, anorexia
- Fever and tachycardia common
- Jaundice seen with obstructive etiology
- Abdominal tenderness to palpation with hypoactive bowel sounds and guarding
- Exam findings (rarely seen but associated with hemorrhagic pancreatitis and poor prognosis)
  1. Grey Turner's sign = ecchymosis on flank
  2. Cullen's sign = ecchymosis around umbilicus

TABLE 1.1.	**Ranson Criteria can be used to predict the severity of acute pancreatitis**	

	Ranson Criteria	
ED Presentation	**48 hr Admission**	
Age >55	HCT drop >10%	
WBC >16,000	BUN rise >5	
Glucose >300	Base deficit >4	
AST >250	Ca <8	
LDH >350	Arterial PaO$_2$ <60	
	Fluid sequestration >6 L	

	Prognosis	
Number of Criteria Met	**Mortality Rate**	
0–2	<5%	
3–4	15%–20%	
5–6	40%	
>6	Almost 100%	

BUN, blood urea nitrogen; HCT, hematocrit; LDH, lactate dehydrogenase.

DIAGNOSTICS
- Lipase: more sensitive and specific than amylase
- Alanine aminotransferase >150 suggests gallstone pancreatitis
- Ultrasound: used to evaluate gallstones, pseudocysts, CBD dilatation
- CT: not necessary unless concerned about complications such as pseudocyst, abscess, necrosis
- MRI: superior to CT for categorizing fluid collections, abscesses, hemorrhage, and pseudocysts

Ranson Criteria
- Predicts the severity of acute pancreatitis, based on 11 signs
- 5 measured on admission and 6 measured 48 hours later (less useful in ED) (Table 1.1)

TREATMENT
- Mainstay treatment is NPO, IVFs, pain control
- Morphine often avoided because of potential to cause spasm of Oddi and worsen symptoms (this is not evidence based and often considered myth)
- Antibiotics only indicated for septic patient
- Most patients require admission, but mild cases may be managed as outpatients if pain controlled and tolerating po

● ESOPHAGEAL DISORDERS
Peptic Ulcer Disease
BASICS
- Include duodenal and gastric ulcers
- Most common cause of acute upper GI bleeding (UGIB)

ETIOLOGY
- Causes: *Helicobacter pylori*, nonsteroidal anti-inflammatory drugs, hypersecretory peptic states

SIGNS AND SYMPTOMS
- Burning, epigastric pain
- Pain worsened by food, suggestive of gastric ulcers
- Pain relieved with food and antacids, suggestive of duodenal ulcers
- Associated with nausea, anorexia, bloating
- Physical exam findings show epigastric tenderness

DIAGNOSTICS
- Endoscopy

TREATMENT
- H2 receptor antagonists (famotidine)
- Proton pump inhibitor (PPI) (omeprazole)
- *H. pylori*: PPI + two antibiotics (tetracycline/Flagyl/clarithromycin/amox) + Bismuth for 7 to 14 days

Esophageal Varices

BASICS
- Dilated submucosal veins causing an upper GI bleed
- Usually caused by portal hypertension
- Highest morbidity and mortality than any other source of UGIB
- Many patients with varices have coagulopathy due to underlying cirrhosis caused by alcohol or hepatitis

SIGNS AND SYMPTOMS
- Most commonly present with hematemesis
  - Bright red blood or coffee grounds
- Jaundice, medusae, angiomata, palm erythema, asterixis, melena (black tarry stools)

DIAGNOSTICS
- Emergent endoscopy

TREATMENT
- ABCs (airway, breathing, circulation), IV fluids, packed red blood cells, PPI, octreotide
- Sclerotherapy, banding under endoscopy
- Balloon tamponade with Sengstaken–Blakemore tube for severe bleeding
- **GI consult and ICU admission**

Mallory–Weiss Tear

BASICS
- Partial-thickness mucosal tear of the distal esophagus caused by vomiting

SIGNS AND SYMPTOMS
- Hematemesis
- Retching and vomiting
- Tachycardia

DIAGNOSTICS
- Endoscopy (can be done outpatient if patient stable)
- Upright chest x-ray to evaluate for free air for **Boerhaave syndrome**
  - Complete esophageal rupture after forceful emesis
  - Most lethal perforation of the GI tract
  - Mortality of 35%
  - Requires emergent surgical repair and broad-spectrum antibiotics

TREATMENT
- Self-limiting, antiemetics, po challenge

GASTROENTERITIS, COLITIS, AND DIVERTICULITIS

Gastroenteritis

BASICS
- Acute inflammation of the intestinal epithelial lining of the GI tract

ETIOLOGY
- Viral: **Norwalk virus** (most common), Rotavirus, Enterovirus
- Bacterial: *Salmonella*, *Shigella*, *E. coli*, *Clostridium difficile*, *Campylobacter* (see Chapter 15)
- Parasites: *Giardia*, *Cryptosporidium*, *Entamoeba*

SIGNS AND SYMPTOMS
- Nausea, vomiting, diarrhea
- Abdominal cramping
- Tachycardia, dehydration

DIAGNOSTICS
- Clinical
- Must have both vomiting and diarrhea
- Consider labs including BMP for electrolyte abnormality
- Consider stool cultures if clinically indicated, such as recent antibiotic use or travel

TREATMENT
- IV fluids, antiemetics, po challenge
- Correction of electrolyte abnormalities
- Anticholinergic agents are not recommended for diarrhea management in children

Colitis

BASICS
- Inflammation of the bowels ranging from mild to moderate to severe
- Inflammatory bowel disease (IBD)
  - Ulcerative colitis: inflammation of the mucosal layer of the colon
    - Bloody diarrhea is hallmark
  - Crohn's disease: transmural inflammation with skip lesions, may involve the entire GI tract (mouth to perianal)
- Antibiotic associated
  - *C. difficile*—can lead to toxic megacolon
    - Causative agents include clindamycin, fluoroquinolones, and penicillins

SIGNS AND SYMPTOMS
- Crampy, lower abdominal pain
- Diarrhea
- Fever

DIAGNOSTICS
- Stool studies
- Elevated WBC especially with *C. difficile*
- CT scan
- Colonoscopy/biopsy

TREATMENT

- IV fluids, pain control
- *C. difficile*
  - Nonsevere infection—po Flagyl 500 mg tid for 10 to 14 days or po vancomycin 125 mg qid
  - Severe infection—indicated by clinical judgment, but many also consider WBC >15,000 or elevated serum Cr ≥1.5 times the premorbid level; po or enema vancomycin may be given in combination with IV Flagyl
  - IV vancomycin has *no* effect on *C. difficile* as it is not excreted in the colon
  - Surgery for toxic megacolon, necrotizing colitis, perforation or impending perforation, or rapidly progressing disease with multi-end organ damage
- IBD: 5-amiosalicylic acid, mesalamine, steroids

Diverticulitis

BASICS

- Inflammation of diverticula, causing micro- or macroscopic perforation
- Most often located in sigmoid colon, with one-third present in proximal colon
- Complications: abscess, obstruction, perforation

ETIOLOGY

- Decreased fecal bulk and increased intraluminal pressures result in thickened colonic diverticula
- Wall weakness and bacterial invasion cause inflammation of diverticular sac
- Incidence increases with age. More than one-third of patients over age of 60 have diverticular disease
- Increased risk in a high-fat/low-fiber diet

SIGNS AND SYMPTOMS

- Most common symptoms: **left lower quadrant abdominal tenderness**
- Nausea, vomiting
- Diarrhea/constipation
- Fifty percent of patients have heme positive stool
- Sterile pyuria due to adjacent inflammation

DIAGNOSTICS

- CT shows localized bowel wall thickening, fat stranding, abscess

TREATMENT

- Conservative: NPO, IVF, antibiotics (Cipro and Flagyl po/IV for 10 to 14 days, alternatives: Augmentin, Clindamycin, Moxifloxacin)
- Surgery is considered in case of perforation
- Colonoscopy is contraindicated in acute diverticulitis but recommended 6 weeks after recovery to rule out cancer
- Prevention of diverticular disease includes high-fiber diet and stool softeners

● GI HEMORRHAGE

GI Bleeds

BASICS

- UGIB
  - proximal to ligament of Treitz
- Lower GI bleed (LGIB)
  - distal to ligament of Treitz

ETIOLOGY

- UGIB
  - Peptic ulcer disease (PUD)
    - *H. pylori*: most common cause of PUD
    - Nonsteroidal anti-inflammatory drug or aspirin use
    - Heavy alcohol
  - Variceal bleeds
  - Mallory–Weiss tear
- LGIB
  - Hemorrhoids and diverticulosis are the most common cause
  - Ischemic colitis
  - Ulcerative colitis

SIGNS AND SYMPTOMS

- UGIB
  - Melena
  - Epigastric pain
  - Hematemesis
- LGIB
  - Bright red blood per rectum
  - Weakness, dizziness
  - Hypotensive

DIAGNOSTICS

- DRE
- Anoscopy
- Complete blood count, LFTs, coags, type, and cross
- Colonoscopy, endoscopy
- Tagged red cell scan
- Upright chest x-ray for free air if perforation is suspected

TREATMENT

- ABCs, resuscitation/supportive: two large-bore IVs, IV fluids, packed red blood cells, telemetry/EKG
- Consider octreotide for varices
- Consider PPI bolus/drip
- GI consult
- Pitfalls
  - Not recognizing signs of shock
  - Delay in GI consult

● HEPATITIS

BASICS

- Inflammation of the liver causing dysfunction
- Can be chronic or acute

ETIOLOGY

- Drugs, alcohol, ingestions (Tylenol and other hepatic toxic, medications, and mushrooms)
- Environmental exposures (industrial chemicals, cleaning material, mushroom picking)

- Autoimmune liver disease, or Wilson's disease (copper toxicity), hemochromatosis, hepatobiliary disease
- Viral:
  - Hepatitis A and E are transmitted via fecal–oral route, contaminated food or water supply, or poor sanitation
  - Hepatitis B, C, and D are transmitted through blood, or sexual contact of infected saliva, semen, vaginal secretions
  - Hepatitis B and C more common with MSM, and hospital employees are at increased risk
  - Hepatitis C seen with history of blood transfusions, IVDU, tattoos

SIGNS AND SYMPTOMS

- Anorexia, nausea, vomiting, fatigue
- Jaundice, hepatomegaly, fever, RUQ tenderness
- Labs may include a normal to low WBC, low platelets, abnormal coags, abnormal/elevated LFTs

DIAGNOSTICS

- Acute or chronic elevations in aspartate aminotransferase (AST), alanine aminotransferase, bilirubin, alkaline phosphatase
- Complications include cirrhosis/liver failure, therefore elevated coagulation factors, pancytopenia
- Hepatitis A: + IgM anti-HAV (acute phase), IgG anti-HAV (previous exposure)
- Hepatitis B:
  - + HBsAg in early and late infection, may remain elevated. + When initially vaccinated
  - + Anti-HBs (antibody) with (–) HBsAg when they have successfully been vaccinated/immune
  - + IgM anti-HBc early phase of acute hepatitis B, + IgG acute phase but also will remain indefinitely and with + HBsAg would indicate chronic hepatitis B
  - + HBeAg and HBV DNA indicate viral infectivity, and replication is present
- Hepatitis D: + anti-HDV and HDV RNA in combination with hepatitis B infection
- Hepatitis C: + anti-HCV, + RIBA, + HCV RNA

TREATMENT

- Symptomatic fluids, antiemetics, pain management, rest
- Avoid, educate and provide treatment for high-risk behaviors (i.e., ETOH abuse, IVDU, high-risk sexual behavior)
- Reverse Tylenol toxicity: *N*-acetylcysteine (NAC), ABCs, supportive
- Hepatitis A: advise not to share food and dishes, and frequently wash hands
  - Immune serum globulin IM if traveling to high-risk locations
- Acute hepatitis B: no recommended antivirals
- Acute hepatitis C: interferon alpha or peginterferon × 6 to 24 weeks. Peginterferon with Ribavirin or with a protease inhibitor
- Arrange for close follow-up, further diagnostic for other associated conditions, including HIV, liver failure

● BOWEL OBSTRUCTIONS

BASICS

- Obstruction of intestine with distal bowel dilation
- Can be divided into small bowel obstruction (SBO) and large bowel obstruction (LBO) depending on location and typically have different causes

ETIOLOGY

- Most common causes of SBO are **adhesions**
- Other causes: hernias, neoplasm, intussusception, Crohn's
- Most common cause of LBO: mass, most often malignant

SIGNS AND SYMPTOMS
- Colicky abdominal pain, nausea and vomiting, distention, lack of flatus
  - Fever in patient with bowel obstruction suggests strangulation and perforation
- Bowel sounds range from high-pitched tinkling (borborygmi) versus absent, which is an ominous sign of perforation or peritonitis
- Perform rectal exam looking for fecal impaction in elderly or occult blood in cases of strangulated obstruction, intussusception, or an obstructing mass

DIAGNOSTICS
- Supine and upright KUB (kidney, ureter, and bladder)
  - Multiple air fluid levels and dilated loops of small bowel
  - More than 3 mm of thickened small bowel, >3 cm of dilated small bowel
  - Air in distal colon and rectum implies early or partial SBO
- Consider CT to exclude diagnosis of closed loop obstruction
  - Ileus distinguished from mechanical obstruction by presence of air fluid levels at uniform heights on upright; various heights with obstruction

TREATMENT
- NPO, bowel rest, IV fluids, pain control, antiemetics
- Gastric decompression with nasogastric tube
- Surgical consultation and admission
- Four categories of LBOs with variable treatment:
  - Mechanical (surgical treatment)
  - Sigmoid volvulus (nonoperative decompression ± rectal tube then elective surgery to prevent recurrence)
  - Cecal volvulus (right colectomy)
  - Pseudo-obstruction (nonsurgical with decompression, colonoscopy, promotility agents, and then surgery if conservative management fails)

● MESENTERIC ISCHEMIA

BASICS
- Insufficient blood supply to mesentery and intestines
- Greater than 50% embolism to SMA, 25% thrombus of SMA, 20% nonocclusive, but in a "low-flow state" such as shock
- Mortality rate 70% (usually from missed or late diagnosis)

ETIOLOGY
- Embolism
  - SMA embolism number one cause
  - Atrial fibrillation
- Hypoperfusion
  - Low-flow states including congestive heart failure, shock
- Thrombosis
  - Hypercoagulable states including cancer or pregnancy
- Blood supply is insufficient → cannot meet metabolic demand → bowel infarction → perforation → sepsis → death

SIGNS AND SYMPTOMS
- Vague diffuse abdominal pain, usually the elderly with history of coronary artery disease, Afib
- If young, consider cocaine or hypercoagulable state
- Postprandial pain

- **Pain out of proportion to exam** (exam may be normal!)
- Late presentation may reveal signs of shock or peritonitis, no bowel sounds
- Leukocytosis, metabolic acidosis, elevated lactic acid, systemic inflammatory response syndrome/*sepsis* criteria

DIAGNOSISTICS
- KUB often normal in early stages, with classic "thumb printing" of bowel in late stages
- CT: bowel wall thickening, pneumatosis
- Gold standard: angiography

TREATMENT
- ABCs, IV fluids, anticoagulation if necessary, broad-spectrum IV antibiotics
- Early surgical evaluation for embolectomy with resection of necrotic bowel
- Pitfalls
  - Not considering the diagnosis
  - Delay in treatment or surgical consult

● NAUSEA AND VOMITING, DIARRHEA, AND CONSTIPATION
Nausea and Vomiting
BASICS
- Upper GI communication with neuro system and lower gut
- Nausea is the unpleasant feeling that one wants/needs to vomit
- Vomiting is the act of expelling gastric contents

ETIOLOGY
- Central (neurologic): associated with motion (motion sickness), dizziness (vertigo)
- Infectious, viral gastro, acute gastritis
- Mechanical: bowel obstruction
- Medication: narcotics, antibiotics, etc.
- Post-op
- Chemo
- Pregnancy
- Gastritis, GERD
- Gastroparesis
- Pancreatitis
- Gastric outlet obstruction
- Cyclic vomiting syndrome (may be marijuana-induced/psychiatric)

SIGNS AND SYMPTOMS
- Upper GI communication with neuro system and lower gut causing nausea with subsequent expulsion of gastric contents

TREATMENT
- Treat dehydration, electrolyte abnormality, metabolic alkalosis, malnutrition if chronic
- Antiemetics (Compazine, Zofran, Phenergan, Reglan)
- Targeted therapy used to treat the underlying cause

Diarrhea
BASICS
- Frequent loose, watery stools often associated with pain, cramping
- Types

- Acute: <14 days
- Persistent: <1 month
- Chronic: >30 days

ETIOLOGY
- Acute/persistent caused by (bacteria, virus, or parasite)
  - Virus: norovirus, rotavirus, adenoviruses
  - Bacteria: *Salmonella*, *Campylobacter*, *Shigella*, enterotoxigenic *E. coli*, *C. difficile*, *Listeria*
  - Parasites/protozoa: *Cryptosporidium*, *Giardia*, *Cyclospora*, *Entamoeba*, and others
- Chronic
  - Caused by (noninfectious)
  - Crohn's, ulcerative colitis, malabsorption syndrome, microscopic colitis, history of cholecystectomy, bowel resection, dumping syndrome, chemo, radiation, laxative abuse, hyperthyroidism, medications, food (lactulose intolerance, fatty foods), celiac disease

SIGNS AND SYMPTOMS
- Watery stools
- Bloody stools
- Lower abdominal cramping
- Fevers
- Diffuse myalgias, or arthralgias

DIAGNOSTICS
- Testing population:
  - Ill-appearing, pregnant women
  - Elderly
  - Bloody diarrhea
  - High fevers
  - Severe abdominal pain
  - Immunosuppression
  - Irritable bowel syndrome (IBS)/Crohn's
- Stool tests
  - Cultures
  - Fecal leukocyte
  - Stool ova and parasites
  - CT abdomen for severe abdominal pain, elderly, immune compromised

TREATMENT
- Oral rehydration with glucose and Na, IV fluids if needed
- Antibiotics if clinically indicated
  - Immunocompromised, recent travel

Constipation
BASICS
- Less than three stools per week
- Change from regular bowel pattern

ETIOLOGY
- Stool moves slowly through GI tract allowing water reabsorption; increased drying to stools → increased difficulty stooling
- Underlying bowel disease (IBS) and anatomical abnormalities (rectocele, fistula, rectal pain, hemorrhoid, prolapse, or rectal mass) may also affect adequate stooling

■ Decreased muscle tone of the muscles to of the lower GI and rectum
■ Dehydration, diet, and activity

SIGNS AND SYMPTOMS
■ Experience a sense of rectal blockage
■ Feeling of incomplete evacuation after stooling
■ Abdominal distention
■ Bloating
■ Fullness and pain

DIAGNOSTICS
■ Rectal exam
■ Anoscopy
■ KUB can reveal heavy stool burden

TREATMENT
■ Fluids
■ High-fiber diet, fiber supplement
■ Stool softeners
  • Colace
■ Laxatives
  • Stimulants: cause rhythmic contractions in the intestines
    ○ Docusate, bisacodyl
  • Lubricants: enable stool to move easier through the colon
    ○ Mineral oil
  • Osmotics: help fluids to move through the colon
    ○ Miralax, Mg citrate
  • Saline laxatives: act like a sponge to draw water into the colon for easier passage of stool
■ Suppositories/enema: locally at the site of the rectum
  • Fleets
■ Manual disimpaction
■ Surgical repair of underlying cause (fistula, rectocele, prolapse)

● PEDIATRIC ABDOMINAL PAIN
Intussusception

BASICS
■ Most common abdominal emergency in children <2 years old, peak 10 to 12 months
■ Occurs when one loop of intestine telescopes into another segment of bowel
  • Ileocolic region most common

ETIOLOGY
■ Likely idiopathic
■ Fifty percent have recent viral illness

SIGNS AND SYMPTOMS
■ Vomiting, episodic, colicky abdominal pain, screaming episodes with hip and knee flexion, ± lethargy
■ Classic triad (>75% have two of these)
  • Vomiting
  • Colicky abdominal pain
  • "Currant jelly" stools

- **Sausage-shaped mass** in RUQ may be present
- Guaiac positive stools, late finding due to bowel ischemia

DIAGNOSTICS
- Barium enema
  - "Coiled spring" = layers of intestine within intestine

TREATMENT
- Barium enemas are both diagnostic and therapeutic
- If barium enema does not work, surgery is needed for reduction
- Ten percent recur within 24 hours and thus admission for 24 hour observation is recommended

Meckel Diverticulum

BASICS
- Most common congenital abnormality of the small intestine
- **Rule of 2s:**
  - 2% of the population
  - 2 feet proximal to the ileocecal valve
  - 2 inches in length
  - 2 types of tissue: gastric and pancreatic
  - 2 years is the most common age
  - 2:1 male: female ratio

ETIOLOGY
- Incomplete obliteration of the vitelline duct, causing an outpouching or bulge in the lower part of the small intestine
- A small number of people have a Meckel diverticulum, but only a few develop symptoms

SIGNS AND SYMPTOMS
- Most are asymptomatic
- **Hematochezia is the most common sign in children**
- Abdominal pain and tenderness

DIAGNOSTICS
- Difficult to diagnose
- Technetium scan and/or colonoscopy

TREATMENT
- Supportive
- Surgery to remove diverticulum if bleeding occurs

Pyloric Stenosis

BASICS
- Thickening of the pylorus, causing obstruction

ETIOLOGY
- Exact cause unknown
- Thought to be genetic and environmental

SIGNS AND SYMPTOMS
- Occurs between 2 and 12 weeks of age
- **Projectile vomiting**
- Weight loss, irritability
- **Olive-shaped mass in RUQ**

DIAGNOSTICS
- Ultrasound

TREATMENT
- Supportive, nasogastric tube
- Surgery

Volvulus

BASICS
- An emergent condition
- Twisting of the bowel, which can lead to necrosis

ETIOLOGY
- Intestinal malrotation, which occurs during fetal development

SIGNS AND SYMPTOMS
- Occurs during first 1 and 3 weeks of life
- Bloody stools, distended abdomen
- Bilious emesis

DIAGNOSTICS
- KUB may show "double bubble" sign
- Barium enema
- Upper GI

TREATMENT
- Surgical emergency

● SPONTANEOUS BACTERIAL PERITONITIS (SBP)

BASICS
- Infection of ascitic fluid
- Commonly seen in patients with severe chronic liver disease, cancer

ETIOLOGY
- Bacterial infection of the intestinal barrier to peritoneum most commonly caused by *E. Coli* or *Klebsiella*

SIGNS AND SYMPTOMS
- Suspect SBP in patients with cirrhosis and one of the following
  - Abdominal pain, fever, encephalopathy, mental status change

DIAGNOSTICS
- High clinical suspicion in patients with cirrhosis as symptoms can be mild
- Paracentesis
  - Send fluid for cell count with differential, culture, pH

TREATMENT
- Third-generation cephalosporin or Unasyn

NOTES

NOTES

Cardiovascular Disorders—11%

Jessica J. Britnell, Kelly Devine, Hannah S. Dodd,
Ashley A. Hughes, and Mary Beth Samborski

● ACUTE CORONARY SYNDROME (ACS)

BASICS
- Unstable angina (UA)
  - Rest angina >20 minutes
  - New onset angina
  - Increasing angina (change from usual pattern of angina)
- Non-ST elevation myocardial infarction (NSTEMI)
  - UA and elevated cardiac markers
- ST elevation myocardial infarction (STEMI)
  - UA and new ST elevation or new left bundle branch block (LBBB)

ETIOLOGY
- Myocardial ischemia resulting from inadequate perfusion to meet oxygen demand
- Coronary artery stenosis
- Thrombus formation
- Vasospasm (Prinzmetal angina)
- Risk factors: age, male sex, diabetes mellitus, hypertension (HTN), hyperlipidemia, smoking, family history of premature coronary artery disease

SIGNS AND SYMPTOMS
- Chest pain: dull, pressure, discomfort, tightness, heaviness
- Gradual onset, substernal, radiating to upper extremity, reproduced with exertion
- Dyspnea, nausea, vomiting, diaphoresis, weakness, dizziness, fatigue, anxiety, neck or jaw pain (diabetic patients and females may present atypically)

DIAGNOSTICS
- Twelve-lead EKG within 10 minutes (Table 2.1)
- Initial EKG often not diagnostic, repeat in 5 to 10 minutes if highly suspicious
- STEMI: new ST elevation at the J point in two anatomically contiguous limb leads
  - ≥1 mm, or ≥2 mm in two anatomically contiguous precordial leads
  - Or new LBBB
- NSTEMI or UA: new horizontal or downsloping ST depression ≥0.5 mm in two anatomically contiguous leads, and /or T-wave inversion ≥ 1mm in two anatomically contiguous leads, with prominent R waves or *R/S ratio* >1
- Cardiac biomarkers: troponin T and I, CK-MB

TABLE 2.1.	**EKG Changes and Vessels Affected in AMI**	
Location of MI	**EKG Leads Affected**	**Vessel Involved**
Anterior wall	V1–V6	LAD
Inferior wall	II, III, AVF	RCA, circumflex
Posterior	V1–V4	RCA, circumflex
Anterolateral	I, AVL, V5, V6	LAD, circumflex
Anteroseptal	I, AVL, V1–V4	LAD

LAD, left anterior descending; RCA, right coronary artery.

TREATMENT

- ABCs (airway, breathing, circulation), O_2, IV
- Cardiac monitoring
- Aspirin 325 mg chewed and swallowed
- Nitrates and morphine
  - Nitrate contraindications include erectile dysfunction drugs and right ventricular (RV) involvement (inferior myocardial infarction [MI]), as preload dependence may cause severe hypotension
  - Use fentanyl for pain if hypotensive
- Consider nitro paste/drip in UA/NSTEMI patients with persistent pain
- β-Blockers
  - **STEMI**
    - Selection and implementation of optimal reperfusion strategy, usually percutaneous coronary intervention (PCI)
    - American Heart Association guidelines recommend maximum "door to balloon" time of 90 minutes
    - Treat with fibrinolysis if PCI unavailable within 90 to 120 minutes, symptoms <12 hours, and no contraindications
  - **NSTEMI and UA**
    - Should *not be treated with fibrinolysis*
    - **Thrombolysis in myocardial infarction risk stratification**
      - Age ≥65
      - At least three risk factors for coronary artery disease: HTN, diabetes mellitus, lipids, smoking, family history of early MI
      - Prior coronary stenosis of ≥50%
      - Presence of ST changes of at least 0.5 mm on ECG
      - At least two anginal episodes in prior 24 hours
      - Elevated serum cardiac biomarkers
      - Use of aspirin in prior 7 days
    - One point for each value present, 0 if absent
    - Low risk = 0 to 2, intermediate risk = 3 to 4, high risk = 5 to 7
    - High and intermediate risk benefit from early coronary revascularization
  - **Other Therapies Used in ACS**
    - Antiplatelet therapy
    - Anticoagulation: unfractionated heparin (or bivalirudin)
    - Statin
    - Maintain serum K above 4.0 mEq per L and serum Mg above 2.0 mEq per L
    - **If cocaine related: benzodiazepines, no β-blockers**

- **Missed MI**
  - ○ 1.9% to 4% with ACS are mistakenly discharged
  - ○ Women <55 years old, nonwhite, shortness of breath (SOB) as major presenting symptoms, or normal/nondiagnostic ECG

AORTIC ANEURYSM AND AORTIC DISSECTION
Aortic Aneurysm
BASICS
- Abnormal dilation of the aorta that has extended 50% beyond normal diameter
- Involves all three layers of vessel wall: the intima, media, and adventitia
- The most common aortic aneurysm is an abdominal aortic aneurysm (AAA)
- **Most AAAs are infrarenal**
- Aortic aneurysms present in the thoracic portion of the aorta and are called thoracic aortic aneurysms (TAAs)
- Aortic aneurysms can be either fusiform or saccular
  - Fusiform: uniform dilation of the entire circumference of the aortic wall
  - Saccular: localized outpouching of the aorta
- Major complications: rupture or dissection, where blood escapes through a tear in the aortic wall
- This leads to significant blood loss, with up to 90% mortality rate
- Other complications: pain, limb ischemia, and compression of adjacent structures

ETIOLOGY
- AAA Risk factors
  - Atherosclerosis, HTN, hyperlipidemia
  - Connective tissue diseases
  - Presence of other aneurysms, family history of aneurysm
  - Male gender, Caucasian race, smoking
  - Advanced age
- Risk factors for AAA rupture
  - Aneurysm with diameter >5.5 cm
  - Aneurysm expanding more than 0.5 cm per year
  - Symptomatic AAA
  - Female gender

SIGNS AND SYMPTOMS
- Most are asymptomatic
- Pulsatile abdominal mass
- Back pain, abdominal or flank pain (may mimic renal colic, including the presence of hematuria)
- Syncope
- May have diminished lower extremities pulses on exam

DIAGNOSTICS
- **Ultrasound is the test of choice both for screening and for rapid assessment in the unstable patient, although not the test of choice for diagnosing rupture**
- Bedside ultrasound: five-point measurement recommended: proximal, mid-aorta, distal (proximal to the bifurcation), common iliacs, and longitudinal view
  - Three centimeters is upper limit of normal (beware of intraluminal clot)
- Transthoracic echocardiography/transesophageal echocardiography can be used to evaluate the aortic root and thoracic aorta, but also cannot determine whether the aneurysm has ruptured
- Abdominal CT scan is the preferred imaging modality to screen for and evaluate AAA (can identify and locate rupture site)

TREATMENT

- If hemodynamically stable, initial treatment should be directed at risk factor modification
  - Smoking cessation, lowering cholesterol, lowering blood pressure, and avoiding activities that require Valsalva maneuvers
  - Medication choices include β-blockers, angiotensin-converting enzyme (ACE) inhibitors, and angiotensin receptor blockers (ARBs)
    - β-Blockers may decrease aneurysm growth
    - ACE inhibitors, statins, and ARBs may decrease risk of rupture
- Refer to vascular surgery for outpatient management and elective surgical repair
- Surgical recommendations
  - Repair of TAA is recommended if ascending TAA >5.5 cm, descending TAA >6 cm, and TAA in Marfan's patient >4.0 to 4.5 cm
  - Repair of AAA is recommended if AAA >5.0 cm or AAA coexistent with peripheral aneurysm or peripheral artery disease
  - Any aneurysm that is rapidly expanding (>0.5 cm per year) should have surgical repair
- Hemodynamically unstable patients require:
  - ABCs, two large-bore IVs, blood transfusion
  - Pain control
  - Reduction of blood pressure (systolic blood pressure [SBP] 80 to 100 mm Hg reduces further aortic damage and blood loss)
  - Emergent operative management via open AAA repair or endovascular repair (EVAR)

Aortic Dissection

BASICS

- Separation of the layers within the aortic wall
- Intimal tears can lead to blood extravasation either proximally or distally
- Can lead to cardiac tamponade, aortic insufficiency, congestive heart failure (CHF), hemothorax, hemoperitoneum, thromboembolic ischemic events, and death
- Classification system includes DeBakey and Sanford
  - **DeBakey:** categorizes the dissection based on where the original intimal tear is located and the extent of the dissection (Figure 2.1)
    - **Type I**
      - Originates in ascending aorta, spreads at least to the aortic arch and often beyond it distally
      - It is most often seen in patients <65 years of age
      - Highest mortality
    - **Type II**
      - Ascending aorta only
    - **Type III**
      - Originates in descending aorta, rarely extends proximally but will extend distally
      - It most often occurs in elderly patients with atherosclerosis and HTN
  - **Sanford:** *characterization based upon whether the ascending aorta is involved*
    - Type A: involves only the ascending aorta
    - Type B: involves the descending aorta

ETIOLOGY

- Congenital aortic anomaly (bicuspid aortic valve, coarctation of the aorta)
- Connective tissue disease (Marfan's, Ehlers–Danlos syndrome)
- Aortitis (giant cell arteritis, endocarditis, lupus)
- Hypertension

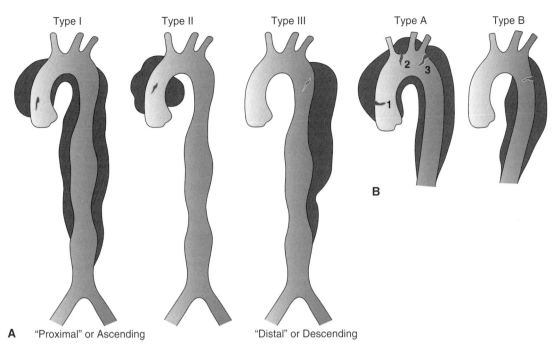

FIGURE 2.1. The DeBakey (**A**) and Stanford (**B**) classification systems of aortic dissection. (From Carey WD, ed. *Cleveland Clinic: Current Clinical Medicine*. 2nd ed. Philadelphia, PA: Saunders/Elsevier; 2010. Figure 3, MD Consult.)

■ Male gender
■ Pregnancy
■ Trauma

SIGNS AND SYMPTOMS
■ Tearing or ripping chest and/or abdominal pain that radiates to the back, neck or jaw pain, syncope, nonspecific back pain, dyspnea, flank pain, hoarse voice, dysphagia, focal neurologic deficits
■ Hypertensive or hypotensive with signs of shock
■ Unequal blood pressures in arms

DIAGNOSTICS
■ EKG may show left ventricular hypertrophy (LVH) or nonspecific ST segment changes
■ Chest x-ray is abnormal in approximately 60% to 80% of those with an aortic dissection
  • May reveal a widened mediastinum and/or left pleural effusion
■ Bedside echo may show an intimal flap (suprasternal notch view may be used to better visualize the aortic arch)
■ **CTA is the preferred study**

TREATMENT
■ Mortality for aortic dissection is ~90%
■ Majority of patients will die before arrival in the emergency department (ED)
■ Hemodynamically unstable patients require the following:
  • Two large-bore IVs placed immediately for fluid resuscitation
  • Blood products
  • Pain control

- Reduction of blood pressure and heart rate to prevent dissection expansion
  - Goal blood pressure is SBP 80 to 100 mm Hg
  - β-Blockers are drug of choice to reduce cardiac contractility (esmolol, labetalol)
  - If bradycardic, may use IV nitroprusside drip to reduce shearing forces
- Immediate vascular surgery consult
  - Type A: require surgical management
  - Type B: treated medically with antihypertensives and pain control

ATRIAL AND VENTRICULAR CONDUCTION DISORDERS

BASICS
- Normal cardiac conduction: sinoatrial (SA) node → atrioventricular (AV) node → bundle branches → Purkinje fibers → cardiac muscle contraction
- Defects in the normal conduction system result in inefficient contractions of the heart

First-Degree Heart Block

BASICS
- Conduction is delayed through the AV node
- The AV node slows electric current from the SA node
- Results in a prolonged PR interval

ETIOLOGY
- Increased parasympathetic tone (sleeping, vomiting, coughing), AV nodal blocking agents (β-blockers, Ca channel blockers, digitalis)
- Myocardial ischemia, infiltrative diseases, myocarditis, congenital structural heart disease

SIGNS AND SYMPTOMS
- Hypotension, diaphoresis, signs of CHF/pulmonary edema
- Chest pain, dyspnea, weakness, fatigue, lightheadedness, near syncope/syncope
- Usually asymptomatic

DIAGNOSTICS
- EKG findings
- PR interval is ≥0.2 seconds

TREATMENT
- Usually benign
- No specific therapy warranted (Figure 2.2)

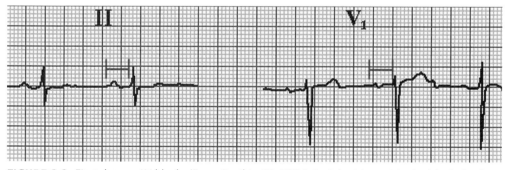

FIGURE 2.2. First-degree AV block. (From Prutkin JM. ECG tutorial: atrioventricular block. In: Post TW, ed. *UpToDate*. Waltham, MA: UpToDate; 2014. Graphic 79990 Version 2.0.)

Second-Degree Heart Block

Mobitz Type I (Wenckebach)

BASICS
- Atrial impulses are intermittently blocked at the level of the AV node, although a small percentage are infranodal blocks
- Block may be reversible, depending on the cause

ETIOLOGY
- Normal finding in some individuals
- Increased parasympathetic tone (sleeping, vomiting, coughing)
- AV nodal blocking agents (β-blockers, Ca channel blockers, digitalis)
- Myocardial ischemia

SIGNS AND SYMPTOMS
- Diaphoresis, signs of CHF/pulmonary edema, hypotension
- Chest pain, dyspnea, weakness, fatigue, lightheadedness, near syncope/syncope
- Usually asymptomatic

DIAGNOSTICS
- EKG findings
- Bradycardia may be present
- Progressive prolongation of the PR interval followed by dropped QRS complex (nonconducted P wave)

TREATMENT
- Usually benign, but symptomatic patients are generally treated when bradycardic
- Attempt to treat reversible causes (Figure 2.3)

Mobitz Type II

BASICS
- Usually due to failure of conduction at the level of the His–Purkinje system (infranodal)
- More frequently due to structural damage, rather than reversible causes
- May progress to complete heart block

ETIOLOGY
- Calcification or fibrosis of the conduction system (Lev disease/Lenegre–Lev syndrome)
- Amyloidosis, sarcoidosis, hemochromatosis
- Hypothyroidism
- Myocardial ischemia

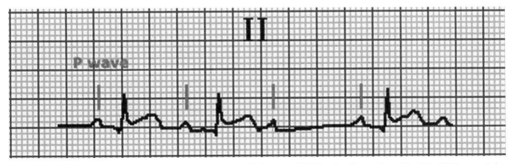

FIGURE 2.3. Wenckebach/Mobitz type I second-degree AV block. (From Prutkin JM. ECG tutorial: atrioventricular block. In: Post TW, ed. *UpToDate*. Waltham, MA: UpToDate; 2014. Graphic 71453 Version 3.0.)

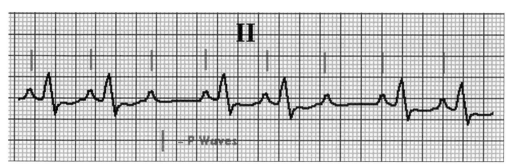

FIGURE 2.4. Mobitz type II second-degree AV block. (From Prutkin JM. ECG tutorial: atrioventricular block. In: Post TW, ed. *UpToDate*. Waltham, MA: UpToDate; 2014. Graphic 58649 Version 3.0.)

SIGNS AND SYMPTOMS
- Hypotension, diaphoresis, signs of CHF/pulmonary edema
- Chest pain, dyspnea, AMS, weakness, fatigue, lightheadedness, presyncope/syncope

DIAGNOSTICS
- EKG findings
- Bradycardia may be present
- Characterized by dropped QRS complexes without prolongation of the PR interval
- Consecutively dropped QRS complexes are a sign of a high-grade block

TREATMENT
- Transcutaneous pacing
- Atropine 0.5 mg IV while awaiting pacer (may repeat to a total dose of 3 mg atropine)
- Consider epinephrine or dopamine infusion while awaiting pacer or if pacing is ineffective
- **Definitive treatment is pacemaker placement** (Figure 2.4)

Third-Degree Complete Heart Block
BASICS
- Supraventricular impulses are unable to be conducted to the ventricles, causing complete AV dissociation
- The atria and ventricles are stimulated by independent pacemakers and thus contract irrespective of each other
- Only escape rhythms allow the heart to contract, and if the escape rhythm fails, death may occur

ETIOLOGY
- Amyloidosis, sarcoidosis, hemochromatosis, hypothyroidism, systemic lupus erythematosus, severe hyperkalemia
- Drug toxicity: β-blocker, Ca channel blocker, other antiarrhythmics
- Myocardial ischemia
- *Lyme disease*, Chagas disease, diphtheria, rheumatic fever, endocarditis, tuberculosis (TB)
- Lev disease/Lenegre–Lev syndrome

SIGNS AND SYMPTOMS
- Hypotension, diaphoresis, signs of CHF/pulmonary edema
- Chest pain, dyspnea, AMS, weakness, fatigue, lightheadedness, near syncope/syncope

DIAGNOSTICS
- EKG findings
  - Bradycardia
  - Complete AV dissociation: the atrial rate is more rapid than the ventricular rate, so P waves appear to "march through" without any relation to the QRS waves

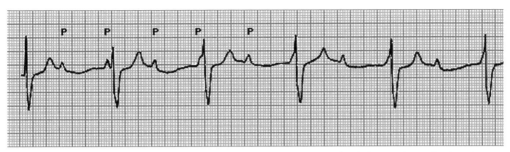

FIGURE 2.5. Third-degree (complete) AV block. (From Sauer WH. Third degree (complete) atrioventricular block. In: Post TW, ed. *UpToDate*. Waltham, MA: UpToDate; 2014. Graphic 72863 Version 5.0. Courtesy of Ary Goldhaber, MD.)

TREATMENT
- Transcutaneous pacing
- Consider transvenous pacing in patients who are unable to tolerate, hemodynamically unstable to sedate, or in those where transcutaneous pacing fails to maintain electrical capture
- Atropine 0.5 mg IV while awaiting pacer (may repeat to a total dose of 3 mg atropine)
- Consider epinephrine or dopamine infusion while awaiting pacer or if pacing is ineffective
- **Definitive treatment is pacemaker placement** (Figure 2.5)

Atrial Fibrillation

BASICS
- Most common arrhythmia

ETIOLOGY
- Caused by progressive fibrosis of the atria, which is due to atrial dilation
- Other causes include:
  - Idiopathic (most common)
  - Ischemia, valvular disease
  - Trauma, toxicity
  - Hypertension, alcohol abuse, hyperthyroidism, family history

SIGNS AND SYMPTOMS
- Pulse is irregularly irregular, tachycardia
- Hypotension, syncope
- Palpitations, exercise intolerance, SOB

DIAGNOSTICS
- EKG

TREATMENT
- Rate control with β-blockers and Ca channel blockers
- Cardioversion with drugs (Flecainide) or electrical
- Anticoagulation
- Based on CHA2DS2-VASc score

AV Node Reentrant Tachycardia (AVNRT)

BASICS
- Most common type of supraventricular tachycardia (SVT)
- Caused by a reentry circuit around the AV node
- Formed by two pathways, a slow and a fast pathway, located within the right atrium
- A premature atrial beat is sent down the slow AV nodal pathway, and rather than continuing down this pathway, it will travel backward up the fast AV nodal pathway, leading to tachycardia

ETIOLOGY
■ Presence of an extra, abnormal pathway in the heart (two AV nodal pathways)

SIGNS AND SYMPTOMS
■ Hypotension, ischemic EKG changes, signs of CHF/pulmonary edema, signs of poor perfusion
■ Palpitations, dyspnea, chest pain, fatigue, near syncope/syncope

DIAGNOSTICS
■ EKG findings
■ Rate >100 bpm (usually >150 bpm) with a regular rhythm
■ Narrow QRS complexes
■ P waves may be embedded within QRS complexes

TREATMENT
■ Vagal maneuvers: carotid sinus massage or Valsalva
■ Adenosine 6 mg IV push
■ If no conversion to normal sinus rhythm, then 12 mg IV push
■ If still no conversion to normal sinus rhythm, may repeat the 12 mg dose one more time
■ Longer-acting AV nodal blocking agents (β-blockers, Ca channel blockers) may be used when adenosine is ineffective
■ **Synchronized cardioversion is first-line treatment for unstable SVT**
■ Catheter ablation: destruction of the slow AV nodal pathway; ultimate treatment for SVT

Wolff–Parkinson–White Syndrome (WPW)

BASICS
■ Accessory conduction pathway causing SVT

SIGNS AND SYMPTOMS
■ Palpitations, diaphoresis
■ Weak pulses, CHF
■ Shock

DIAGNOSTICS
■ EKG: short PR interval, widened QRS, *delta wave (slurring upstroke of QRS)*
■ Heart rate above 200 (Figure 2.6)

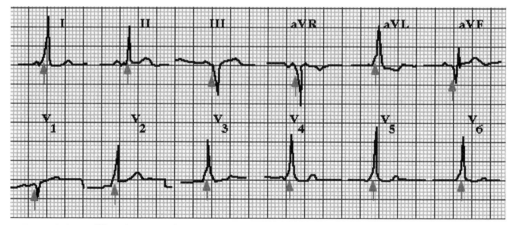

FIGURE 2.6. Wolff–Parkinson–White pattern, arrow indicates a delta wave. (From Prutkin JM. ECG tutorial: preexcitation syndromes. In: Post TW, ed. *UpToDate*. Waltham, MA: UpToDate; 2014. Graphic 75578 Version 4.0.)

TREATMENT
- ABCs, monitor, IV
- Stable: treat with amiodarone, flecainide
- Unstable: emergent cardioversion
- Do *not* give the following medications (with WPW-associated a-fib, a-flutter, or wide complex tachycardia):
  - **A**denosine
  - β-Blockers
  - **C**a channel blockers
  - **D**igoxin

Torsade De Pointes
BASICS
- Variation of ventricular tachycardia
- QRS axis swings from positive to negative in single lead

ETIOLOGY
- Often caused by R-on-T phenomenon
- Medications, idiopathic, electrolyte abnormality, intracranial bleeds

DIAGNOSTICS
- EKG (Figure 2.7)

TREATMENT
- IV Mg
- Cardioversion

Sick Sinus Syndrome (SSS)
BASICS
- Tachy–brady syndrome

SIGNS AND SYMPTOMS
- Palpitations, dyspnea
- Syncope
- Fatigue, weakness

DIAGNOSTICS
- EKG

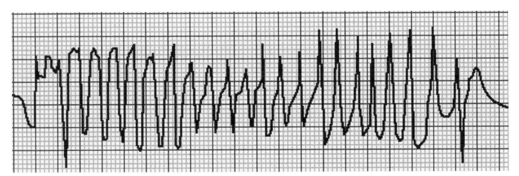

FIGURE 2.7. Torsades de pointes. (From Berul CL, Seslar SP, Zimetbaum PJ, Josephson ME. Acquired long QT syndrome. In: Post TW, ed. *UpToDate*. Waltham, MA: UpToDate; 2014. Graphic 53891 Version 4.0.)

TREATMENT
- ABCs, IV, monitor
- Follow advanced cardiac life support protocol
- Pacemaker

● CARDIAC TAMPONADE AND CARDIOGENIC SHOCK

Cardiac Tamponade

BASICS
- Compression of myocardium by accumulation of fluid in the pericardial space
- May be acute (trauma) or subacute/chronic (malignancy, uremia)
- With trauma, as little as 60 to 100 mL of blood can produce tamponade
- Suspect in any patient with penetrating wound or blunt trauma to thorax or upper abdomen
- High mortality

ETIOLOGY
- Intrapericardial pressure and volume limit capacity of atria and ventricles to fill
- Ventricular filling mechanically reduced, resulting in decreased stroke volume
- Compensatory mechanism: heart rate and peripheral resistance rise to maintain cardiac output (CO) and BP

SIGNS AND SYMPTOMS
- Chest pain, cough, dyspnea
  - Beck's triad
    - Hypotension
    - Distended neck veins
    - Muffled heart sounds
  - Most reliable signs: elevated central venous pressure >15 cm H_2O with hypotension and tachycardia
  - Pulsus paradoxus: an excessive drop in SBP during inspiration

DIAGNOSTICS
- Chest x-ray shows cardiomegaly only if large accumulation of fluid (250 mL)
- EKG: decreased voltage (amplitude) or electrical alternans (beat-to-beat alteration in amplitude of the QRS complex)
- Echo confirms an effusion
  - Tamponade physiology: systolic right atrium collapse, diastolic RV collapse
  - "Swinging heart": all four chambers floating in the pericardial space in a phasic manner

TREATMENT
- Initial treatment: IV fluids to maintain intravascular volume
  - Increases the filling pressure to overcome pericardial constriction
- Pericardiocentesis (treatment of choice): preferably in the cath lab
- Remove enough fluid to stabilize the patient, consider drainage catheter
- May need surgical procedure (pericardial window)

Cardiogenic Shock

BASICS
- Systemic signs of hypoperfusion due to inability of the heart to pump an adequate amount of blood
- Arterial SBP <90% or 30% below known baseline
- Immediate treatment focuses on improving myocardium contractility and pump function

ETIOLOGY
- Acute myocardial infarction (AMI) (most common)
- Greater than 40% myocardium involved
- Acute, severe mitral regurgitation (MR)
- Interventricular septum rupture, papillary muscle rupture
- Cardiac tamponade
- Mortality approaches 50%

SIGNS AND SYMPTOMS
- Ill appearing, AMS, diaphoresis, cool extremities
- New murmur from ruptured papillary muscle
- High systemic vascular resistance
- Tachycardia, hypotension
- Respiratory rate >20 breath per minute or partial pressure of carbon dioxide <32 mm Hg
- Arterial base deficit <−4 mEq per L or lactate >4 mm per L
- Urine output <0.5 mL/kg/hr

DIAGNOSTICS
- EKG: may have ST elevation
  - Consider right-sided leads to evaluate for RV infarct pattern
- Echocardiogram
- Labs: complete blood count (CBC), basic metabolic panel, prothrombin time/partial thromboplastin time, serial troponins
- Chest x-ray

TREATMENT
- Hemodynamic monitoring, including pulmonary artery catheterization
- Do not delay transfer to catheterization lab
- Adequate ventilation and oxygenation (O_2, positive-end expiratory pressure)
- IV fluids if no evidence of overt CHF
- Treat emergent dysrhythmias
- Vasopressor/inotropic support (dopamine and dobutamine are first line)
- May consider norepinephrine if additional blood pressure support needed
- Withhold β-blockers
- Aspirin
- Heparin and arrangement for emergent PCI (possible coronary artery bypass grafting, if mechanical complication)
- Consider intra-aortic balloon pump counterpulsation as bridge for refractory shock

● CARDIOMYOPATHIES, MYOCARDITIS, AND PERICARDITIS
Dilated Cardiomyopathy

BASICS
- Dilation and impaired contraction of one or both ventricles
- Generally with decreased systolic function, measured by ejection fraction (EF)

ETIOLOGY
- Approximately one-third of cases of CHF are due to dilated cardiomyopathy
- L/R ventricular systolic pump function is impaired, causing progressive cardiac enlargement/hypertrophy
- **Most common cause is idiopathic** (Fifty percent of these have a familial component)
- Commonly caused by myocardial damage produced by a variety of toxic metabolic (doxorubicin), or infectious agents (HIV, viral myocarditis)

- Reversible causes: ETOH abuse, pregnancy, thyroid disease, cocaine use, and chronic uncontrolled tachycardia
- Associated with ischemic heart disease, HTN, connective tissue disease, obstructive sleep apnea
- Most common in middle-aged men and African American

SIGNS AND SYMPTOMS
- May be asymptomatic
- Vague CP
- Syncope due to atrial/ventricular arrhythmias
- Cerebral or systemic embolic phenomena due to mural thrombus
- Elevated jugular venous pressure (JVP)

DIAGNOSTICS
- EKG
- Chest x-ray:
  - Cardiac silhouette enlargement from LVH
  - Pulmonary venous HTN and interstitial edema
- Echocardiogram
- Elevated B-type natriuretic peptide

TREATMENT
- Spontaneous improvement in 25% (depending on cause)
- Poor prognosis if age >55 years, ventricular tachycardia or bradyarrhythmia
- Anticoagulation
- Salt restriction, ACE inhibitors, diuretics, and digitalis
- *Avoid:* ETOH, Ca channel blockers (reduce inotropy and stroke volume), nonsteroidal anti-inflammatory drugs (NSAIDs)
- Implantable cardioverter defibrillator for symptomatic ventricular arrhythmias
- Cardiac transplantation

Hypertrophic Cardiomyopathy

BASICS
- Characterized by LVH, usually of a nondilated chamber, without obvious cause such as HTN or aortic stenosis
- Termed idiopathic hypertrophic subaortic stenosis and hypertrophic obstructive cardiomyopathy (HOCM)
- Diastolic dysfunction characterized by increased stiffness of the hypertrophic muscle, causing elevated diastolic filling pressures

ETIOLOGY
- Approximately 50% positive family history
- Outflow obstruction from narrowing of an already small left ventricular outflow tract by systolic anterior motion of the mitral valve against a hypertrophic septum

SIGNS AND SYMPTOMS
- Clinical course is highly variable
- **Sudden death, commonly occurring in children/young adults, during/after physical exertion**
- Dyspnea (most common)
- Angina pectoris, fatigue, and syncope
- Systolic murmur that may be accentuated with Valsalva, standing from a squatting position, and administration of nitroglycerin

DIAGNOSTICS

- EKG: LVH, deep, inferolateral Q waves; arrhythmias (SVT, A-fib, V-tach)
- Chest x-ray
- Echo

TREATMENT

- Physical exertion restriction
- Avoid dehydration; diuretics should be used with caution
- β-Blockers may be utilized in treating angina pectoris and syncope
- Implantable cardioverter defibrillator in patients with high risk of sudden cardiac death
- Septal myectomy in severe cases

Restrictive Cardiomyopathy

BASICS

- Abnormal diastolic function; rigid ventricular walls impairing ventricular filling, resulting in diminished CO and elevated filling pressures

ETIOLOGY

- Least common of the triad of cardiomyopathies
- Myocardial fibrosis, hypertrophy, or infiltration
- Amyloidosis, hemochromatosis, sarcoidosis, scleroderma, neoplastic infiltration
- Complication of cardiac transplant, mediastinal radiation

SIGNS AND SYMPTOMS

- Exercise intolerance, dyspnea, orthopnea, paroxysmal nocturnal dyspnea (PND)
- Dependent edema, ascites, and enlarged, tender liver
- **Paradoxical rise in JVP on inspiration (*Kussmaul sign*)**
- Distant heart sounds, S3 and S4 present

DIAGNOSTICS

- EKG: low-voltage, nonspecific ST-T-wave changes, various arrhythmias including AF
- Echocardiogram may show thickening of the ventricular walls

TREATMENT

- Diuretics, vasodilators (ACE inhibitors, nitrates), antiarrhythmics
- Anticoagulation in patients with a-fib
- Endomyocardectomy and cardiac transplant for refractory cases

Myocarditis

DEFINITION

- Inflammatory/infectious process causing necrosis that involves the myocardium

ETIOLOGY

- **Most common etiology in the United States is viral (coxsackie virus most common)**
- Bacterial causes: diphtheria, TB, staphylococci, meningococci, group A streptococci (acute rheumatic fever) and Lyme (*Borrelia burgdorferi*)
- Other causes: drugs, toxins, radiation, hypersensitivity reactions, immunologic (Kawasaki disease, giant cell myocarditis)
- Peripartum cardiomyopathy

SIGNS AND SYMPTOMS

- Commonly asymptomatic
- CHF may present days to weeks after infection

- Chest pain, dyspnea, fatigue, decreased exercise tolerance, palpitations, fever, syncope, palpitations, sudden death
- Atrial/ventricular arrhythmias, conduction disturbances
- MR and tricuspid regurgitation murmurs, muffled S1 and S3 present
- Peripheral edema, rales, JVP
- Pleural and pericardial rubs

DIAGNOSTICS
- EKG: nonspecific ST changes and diffuse ST elevations if accompanying pericarditis
- Chest x-ray may show evidence of CHF
- Labs: CBC, erythrocyte sedimentation rate (ESR), C-reactive protein (CRP), viral AB titers, cardiac enzymes, rheumatologic testing
- Echocardiogram

TREATMENT
- Generally self-limited, occasionally progresses to chronic form with dilated cardiomyopathy
- Acute illness requires hospitalization, monitoring
- Antipyretics and analgesics (avoid NSAIDs in the acute phase)
- Antiarrhythmics, diuretics in the event of CHF

Pericarditis

BASICS
- Inflammation of the pericardium that may be characterized by chest pain, pericardial friction rub, and ECG changes
- Most common in young adults

ETIOLOGY
- Infectious (viral, TB, bacterial), uremia, autoimmune, radiation, drug toxicity, post-MI (Dressler syndrome), malignancy

SIGNS AND SYMPTOMS
- Chest pain (often pleuritic) worse with lying flat, improved when leaning forward, cough, dyspnea
- Pericardial friction rub, fever, leukocytosis

DIAGNOSTICS
- EKG may demonstrate diffuse ST elevation, PR depression, electrical alternans in cardiac tamponade
- Chest x-ray
- CBC, ESR/CRP, cardiac enzymes (elevated in myopericarditis)
- Echocardiogram: pericardial effusion may be present

TREATMENT
- Anti-inflammatory drugs (NSAIDs, colchicine, corticosteroids)
- Avoid anticoagulants
- Pericardiocentesis or pericardial window placement in patients with tamponade

● CHF AND PULMONARY EDEMA
Congestive Heart Failure

BASICS
- Clinical syndrome in which an abnormality of cardiac structure or function is responsible for the inability of the heart to eject or fill, leading to dyspnea, fatigue, and edema

TYPES

- Systolic or diastolic
  - **Systolic:** the inability of the ventricle to contract and eject sufficient blood to meet metabolic demands
  - **Diastolic:** the inability of the ventricle to relax and fill appropriately
- Right-sided or left-sided
  - **Left-sided:** LV is hemodynamically overloaded or weakened, more frequently causing pulmonary vascular congestion
  - **Right-sided:** underlying abnormality affects RV primarily, causing edema, congestive hepatomegaly, and systemic venous distention
  - High-output heart failure: results from excessive demand for CO (anemia, hyperthyroidism)

ETIOLOGY

- Causes include infection, arrhythmia, AMI, anemia, thyrotoxicosis, pregnancy, HTN, myocarditis, infective endocarditis
- Causes of left HF: HTN, MI, mitral valve disease, aortic valve disease
- Causes of right HF: left HF, Cor pulmonale, pulmonary HTN, pulmonic valve disease, tricuspid valve disease, congenital heart disease

SIGNS AND SYMPTOMS

- Dyspnea, orthopnea, and PND
- Fatigue, weakness, abdominal pain/fullness, AMS (confusion, memory loss)
- Tachycardia, S3 and S4 (audible but not specific for HF)
- Pulsus alternans: arterial pulse alternates between strong and weak beats
- Distended jugular veins, dependent edema, ventricular arrhythmias, sudden death
- Rales, wheezes, ascites, congestive hepatomegaly, cool, pale and diaphoretic skin
- Severe acute CHF: sinus tachycardia and systolic hypotension may be present with cool, diaphoretic extremities, cyanosis of lips and nail beds, Cheyne–Stokes respiration (oscillation between hyperpnea and apnea)

DIAGNOSTICS

- EKG
- Labs including B-type natriuretic peptide, cardiac enzymes
- Chest x-ray reveals pulmonary edema, pleural effusions, cardiomegaly, Kerley B lines
- Echocardiogram

TREATMENT

- Outpatient management: monitor Na intake, daily weight, avoid ETOH
- Medication management with diuretics (thiazides, loop diuretics, ACE/ARBs, β-blockers, digitalis)
- ED CHF management: IV furosemide, sublingual nitroglycerin, nitroglycerin drip for refractory CHF
- Airway management: noninvasive positive pressure ventilation helpful for those in acute respiratory distress
- Patients with persistent hypoxia may require intubation

Pulmonary Edema

BASICS

- Increase in pulmonary venous pressure, which results in engorgement of pulmonary vasculature, decreasing lung compliance

ETIOLOGY

- Elevated pulmonary capillary hydrostatic pressure, leading to transudation of fluid into the pulmonary interstitium and alveoli
- Most common cause is severe LV dysfunction

- Imbalance of Starling forces: increased pulmonary capillary pressure, decreased plasma oncotic pressure, increased negative interstitial pressure
- Noncardiogenic pulmonary edema (acute lung injury or acute respiratory distress syndrome): may be caused by pulmonary contusion, reexpansion s/p thoracentesis, heroin overdose, aspiration, severe infection

SIGNS AND SYMPTOMS
- SOB, dyspnea on exertion, orthopnea, PND, cough, chest pain
- Tachypnea, tachycardia, HTN, or hypotension in severe LV dysfunction
- Jugular venous distention (JVD), rales/rhonchi/wheezes

DIAGNOSTICS
- EKG: left atrial enlargement, LVH, brady/tachyarrhythmia
- Chest x-ray: diffuse haziness of lung fields with greater density in more proximal hilar regions, Kerley B lines, and loss of distinct vascular margins, cardiomegaly, pleural effusions
- Echocardiogram

TREATMENT
- ABCs
- Preload reduction: nitro, diuretics, morphine
- Continuous positive airway pressure or bi-level positive airway pressure for respiratory distress, maintains fluid-filled alveoli patency, and prevents collapse during exhalation
- Afterload reduction: nitroprusside, catecholamines, and dopamine/dobutamine stimulate myocardial contractility while promoting peripheral and pulmonary vasodilation

● HYPERTENSIVE URGENCY AND HYPERTENSIVE EMERGENCY
Hypertensive Urgency

BASICS
- HTN is SBP ≥140 mm Hg and/or diastolic blood pressure (DBP) ≥90 mm Hg
- Significant HTN without evidence of end-organ damage

ETIOLOGY
- Nonadherence with antihypertensive medications or dietary restrictions

SIGNS AND SYMPTOMS
- Typically, those with hypertensive urgency are asymptomatic
- When symptomatic, the primary complaint is headache

DIAGNOSTICS
- SBP ≥140 mm Hg and/or DBP ≥90 mm Hg
- There is no benefit to ordering laboratory tests, unless patient is truly symptomatic and there is concern for end-organ damage

TREATMENT
- If patient has follow-up, initiating treatment for asymptomatic HTN in the ED is not necessary
- Reduce blood pressure slowly to a goal blood pressure of SBP ≤160 mm Hg and DBP ≤100 mm Hg
- Lower BP slowly over a period of several hours or several days
- Reducing blood pressure quickly is unsafe, as this can lead to cerebral or myocardial ischemia
- First attempt to lower blood pressure should include placing the patient in a quiet room and allowing them to rest and then repeating the blood pressure

- Restart antihypertensive medications
- Reinforce the necessity for a low-salt diet
- Increase the dose of current antihypertensive, or add second agent
■ Untreated HTN
  - Blood pressure reduction over a period of 1 to 2 days with oral medications
  - Initial medications of choice include thiazides, Ca channel blockers, β-blockers, ACE inhibitors, or ARBs
    - ○ Medication of choice depends on underlying health conditions (although thiazides are generally first line)

Hypertensive Emergency

BASICS
■ SBP of 180 mm Hg or higher and DBP of 115 mm Hg with signs of end-organ damage
■ Organ systems that are affected in hypertensive emergencies are the central nervous system, cardiovascular, renal, and ophthalmologic

ETIOLOGY, SIGNS AND SYMPTOMS, DIAGNOSTICS
See Table 2.2

TREATMENT
■ Goal of treatment is to lower blood pressure to avoid end-organ damage
■ **Reduce blood pressure by 25%, to reduce risk of myocardial or cerebral ischemia**
■ Ultimate goal is to bring DBP down to 100 to 110 mm Hg over several hours
■ Posterior reversible encephalopathy syndrome (PRES): characterized by headache, AMS, and seizures in the setting of significant HTN and diagnosed by MRI
■ Patients with end-organ damage generally require ICU level of care (Table 2.3)

TABLE 2.2. Hypertensive Emergencies by Organ Systems Affected				
	Predisposing Factors	**Symptoms**	**Physical Exam Findings**	**Evaluation**
Neurologic	SAH ICH Ischemic stroke TIA Head trauma Encephalopathy	Headache Confusion Nausea Vomiting	Stroke Encephalopathy Seizure Coma Mental status change Focal neurologic deficits	Head CT scan ➢ Ischemic infarct or ICH
Cardiovascular	Aortic dissection Myocardial infarction Unstable angina Medication noncompliance	Chest pain Abdominal pain Back pain Shortness of breath Palpitations	Aortic dissection ACS CHF/pulmonary edema JVD Peripheral edema Cardiac bruit Murmurs Extra heart sounds (S3 or S4)	EKG, troponin ➢ Ischemia, infarction, and LVH CXR ➢ Widened mediastinum and pulmonary edema

(continued)

TABLE 2.2.	**Hypertensive Emergencies By Organ Systems Affected (Continued)**			
	Predisposing Factors	Symptoms	Physical Exam Findings	Evaluation
Renal	Acute renal failure Acute glomerulonephritis Scleroderma Preeclampsia Eclampsia	Weakness Oliguria Hematuria Peripheral edema	None	CBC ➢ Anemia Electrolytes ➢ Increased BUN & creatinine and hyperkalemia Urinalysis ➢ Proteinuria and hematuria
Ophthalmologic	None	Blurred vision Diplopia	Retinal hemorrhages Cotton wool spots Papilledema	None

Hypertensive emergencies can also be the result of illicit drug use (cocaine and amphetamines) and excessive catecholamine states (pheochromocytoma, MAOI drug–drug interactions) and rebound after cessation of antihypertensive medications.

SAH, subarachnoid hemorrhage; ICH, intracerebral hemorrhage; CXR, chest x-ray; BUN, blood urea nitrogen; TIA, transient ischemic attack.

TABLE 2.3.	**Antihypertensive Drugs for Hypertensive Emergency**		
	Uses	Rationale	Contraindication
Nitroprusside	Aortic dissection	Rapid onset of action Short duration of action (~10 min)	
Nitroglycerin	Myocardial ischemia CHF	Causes venodilation and arteriolar dilation	
Nicardipine	SAH		
Hydralazine	Eclampsia, preeclampsia	Arteriolar vasodilator	
Phentolamine	Excessive catecholamine state	α-Adrenergic blocker	
Labetalol	Aortic dissection	Rapid onset of action	Bradycardia Heart block Excessive catecholamine state

THROMBOEMBOLIC DISEASE

BASICS
- Syndrome in which blood clot forms in the deep veins

ETIOLOGY
- **Virchow triad**
  - Venous stasis
  - Hypercoagulability
  - Vessel intimal injury
- General risk factors
  - Age
  - Immobilization longer than 3 days
  - Pregnancy and postpartum period
  - Major surgery in previous 4 weeks
  - Long plane or car trips (>4 hours) in previous 4 weeks
- Medical
  - Cancer, previous deep vein thrombosis (DVT), stroke, AMI, CHF, sepsis, nephrotic syndrome, ulcerative colitis, systemic lupus erythematosus, lupus anticoagulant
- Trauma
- Hematologic
  - Inherited disorders of coagulation/fibrinolysis
  - Antithrombin III deficiency, factor V Leiden, protein C and protein S deficiency
- Drugs/medications
  - Intravenous drug use (IVDU)
  - Oral contraceptives
  - Estrogens

SIGNS AND SYMPTOMS
- Many asymptomatic
- Unilateral edema, leg pain in 50%
- **Homan sign**
  - Pain with foot dorsiflexion
  - Not sensitive or specific
- Calf tenderness, warmth, or erythema
- Phlegmasia cerulea dolens: "painful blue edema" from venous engorgement and obstruction
- Phlegmasia alba dolens: "painful white edema" often with poor or even absent distal pulses

DIAGNOSTICS
- D-dimer
  - A negative D-dimer rules out DVT in points with low risk and a Wells DVT score <2
  - All patients with a positive D-dimer and all patients with a moderate-to-high risk of DVT (Wells score >2) require a diagnostic study (although) (Table 2.4)
  - D-dimer level is elevated in trauma, pregnancy, recent surgery, hemorrhage, cancer, and sepsis
- Duplex ultrasound, MR venography, or contrast venography
- Consider repeat ultrasound in 7 days if symptoms persist
- Labs including CBC, prothrombin time, partial thromboplastin time, INR
- Outpatient labs include protein S and protein C, antithrombin III, factor V Leiden, prothrombin 20210A mutation, antiphospholipid antibodies, and homocysteine levels can be measured (often not particularly helpful during acute phase of DVT)
  - Deficiencies of these factors or the presence of these abnormalities all produce a hypercoagulable state

TABLE 2.4. Wells Clinical Score for DVT	
Clinical Parameter Score	**Score**
Active cancer (treat ongoing, or within 6 mo)	+1
Paralysis or recent plaster immobilization of the lower extremities	+1
Recently bedridden for >3 d or major surgery <4 wk	+1
Localized tenderness along the distribution of the deep venous system	+1
Entire leg swelling	+1
Calf swelling >3 cm compared with the asymptomatic leg	+1
Pitting edema (greater in the symptomatic leg)	+1
Previous DVT documented	+1
Collateral superficial veins (nonvaricose)	+1
Alternative diagnosis (as likely as or greater than that of DVT)	−2
Total of Above Score	
High probability	≥3
Moderate probability	1 or 2
Low probability	≤0

TREATMENT

- Distal DVT (calf) does not pose significant risk of PE
- Decision to anticoagulate, as well as duration of therapy, is highly variable
- Superficial thrombophlebitis: warm compresses, NSAIDs, elevation, compression
- Heparin, low molecular weight heparin (enoxaparin)
- Warfarin with target INR 2.0 to 3.0
- Factor Xa inhibitors (fondaparinux, rivaroxaban)

● VALVULAR DISORDERS

Infectious Endocarditis

BASICS

- Preexisting cardiac pathology
  - Elderly: calcific or degenerative disease of aortic or mitral valve
  - Developing countries: rheumatic heart disease
  - Congenital cardiac lesions with high pressure gradients
  - Previous infectious endocarditis (IE)
- Recent sources of bacteremia: intravenous drug abuse, indwelling lines, dental or invasive procedures
- Most ED procedures do not require prophylaxis

ETIOLOGY

- Vegetation: sterile thrombus, then microorganisms adhere and colonize
- Typically, staphylococci (42%) and streptococci (40%), HACEK group (*Haemophilus parainfluenzae, Actinobacillus, Cardiobacterium, Eikenella, Kingella*)
- Native valve: typically, *Streptococcus* (*viridans, bovis*)
- Prosthetic valve: typically, *Staphylococcus* (*aureus, epidermidis*)
- **IVDU:** *S. aureus*

SIGNS AND SYMPTOMS

- Nonspecific, difficult to distinguish from febrile viral illness
- Most common: intermittent fever (85%), malaise (80%)
  - Also weakness, myalgias, back pain, dyspnea, chest pain, cough, headache, anorexia

TABLE 2.5.	Modified Duke Criteria	
Major	**Minor**
Bacteremia of an organism known to cause endocarditis	Predisposing condition
Endocardial involvement on echo or new valve regurgitation	Vascular phenomenon
	Fever
Definitive: 2 major or 1 major + 3 minor or 5 minor	Immunologic phenomenon + BCx (not meeting major criteria)
Possible: 1 major + 1 minor or 3 minor	

- Fever, murmur
- Vasculitic lesions
  - Petechiae
  - Splinter hemorrhages
  - Janeway lesions (painless)
- Immunologic phenomena
  - Glomerulonephritis
  - Osler nodes (painful)
- Ocular findings:
  - Roth spots (conjunctival or retinal hemorrhages)

DIAGNOSTICS
- Blood cultures ×3
- Echocardiogram
- Duke criteria (Table 2.5)

TREATMENT
- Antibiotics
  - Prosthetic valve/IVDU—Vancomycin (methicillin-resistant *S. aureus*) and gentamicin
  - Native valve—Gentamicin plus penicillin (PCN) *or* nafcillin
- Admit, infectious disease and cardiology consultation

Rheumatic Fever

BASICS
- Leading cause of childhood mortality in developing nations

ETIOLOGY
- Delayed complications of group A β-hemolytic streptococcal pharyngitis
- Latency of 1 to 5 weeks (average 18 days) after pharyngitis

SIGNS AND SYMPTOMS
- See Jones criteria below

DIAGNOSTICS
- **Jones criteria**
  - Evidence of antecedent strep (throat culture, or antistreptolysin titers, which remain positive for 4 to 6 weeks)
  - Two major or one major and two minor criteria
    - Major: carditis, polyarthritis, chorea, erythema marginatum, subcutaneous nodules
    - Minor: arthralgias, fever, increased ESR/CRP, prolonged PR interval

TREATMENT
- Adults
  - PCN 500 mg bid-tid po × 10 days
  - Benzathine PCN 1.2 million units IM × 1
- Children
  - PCN 250 mg bid-tid po × 10 days
  - Benzathine PCN 600,000 units IM × 1 <25 kg

Mitral Stenosis

BASICS
- Flow from left atrium to left ventricle impeded
  - Left atrial HTN
  - Restricted CO
  - Pulmonary congestion
  - Pulmonary HTN and RV failure

ETIOLOGY
- Rheumatic fever is the most common cause (globally)
- A-fib (common complication)
- Decompensate with increased cardiac demand and reduced ventricular filling (e.g., pregnancy, anemia, infection, hyperthyroidism)

SIGNS AND SYMPTOMS
- Early: reduced exercise tolerance, dyspnea on exertion
- Advanced: orthopnea and peripheral edema
- Hemoptysis and hoarseness (classic, but rare)
- Heart sounds
  - Loud S1
  - Opening snap in early diastole
  - Low-pitched rumbling diastolic apical murmur

DIAGNOSTICS
- Echocardiogram: confirms and assesses severity
- Chest x-ray: may show left atrial enlargement
- EKG: A-fib, left atrial enlargement, RV hypertrophy

TREATMENT
- Identify and treat precipitants (e.g., A-fib or anemia)
- Diuresis, anticoagulation (if arrhythmia), and refer for definitive surgical management

Mitral Regurgitation

BASICS
- Results in dilatation of left atrium and increase in left atrial pressure, which leads to pulmonary edema

ETIOLOGY
- Acute (true emergency)
  - Papillary muscle dysfunction with acute ischemia
  - Ruptured chordae tendineae
  - Perforation of valve leaflet with IE

- Chronic
  - Dilated cardiomyopathy
  - Rheumatic heart disease
  - Mitral valve prolapse
  - Connective tissue disorders (Marfan's, Ehlers–Danlos)

SIGNS AND SYMPTOMS
- Acute
  - Fulminant pulmonary edema
  - Harsh midsystolic murmur that radiates to base, not axilla
  - Low left atrial compliance
  - Sharply elevated left atrial pressure
  - Acute pulmonary congestion
- Chronic
  - CHF with decompensated congestion
  - Holosystolic murmur, heard at apex and radiates to axilla
  - High left atrial compliance
  - Near-normal left atrial pressures
  - Decompensation with volume overload

DIAGNOSTICS
- Acute
  - EKG: may show ischemia or infarction
  - Emergent echo and cardiac cath
- Chronic
  - EKG: left atrial and ventricular hypertrophy, A-fib (common)
  - Normal or above normal EF
  - Chest x-ray: may show left atrial enlargement

TREATMENT
- Acute
  - Assess degree and urgency for surgery
  - Treat pulmonary edema with nitrates and diuretics
  - Consider counterpulsation with intra-aortic balloon pump if hypotensive
- Chronic
  - Diuresis and afterload-reducing agents
  - Value replacement or repair if EF <60%

Aortic Stenosis

BASICS
- Most common: calcific degeneration
- Bicuspid aortic valve
- Rheumatic heart disease

ETIOLOGY
- Significant obstruction if valve area reduced >50%
- LVH maintains CO until stenosis severe
- Left ventricular dysfunction, left atrial enlargement, A-fib
- Preload dependent, very little cardiovascular reserve
- Decompensate with ischemia, rapid A-fib, dehydration, and acute blood loss

SIGNS AND SYMPTOMS
- Classic: **angina → exertional syncope → CHF**
- Heart sounds
  - **Crescendo–decrescendo systolic murmur,** heard best at base that radiates to carotids
  - S4 gallop
- Carotid pulses: delayed and diminished

DIAGNOSTICS
- EKG: LVH
- Echocardiogram: assess severity and left ventricular dysfunction

TREATMENT
- If decompensated
  - Fluid resuscitation, blood transfusion, restoration of sinus rhythm
  - Avoid vasodilators, diuretics, and inotropic agents
- Consider intra-aortic balloon pump bridge

Aortic Insufficiency

BASICS
- Regurgitation of blood back into ventricle, leading to dilated cardiomyopathy and heart failure

ETIOLOGY
- Valvular abnormalities
  - Congenital bicuspid valve, rheumatic heart disease, IE
- Aortic root abnormalities
  - Ectasia, aneurysm, or dissection
  - Connective tissue diseases (Marfan's)
- Acute
  - Left ventricular compliance low
  - LV pressure increases rapidly
  - Acute pulmonary congestion
- Chronic
  - LV dilatation
  - Normal/near-normal CO
  - Significant regurgitation
  - Volume overload causes congestion

SIGNS AND SYMPTOMS
- Acute
  - History of aortic dissection, aneurysm, severe respiratory distress or shock
  - May have subtle physical findings
    - Short, soft diastolic murmur
- Chronic
  - Widened pulse pressure
    - Rapidly rising and falling carotid pulses
  - Heart sounds
    - High-pitched, blowing, diastolic murmur at left sternal border
    - Austin flint murmur: soft, diastolic rumble caused by regurgitant stream against mitral valve

DIAGNOSTICS
- Echocardiogram

TREATMENT
- Acute
  - Surgical emergency, immediate valve replacement
  - Medical stabilization: cautious vasodilation and diuretics
  - Intra-aortic balloon counterpulsation is contraindicated
- Chronic
  - Similar to other decompensated CHF

NOTES

Dermatologic Disorders—2%

Matthew Brochu, Hannah S. Dodd, and Donna Collins

● CUTANEOUS MANIFESTATIONS OF SYSTEMIC DISEASES

Stevens–Johnson Syndrome/Toxic Epidermal Necrolysis

BASICS
- A rare, life-threatening disorder of skin and mucous membranes
- Most commonly a reaction to a medication or an infection
- Toxic epidermal necrolysis involves more than 30% of the body surface, whereas Stevens–Johnson syndrome involves less than 10%

ETIOLOGY
- Usually drug related (sulfa, nonsteroidal anti-inflammatory drug, antiepileptics)
- Postinfectious

SIGNS AND SYMPTOMS
- Flu-like symptoms, pruritus
- **Nikolsky sign:** slight pressure of the skin results in exfoliation of the dermis, leaving a blister
- Mucosal involvement (oropharynx, eyes, genitals, anus)
- Can lead to respiratory distress

DIAGNOSTICS
- Based on clinical exam findings
- Skin biopsy shows keratinocytes

TREATMENT
- Airway, breathing, circulation (ABCs), supportive, IV fluids, pain control
- Withdrawal of causative agent
- Systemic corticosteroids
- Transfer to ICU or *burn* center

Necrotizing Fasciitis

BASICS
- A rapidly progressive bacterial infection of the fascia, with secondary necrosis of the subcutaneous tissues
- How quickly the disease spreads is directly proportional to the thickness of the subcutaneous layer
- High mortality rate

ETIOLOGY
- Polymicrobial or streptococcal (aka flesh eating)
- *Streptococcus pyogenes* (group A) is most common cause
- Infection of fascial planes causing thrombosis of blood vessels

SIGNS AND SYMPTOMS
- Initial cellulitic appearance
- Red tissue turns to dusky blue with rapid necrosis
- Pain out of proportion to exam
- Gangrenous tissue within 36 to 72 hours

DIAGNOSTICS
- Imaging to evaluate for gas in soft tissue (although gas is a late finding)
- Blood cultures
- Wound cultures

TREATMENT
- ABCs, supportive, IV fluids
- Broad-spectrum antibiotics
- Immediate surgical consult for surgical debridement

Toxic Shock Syndrome

BASICS
- Uncommon, life-threatening disease caused by bacterial toxin

ETIOLOGY
- *Staphylococcus aureus* infections caused from tampons or nasal packing
- Superficial skin infection or surgical wound infections

SIGNS AND SYMPTOMS
- Rash initially on trunk and spreads peripherally to palms and soles
- Generalized erythema with desquamation especially of palms and soles within 1 to 2 weeks
- Fever, hypotension, and potential multiorgan failure
- Systemic involvement can include vomiting and diarrhea, myalgias, involvement of mucous membranes, renal failure, hepatic inflammation, thrombocytopenia, central nervous system involvement

DIAGNOSTICS
- Physical exam findings and multisystem organ involvement
- Complete blood count, blood cultures

TREATMENT
- ABCs, intravenous fluids, supportive management
- Broad-spectrum antibiotics
- Remove tampon if that is the culprit
- Admit to ICU

● FUNGAL, BACTERIAL, AND VIRAL SKIN INFECTIONS
Fungal
Tinea
BASICS
- Tinea capitis: tinea of the scalp
- Tinea pedis: athlete's foot

- Tinea manuum: tinea of the hands
- Tinea unguium (onychomycosis): nail infection
- Tinea barbae: tinea of the beard area
- Tinea cruris (jock itch): tinea of the groin
- Tinea corporis (ring worm): tinea of the body

ETIOLOGY
- Fungal superficial dermatophyte infection
- Highly contagious

SIGNS AND SYMPTOMS
- Erythematous, pruritic, scaly, well demarcated plaques
- Thickened, yellow discoloration of the nails
- Spots with no hair on scalp

DIAGNOSTICS
- Clinical exam findings
- KOH preparation

TREATMENT
- Topical antifungal
- Oral antifungal is needed for tinea capitis

Candidiasis
BASICS
- Fungal infection which can cause a range of diseases from superficial to systemic

ETIOLOGY
- *Candida albicans*

SIGNS AND SYMPTOMS
- Erythematous, scaly plaques
- Commonly seen in intertriginous areas
- Oral thrush: white plaques on mucosal surface that easily scrape off

DIAGNOSTICS
- Clinical exam findings
- KOH preparations: budding yeast

TREATMENT
- Topical Nystatin
- Oral fluconazole

BACTERIAL
Impetigo
BASICS
- Highly contagious, superficial skin infection

ETIOLOGY
- *Staphylococcus aureus*
- *Streptococcus pyogenes*

SIGNS AND SYMPTOMS
- **Honey-crusted lesions**, usually around the mouth
- Usually affecting children

DIAGNOSTICS
- Clinical exam findings

TREATMENT
- Topical - Mupirocin
- Systemic - Cephalexin, amoxicillin-clavulanate.
  - If suspect MRSA, trimethoprim-sulfamethoxazole or clindamycin.

Abscesses

BASICS
- Pocket of pus from skin flora

ETIOLOGY
- *S. aureus* is the most common
- *Pseudomonas aeruginosa* from hot tubs or swimming pools

SIGNS AND SYMPTOMS
- Fluctuant, erythematous, painful, warm area
- Often seen around areas with increased hair follicles

DIAGNOSTICS
- Clinical exam findings
- Culture can confirm species, but not necessary

TREATMENT
- Incision and drainage
- If surrounding cellulitis or immunocompromised: Keflex, add Bactrim or Clinda if concerning for Methicillin-resistant *S. aureus*

Erysipelas

BASICS
- Bacterial skin infection

ETIOLOGY
- **Group A streptococcus** is the most common pathogen

SIGNS AND SYMPTOMS
- Tender, well-defined, shiny, erythematous, indurated plaque on the face or legs
- Fevers, lymphadenopathy

DIAGNOSTICS
- Clinical exam findings

TREATMENT
- IV antibiotics, most often penicillin, Ancef

Scarlet Fever

BASICS
- Common in 4 to 8 year olds
- Spread through inhalation

ETIOLOGY
- Caused by group A streptococcus

SIGNS AND SYMPTOMS
- Fever, sore throat, swollen glands, strawberry tongue, rash
- Erythematous rash, rough textured like sand paper that blanches upon pressure
- Most prominent in folds of skin such as armpits, neck, groin, chest

DIAGNOSTICS
- Clinical exam findings
- Throat culture for streptococcus

TREATMENT
- Antibiotics: first-line penicillin
- Complications include sepsis, glomerulonephritis, rheumatic fever, erythema nodosum

Viral

Herpes Zoster (Shingles)

BASICS
- Reactivation of varicella zoster virus in sensory nerve endings

ETIOLOGY
- Caused by varicella zoster virus
- Over half the cases appear in adults over 50 years

SIGNS AND SYMPTOMS
- Painful, **vesicular skin rash in a dermatomal pattern** that does not cross midline
- Headache, fevers, malaise
- Complications: motor involvement, secondary bacterial infections, eye involvement which could lead to blindness, postherpetic neuralgia

DIAGNOSTICS
- Clinical exam findings
- Confirmatory is polymerase chain reaction

TREATMENT
- Antiviral therapy within 72 hours onset of rash for 7 to 10 days may help lessen severity and length of illness
- Pain management

Measles (Rubeola)

BASICS
- Highly contagious virus spread through respiratory secretions

ETIOLOGY
- Paramyxovirus

SIGNS AND SYMPTOMS
- Fever, cough, coryza, conjunctivitis
- Maculopapular, erythematous rash starts in back of ears, spreads to face and trunk, and then extremities
- **Koplik spots in mouth:** white lesions on buccal mucosa

DIAGNOSTICS
- Clinical exam findings
- Confirmatory with enzyme immunoassay serologic test

TREATMENT
- Symptomatic treatment
- Prevention with MMR vaccine
- Complications include pneumonia, otitis media, corneal ulceration, encephalitis

Infestations

Scabies

BASICS
- Contagious skin infection caused by mites

ETIOLOGY
- *Sarcoptes scabiei*
- Mites burrow into the skin and lay eggs

SIGNS AND SYMPTOMS
- Intensely pruritic rash classically between web spaces, genitalia with excoriations in a linear pattern

DIAGNOSTICS
- Clinical

TREATMENT
- Permethrin, lindane
- Treat household members, and wash all clothing and bedding in high heat

Lice

BASICS
- Contagious, parasitic infection
- Lives on human hairs and feeds on human blood

ETIOLOGY
- Mites and nits (eggs) are spread through direct contact
- Usually school-aged children

SIGNS AND SYMPTOMS
- Itchy scalp is a reaction to lice saliva
- Papules often seen on neck and scalp

DIAGNOSTICS
- Clinical exam findings and visualization of lice or nits in hair

TREATMENT
- Permethrin, lindane
- Fine-toothed comb to manually remove nits

NOTES

NOTES

Endocrine, Metabolic, and Nutritional Disorders—4%

Erin Bradley, Sabrina E. Serino, Hannah S. Dodd, Kristen Vella Gray, and Fred Won

● ACID-BASE DISORDERS

BASICS
- Determine the primary disorder (Table 4.1)
  - Respiratory alkalosis
    - Central nervous system disorders
    - Hypoxia
    - Asthma, pneumonia, pulmonary edema, pulmonary embolism, anxiety hyperventilation
  - Respiratory acidosis
    - Respiratory center inhibition (opiates)
    - Neuromuscular disorder (Guillain–Barré, Myasthenia Gravis, hypokalemia)
    - Chest wall disorder (obesity)
    - Airway obstruction (chronic obstructive pulmonary disease)
  - Metabolic alkalosis
    - Chloride responsive (vomiting)
    - Nasogastric drainage, diuretics, posthypercapnia
    - Chloride resistant (primary or secondary aldosteronism)
  - Metabolic Acidosis: anion gap (AG)
    - **MUDPILES**
      - **M**ethanol/ethanol intoxication
      - **U**remia
      - **D**iabetic ketoacidosis (DKA)
      - **P**araldehydes
      - **I**soniazid
      - **L**actic acidosis
      - **E**thylene glycol intoxication
      - **S**alicylates

TABLE 4.1.   Primary Acid-Base Disorders

Disorder	pH (7.4)	pCO_2 mm Hg	HCO_3 mEq/L
Respiratory alkalosis	High	<40	—
Respiratory acidosis	Low	>40	—
Metabolic alkalosis	High	—	>24
Metabolic acidosis	Low	—	<24

TABLE 4.2.	Acid-Base Disorders Primary Defect and Compensatory Response	
Disorder	**Primary Defect**	**Compensatory Response**
Respiratory acidosis: *acute*	↑ pCO_2	↑ HCO_3
Respiratory acidosis: *chronic*	↑ pCO_2	↑ HCO_3
Respiratory alkalosis: *acute*	↓ pCO_2	↓ HCO_3
Respiratory alkalosis: *chronic*	↓ pCO_2	↓ HCO_3
Metabolic acidosis	↓ HCO_3	↓ pCO_2
Metabolic alkalosis	↑ HCO_3	↑ pCO_2

- Metabolic acidosis: non-anion gap
  - Appropriate renal response to acidemia
    - Diarrhea, type 2 RTA, dilutional
  - **Kussmaul breathing:** deep and labored breathing pattern
- **Evaluate for compensation**
  - Respiratory disorders depend on being chronic in order to compensate
  - If compensation does not match expected values, there is a mixed acid-base disorder
- **Determine the anion gap**
  - $Na - Cl + HCO_3$ = anion gap (normal 5 to 17)
  - If ≥20, then a metabolic acidosis almost always exists regardless of pH or HCO_3 (Table 4.2)

●ADRENAL INSUFFICIENCY AND CRISIS
Adrenal Insufficiency
BASICS
- Deficiency in cortisol and aldosterone
- Two types:
  - Primary is caused by impairment of adrenal gland
  - Secondary is caused by impairment of pituitary gland or hypothalamus

ETIOLOGY
- Autoimmune, adrenal hemorrhage or thrombosis, drugs, infection, sarcoidosis, metastatic cancer, surgery on adrenals, hereditary
- Sudden steroid withdrawal

SIGNS AND SYMPTOMS
- Weakness, dehydration, hypotension, nausea, vomiting, weight loss, abdominal pain, fever, confusion, lethargy
- Hypoglycemia, hyponatremia, hyperkalemia, hypercalcemia
- Hyperpigmentation is seen in primary adrenal insufficiency

DIAGNOSTICS
- **Adrenocorticotropic hormone stimulation test**

TREATMENT
- ABCs (airway, breathing, circulation), IV fluids
- Steroids
- Identifying cause

Adrenal Crisis
BASICS
- Acute life-threatening form of adrenal insufficiency

ETIOLOGY
- Most commonly caused by exogenous glucocorticoid intake
- Leading to mineralocorticoid deficiency

SIGNS AND SYMPTOMS
- Shock and altered mental status (AMS), acute pain in the abdomen or back, vomiting, diarrhea
- Hypotension refractory to fluid bolus

DIAGNOSTICS
- Adrenocorticotropic hormone stimulation test

TREATMENT
- ABCs, IV fluids, supportive
- **Hydrocortisone 100 mg IV bolus** is first-line therapy

DIABETIC KETOACIDOSIS

BASICS
- Hyperglycemia associated with ketosis and high AG metabolic acidosis
- Results from uncontrolled diabetes, typically type one; type two when acutely ill

ETIOLOGY
- Inadequate insulin treatment or noncompliance
- New onset diabetes (20% to 25%)
- Acute illness
  - Infection (30% to 40%)
  - Stroke
  - Myocardial infarction
  - Acute pancreatitis
- Drugs: glucocorticoids, higher-dose thiazide diuretics, clozapine or olanzapine, cocaine, second-generation antipsychotic agents

SIGNS AND SYMPTOMS
- Early: polyuria, polydipsia, nocturia, fatigue, weight loss, abdominal pain, nausea, and vomiting
- Severe: orthostatic hypotension, tachycardia, poor skin turgor decreased level of consciousness, and Kussmaul breathing and **acetone breath** (fruity odor) (Table 4.3)

DIAGNOSTICS
- Diagnostic criteria: hyperglycemia, AG metabolic acidosis, ketonemia
- Metabolic acidosis is often the major finding
- Serum glucose concentration is usually >250

TABLE 4.3. Diagnostic Features				
	Mild DKA	**Moderate DKA**	**Severe DKA**	**HHS**
Glucose	>250	>250	>250	>600
Arterial pH	7.25–7.30	7.00–7.24	<7.00	>7.30
Serum bicarb	15–18	10–<15	<10	>18
Urine ketones	+	+	+	Small
Serum ketones	+	+	+	Small
Serum os	Variable	Variable	Variable	>320
AG	>10	>12	>12	Variable
Mental status	Alert	Alert/drowsy	Stupor/coma	Stupor/coma

TREATMENT
- First priority: *fluid repletion!* while monitoring pH, K, and glucose
- Regular insulin as needed based on glucose either IV or subcutaneous with close monitoring and repletion of K
- Identify and treat underlying infection

● ELECTOLYTE DISORDERS AND SIADH

Hypokalemia

BASICS
- Serum K <3.5

ETIOLOGY
- Loop diuretics, gastrointestinal (GI) losses, malabsorption, lithium, insulin

SIGNS AND SYMPTOMS
- Weakness, cramps, hyporeflexia, ileus, metabolic alkalosis

DIAGNOSTICS
- Serum K <3.5
- EKG: U waves, ST depression, prolonged QT (Figure 4.1)

TREATMENT
- 20 meq K+ will raise K by 0.25 meq
  - 20 to 40 meq po or 10 to 20 meq IV (only able to give 10 meq per hour through peripheral IV)
- Replete Mg, normal Mg is required for maintenance of serum K levels
- In renal failure, small doses of oral or IV K dramatically increase serum K

Hyperkalemia

BASICS
- Serum K >5.5

ETIOLOGY
- Renal failure, medications, muscle breakdown

SIGN AND SYMPTOMS
- Vomiting, diarrhea, weakness

DIAGNOSTICS
- Serum K >5.5
- EKG: peaked T waves, prolonged PR, wide QRS, short QT interval (Vfib or sine wave pattern if K>8) (Figure 4.2)

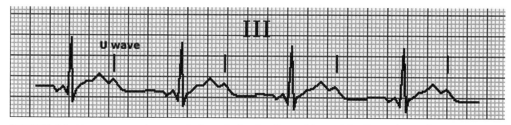

FIGURE 4.1. U waves may be seen in hypokalemia. (From Mount DB. Clinical manifestations and treatment of hypokalemia in adults. In: Post TW, ed. *UpToDate.* Waltham, MA: UpToDate; 2014. Graphic 73888 Version 2.0.)

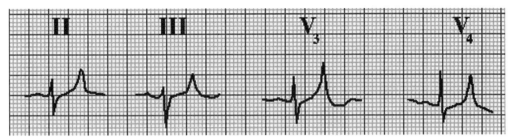

FIGURE 4.2. Tall peaked and symmetric T waves may be seen in hyperkalemia. (From Mount DB. Clinical manifestations and treatment of hyperkalemia in adults. In: Post TW, ed. *UpToDate.* Waltham, MA: UpToDate; 2014. Graphic 80441 Version 4.0.)

TREATMENT
- Calcium chloride or Calcium gluconate
- Bicarbonate or β-agonist (albuterol)
- Kayexalate
- Insulin (with D50 in euglycemic patients)

Hypomagnesemia

BASICS
- Serum Mg <1.5

ETIOLOGY
- Alcoholism, poor nutrition, cirrhosis, pancreatitis, correction of DKA, excessive GI losses, diuretic use

SIGNS AND SYMPTOMS
- Depression, vertigo, ataxia, seizures, increased deep tendon reflex, arrhythmia
- Hyperreflexia, tetany

DIAGNOSTICS
- Serum Mg <1.5
- EKG: prolonged PR, QT and QRS, **torsades de pointes** (Figure 4.3)

TREATMENT
- Oral/IV Mg

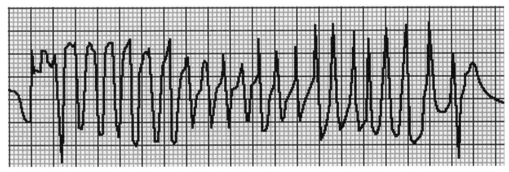

FIGURE 4.3. Torsades de pointes. (From Berul CL, Seslar SP, Zimetbaum PJ, Josephson ME. Acquired long QT syndrome. In: Post TW, ed. *UpToDate.* Waltham, MA: UpToDate; 2014. Graphic 53891 Version 4.0.)

Hypermagnesemia

BASICS
- Serum Mg >2.5

ETIOLOGY
- laxative or antacid use, iatrogenic, chronic renal impairment

SIGNS AND SYMPTOMS
- Nausea, vomiting, somnolence, muscle weakness respiratory depression, cardiac arrest

DIAGNOSTICS
- Serum Mg >2.5
- Often present with hyperkalemia as Mg and K move together intra/extra-cellularly
- EKG: wide QRS, prolonged PR

TREATMENT
- IV Ca chloride to antagonize effects of Mg
- IV Lasix
- Dialysis

Hypernatremia

BASICS
- Serum Na >145
- Excess water loss or increased Na intake

ETIOLOGY
- Fluid loss, steroid use
- Diuretics, dehydration, diabetes insipidus, iatrogenic, diarrhea, kidney disease, sickle cell disease

SIGNS AND SYMPTOMS
- Irritability, tremulousness, ataxia, lethargy, coma, seizures
- Impaired thirst mechanism

DIAGNOSTICS
- Serum Na >145
- Use urine osmoles to determine cause

TREATMENT
- Replace free water deficit with hypotonic saline
- Correct gradually over 48 to 72 hours
- Diuretics
- Desmopressin: if diabetes insipidus

Hyponatremia

BASICS
- Serum Na <130
- Most common electrolyte abnormality
- Three types: Hypovolemic, euvolemic, hypervolemic

ETIOLOGY
- GI loss, adrenal insufficiency, high-output ileostomy , medications, SIADH, paraneoplastic syndromes

SIGNS AND SYMPTOMS
- May be asymptomatic
- Nausea, vomiting, seizures, coma

DIAGNOSTICS
- Serum Na <130
- Urine Na can help distinguish from renal versus nonrenal causes

TREATMENT
- Water restriction
- Hypertonic saline IV (only for profound cases in patients who are symptomatic)
  - Caution with rapid correction of hyponatremia to avoid **central pontine myelinolysis**
- Loop diuretics

SIADH (Syndrome of Inappropriate Antidiuretic Hormone)

BASICS
- Defined as hypotonic hyponatremia

ETIOLOGY
- Excess antidiuretic hormone produces euvolemic hyponatremia
- Trauma, tumor, pneumonia, drugs, hypothyroidism

SIGNS AND SYMPOMS
- Anorexia, nausea, headache (HA), AMS, seizures

DIAGNOSTICS
- Hyponatremia
- Urine osmolality >100, urine Na >40

TREATMENT
- Fluid restriction
- Loop diuretics plus normal saline infusion
- Hypertonic saline for profound hyponatremia (<120 and moderate to severe neurologic symptoms)

Hypercalcemia

BASICS
- Serum Ca >11

ETIOLOGY
- Malignancy is number one cause
- Hyperparathyroidism

SIGNS AND SYMPTOMS
- **Stones, bones, moans, and psychiatric overtones**
- AMS, muscle weakness, nausea, vomiting

DIAGNOSTICS
- Serum Ca >11
- Ionized serum Ca >6 mg per dL
- ECG may show shortened QT interval

TREATMENT
- Must identify primary cause
- Ca restriction
- Loop diuretics, hydration
- Dialysis in severe cases

Hypocalcemia

BASICS
- Serum Ca <8

ETIOLOGY
- Renal failure, sepsis, pancreatitis
- Hypoparathyroidism

SIGNS AND SYMPTOMS
- **Chvostek sign**
  - Early sign
  - Tapping of the facial nerve causes muscle contraction on same side of face
- **Trousseau sign**
  - Late sign
  - Inflation of blood pressure cuff for 3 minutes will induce hand and arm spasm
- Usually asymptomatic, although many patients will experience perioral paresthesias, and generalized tetany

DIAGNOSTICS
- Serum Ca <8
- Ionized Ca <4.0 mg per dL
- EKG may show prolonged QT

TREATMENT
- Calcium gluconate
- Vitamin D

● HYPOTHYROIDISM, HYPERTHYROIDISM, THYROID STORM, AND MYXEDEMA

Hypothyroidism

BASICS
- Decreased levels of effective circulating thyroid hormone
- Myxedema coma is a rare extreme form characterized by AMS and defective thermoregulation

ETIOLOGY
- Autoimmune
  - Hashimoto thyroiditis
  - Postpartum thyroiditis
- Iodine deficiency
- Iatrogenic
  - Radiation, postsurgical, antithyroid drugs

SIGNS AND SYMPTOMS
- Hypothyroid
  - Weakness, fatigue, drowsiness, cold intolerance, menorrhagia, constipation
  - Absent lateral one-third eyebrows, prolonged deep tendon reflexes, swelling of hands and feet
- Myxedema coma:
  - Extreme form triggered by stress or illness
  - Profound lethargy, hypothermia
  - Bradycardia or circulatory collapse
  - Hyponatremia, hypoglycemia

DIAGNOSTICS
- Thyroid function testing (thyroid-stimulating hormone [TSH] increased, free T4 decreased)

TREATMENT
- Hypothyroidism without myxedema
  - Outpatient referral for oral replacement
- Myxedema coma
  - ABCs, supportive care
  - Correct hypothermia with passive warming
    - Active warming may cause hypotension from vasodilation
  - Thyroid replacement (levothyroxine 200 to 500 μg IV)
  - Glucocorticoids to prevent Addisonian crisis
  - Dextrose for hypoglycemia
  - Treat underlying precipitant

Hyperthyroidism

BASICS
- Excessive thyroid hormone production
- Can have mild disease to life-threatening manifestations
- 1% to 2% of patient progress to thyroid storm

ETIOLOGY
- **Graves disease** (autoimmune stimulation of TSH receptors)
- Toxic multinodular goiter
- Hashimoto thyroiditis
- Excessive iodine
- Postpartum thyroiditis
- Drug induced (amiodarone, lithium, levothyroxine)

SIGNS AND SYMPTOMS
- Sweating, tremor, weight loss, diarrhea
- **Thyroid storm**
  - A life-threatening condition that may be precipitated by
    - Infection, trauma, DKA, myocardial infarction/costovertebral angle, abrupt withdrawal, or acute injection of thyroid medication
  - Fever, tachycardia, dysrhythmias, high output congestive heart failure, shock, AMS

DIAGNOSTICS
- Clinical diagnosis for thyroid storm (fever, altered mental status, respiratory distress, seizure, nausea/vomiting, tachycardia disproportionate to fever)
- TSH (usually decreased), free T4 (usually increased)

TREATMENT
- Usually outpatient therapy unless thyroid storm
- Propylthiouracil, methimazole, iodine, β-blockers

⬤ HYPOGLYCEMIA

BASICS
- Abnormally low blood glucose levels

ETIOLOGY
- Iatrogenic hypoglycemia
  - Type 1 diabetic: injected too much insulin
  - Type 2 diabetic: side effect of sulfonylurea

- Fasting hypoglycemia: caused by hepatic failure, adrenocortical insufficiency, ethanol, insulinomas
- Postprandial: rare and occur several hours after eating and presents with adrenergic symptoms

SIGNS AND SYMPTOMS
- Coma and death can develop rapidly
- Autonomic response:
  - Hunger, diaphoresis, anxiety
  - Tremors, palpitation, tachycardia
  - Weakness, tingling around mouth/hands
- Neurologic response:
  - Blurred vision and HA
  - AMS with focal neuro deficits
  - Difficulty speaking and ambulating
  - Seizure and coma

DIAGNOSTICS
- Low serum glucose levels <60 mg per dL
- Brain function often impaired at 50 mg per dL

TREATMENT
- This is life-threatening
- Conscious patient: administer rapidly absorbed glucose (tablets, fruit juice)
- AMS, unable to swallow: give a IV bolus of an amp of D50

● HYPEROSMOLAR COMA

BASICS
- Also called hyperosmolar hyperglycemic state (HHS)
- Complication of diabetes, occurs almost exclusively in type 2 DM

ETIOLOGY
- Severe hyperosmolality and intense dehydration
- Severe hyperglycemia in absence of ketosis/acidosis
- Profound dehydration due to intense osmotic diuresis from high level hyperglycemia
- Precipitating factors often include infection or patients with limited access to water

SIGNS AND SYMPTOMS
- Insidious onset
- Polyuria, polydipsia, nocturia, weight loss, and malaise
- Altered sensorium, progressive to coma.
- Severely ill, dry oral mucosa, poor skin turgor
- Mortality rate >50%

DIAGNOSTICS
- Glucose often >1,000
- Renal failure, no acidosis, hypokalemia

TREATMENT
- ABCs, IV fluids, and electrolyte repletion are mainstay of treatment
- Insulin is required

HYPOPARATHYROIDISM

BASICS

- Occurs when the body secretes abnormally low levels of parathyroid hormone (PTH)
  - PTH plays a key role in regulating and maintaining a balance of Ca and P
- Four parathyroid glands in neck, adjacent to thyroid gland

ETIOLOGY

- Acquired
  - Most common cause
  - Occurs after accidental damage to or removal of the parathyroid glands during surgery
- Hereditary
  - Either the parathyroid glands are not present at birth or they do not work properly
  - Autoimmune disease
  - Immune system creates antibodies against the parathyroid tissues
  - Extensive cancer radiation treatment
  - Can result in destruction of parathyroid glands
  - Occasionally because of radioactive iodine treatment for hyperthyroidism
  - Hypomagnesemia

SIGNS AND SYMPTOMS

- Paresthesias in fingertips, toes, and lips
- Muscles aches and cramps
- Twitching or spasms around mouth, hands, arms
- Fatigue
- Patchy hair loss, dry, coarse skin
- HAs, memory problems

DIAGNOSTICS

- Clinical exam findings
- Serum testing of PTH, Ca, albumin, and vitamin D

TREATMENT

- Ca and vitamin D tablets
- Treatment is generally lifelong

NOTES

Environmental Disorders—2%

Hannah S. Dodd, Tara Itrich, Nicole Kostarellas, and Kristen Vella Gray

● ALTITUDE AND DIVE EMERGENCIES
High Altitude Syndrome

BASICS
- A broad spectrum of symptoms ranging from acute mountain sickness (AMS) to the more severe high altitude cerebral edema (HACE) and high altitude pulmonary edema (HAPE)
- High altitude syndrome typically appears on rapid ascent to altitude above 2,500 m (8,000+ feet)
- Caused by acute exposure to low partial pressure of oxygen at high altitude

MILD AMS
- **Signs and Symptoms**
  - No appetite, nausea, vomiting, fatigue, lightheadedness, tachycardia, headache
- **Treatment**
  - Stop ascent
  - Descend to lower altitude or acclimatize at same altitude
  - Symptomatic treatment as necessary

MODERATE AMS
- Signs and Symptoms
  - More intense than mild and are not relieved by over-the-counter medicines
  - Fatigue, weakness, and shortness of breath (SOB) worsen instead of improving over time
  - Loss of coordination, difficulty walking, severe headache, nausea and vomiting, and chest tightness
  - Normal activity is difficult, although the person may still be able to walk on his or her own
- Treatment
  - Immediate descent
  - Low-flow O_2 if available
  - Acetazolamide and/or dexamethasone
  - Hyperbaric therapy

High Altitude Cerebral Edema

BASICS
- A potentially life-threatening form of AMS characterized by swelling in the brain

ETIOLOGY
- Caused by the physiological effects of traveling to a high altitude
- Those patients with brain tumor, hydrocephalus, or recent bleeding are at an increased risk for HACE as there is less room for brain swelling

SIGNS AND SYMPTOMS
- Headache, confusion, behavior change, ataxia, speech difficulty, vomiting, seizures, coma, paralysis

DIAGNOSTICS
- Clinical evaluation

TREATMENT
- Immediate descent or evacuation
- Oxygen 2 to 4 L per minute or titrated to SaO_2 >90%
- Dexamethasone
- Hyperbaric therapy

High Altitude Pulmonary Edema

BASICS
- A life-threatening form of noncardiogenic pulmonary edema occurs at altitudes typically above 2,500 m

ETIOLOGY
- Caused by the physiological effects of traveling to a high altitude
- Seen with:
  - Rapid ascent
  - Physical exertion at high altitude
  - Exposure to cold

SIGNS AND SYMPTOMS
- Dyspnea, cough, chest tightness, central cyanosis, tachypnea, tachycardia, crackles or wheezing on exam

DIAGNOSTICS
- At least two of the following symptoms: SOB at rest, cough, weakness and decreased exercise performance, chest tightness or congestion
- *And* at least two of the following signs on physical exam: tachycardia, tachypnea, crackles or wheezing heard in the lungs, or hypoxia
- Chest x-ray pulmonary edema

TREATMENT
- Immediate descent or evacuation
- Oxygen 4 L per minute or titrated to SaO_2 >90%
- Dexamethasone
- Nifedipine
- Hyperbaric therapy; this can be simulated with a Gamow bag, which is a portable hyperbaric oxygen chamber
- Continuous positive airway pressure

PREVENTION
- Graded ascent with adequate time for acclimatization
- Avoid overexertion, alcohol, respiratory depressants
- **Acetazolamide prophylactically** for those with history of AMS or for forced ascent

● DECOMPRESSION ILLNESS

BASICS
- Results from a reduction in the ambient pressure surrounding a body, causing decompression
- Encompasses two diseases: decompression sickness (DCS) and arterial gas embolism (AGE)

Decompression Sickness

BASICS
- Also called "the bends"

ETIOLOGY
- Gas dissolved in body tissue under pressure precipitating out of solution and forming bubbles on decompression
- Typically affects scuba divers on poorly managed ascent from depth

SIGNS AND SYMPTOMS
- Usually appears within 15 minutes to 12 hours after surfacing
- Fatigue, pruritus, joint pains, vertigo, numbness, SOB, paralysis, rash, confusion, amnesia, tremors, personality changes, coughing up bloody, frothy sputum

DIAGNOSTICS
- Clinical evaluation

TREATMENT
- Oxygen, intravenous fluids (IVFs), hyperbaric chamber

Arterial Gas Embolism

BASICS
- Occurs within 10 minutes of surfacing from diving

ETIOLOGY
- Results from bubbles entering the lung circulation, traveling through the arteries, and causing tissue damage

SIGNS AND SYMPTOMS
- Dizziness, blurred vision, chest pain, confusion, paralysis, convulsion, respiratory arrest, death
- Symptoms of other consequences of lung overexpansion such as pneumothorax, subcutaneous or mediastinal emphysema

DIAGNOSTICS
- Clinical evaluation

TREATMENT
- Trendelenburg or left lateral positioning
- Oxygen
- Hyperbaric chamber

● ANIMAL BITES AND TOXIC ENVENOMATION

Hymenoptera (Wasps, Bees, and Ants)

ETIOLOGY
- Venom from wasps and bees contains histamine
- Ant venom is more alkaloid, but has cross-reactivity with venom from bees/wasps

SIGNS AND SYMPTOMS
- Redness, swelling, pain at local site
- Nausea, vomiting, and diarrhea
- Typically IgE-mediated symptoms
- Anaphylaxis
- Muscle spasms

TREATMENT
- Remove stinger! (scoop with credit card technique)
- Thoroughly irrigate wound with soap and water
- Oral antihistamines, ice, nonsteroidal anti-inflammatory drugs, as conservative management
- Anaphylaxis treatment
  - Epinephrine 1:1,000 0.3 to 0.5 mL SQ in adults

Brown Recluse Spider

BASICS
- Anatomy: **violin or fiddle back appearance**
- Distribution: North and South America, Africa, Mediterranean, Brazil, South Africa

SIGNS AND SYMPTOMS
- **Initially painless** with erythematous area
- Blister blue discoloration within 24 hours and pain
- Necrotic lesion in 3 to 4 days and eschar formation with 1 week
- Systemic illness is rare, more often in children and occurs 1 to 3 days after bite
- Nausea, vomiting, chills, arthralgias, hemolysis, thrombocytopenia, hemoglobinuria
- Acute renal failure, disseminated intravascular coagulation, death

TREATMENT
- ABCs (airway, breathing, circulation)
- Nonsteroidal anti-inflammatory drugs, steroids, pain control
- Infection management, including antibiotics
- Consider Dapsone leukocyte inhibitor

Black Widow Spider

BASICS
- Anatomy: red/orange hour glass marking on abdomen of spider
- Distribution: North America, Australia, Africa
- Neurotoxic protein in venom releases acetylcholine and norepinephrine
- April–October are more commons months

SIGNS AND SYMPTOMS
- Feel pinprick, **immediate pain,** and erythema that spreads quickly
- Within 20 to 60 minutes, it can extend to whole limb
- Then becomes target lesion 2 to 6 hours
- Muscle cramps and spasm, generalized trunk, back and abdominal pain for 24 hours or more

TREATMENT
- ABCs, tetanus, local wound care
- Pain management
- Benzodiazepines and consider Calcium gluconate for muscle spasm
- Latrodectus antivenom vial

Scorpions

BASICS
- Distribution: nocturnal stingers and highly toxic species found in Middle East, India, North Africa, South America, Mexico, Trinidad

SIGNS AND SYMPTOMS
- Immediate, severe pain, cranial and somatic motor dysfunction
- Usually no visible local injury

- Can develop rolling eye movements, blurred vision, pharyngeal muscle disorder, drooling, restlessness, myoclonic jerking, nausea, vomiting, tachycardia
- Can last 24 to 48 hours

TREATMENT
- ABCs, tetanus, local wound care
- Benzodiazepines for muscle spasm, pain control
- If severe: scorpion antivenin (in Arizona only)

Pit Vipers

BASICS
- Rattlesnakes, Copperheads, Water Moccasins, Mississauga
- Crotaline venom alters blood vessel permeability and causes hypovolemia
- It activates fibrinogen and platelets, which causes coagulopathy
- Blocks neuromuscular transmission: central nervous system weakness (ptosis), respiratory failure

SIGNS AND SYMPTOMS
- One or more fang marks, pain, edema extending from site
- Nausea, vomiting, weakness, oral numbness/tingling of tongue/mouth, tachycardia, dizziness, muscle fasciculation
- Tachypnea, tachycardia, hypotension, AMS
- Cellulitis, compartment syndrome, and shock

TREATMENT
- ABCs, supportive, tetanus, wound care
- Antivenin is the mainstay
- Before ED care, rest the affected limb, below the heart level with minimal activity
- A constriction band may be helpful to prevent venom from absorbing further along area
- If evidence of compartment syndrome, consider additional antivenom and fasciotomy
- Monitor for at least 8 hours

Coral Snake

BASICS
- Corals, cobras, kraits, mambas
- Anatomy: **bright colored with black, red, yellow rings**
- If poisonous the red and yellow rings touch (*"Red on yellow, kill a fellow; red on black, venom lack"*)
- Distribution: Southern US
- Venom is a neurotoxin

SIGNS AND SYMPTOMS
- Primarily neurologic effects
  - Diplopia, dysarthria, tremors, salivation, bulbar paralysis with ptosis, fixed/contracted pupils, dysphagia, dyspnea, seizures
- Caution respiratory muscle paralysis and death
- May be delayed for 12 hours and most have local and minimal reactions

TREATMENT
- ABCs, supportive, tetanus, wound care
- Antivenin is mainstay
- Admission for observation, consider ICU

Cat Bite

BASICS
- *Pasteurella multocida* most common pathogen
- High rate of infection despite antibiotics

SIGNS AND SYMPTOMS
- Puncture wounds 50% to 80% of the time

TREATMENT
- Consider x-ray to evaluate for retained tooth fragment
- Copious irrigation, tetanus
- Augmentin

● BURNS

BASICS
- First degree: superficial, epidermis only, painful (think sunburn)
- Second degree: partial thickness, epidermis and into the dermis, painful (blisters, red and deep second may be white)
- Third degree: full thickness, complete destruction of epidermis and dermis including nerve endings, **painless** (white, leathery to charred)
- Fourth degree: the existence of this degree is now being debated, may involve muscle or bones
- Classification of percentage total body surface area (TBSA)
  - Does not include first-degree burns
  - **Rule of nines**
    - 9% each: head/neck, each upper extremity
    - 18% each: anterior torso, posterior torso and buttocks, each lower extremity
    - 1%: genitalia/perineum
  - Palmar method: the patient's palmar hand equals 1% of his or her TBSA (Figure 5.1)
- Inhalation injuries
  - 100% oxygen non-rebreather mask prior to evaluation
  - Signs: soot in nares or oropharynx, oropharyngeal, or uvula edema
  - Order **HbCO to assess CO level** and cyanide levels
  - Treatment: airway protection by endotracheal tube
- Electrical burns
  - There is more damage than can be seen, high risk for internal injuries (order complete blood count, comprehensive metabolic panel, cardiac enzymes, lipase)
  - Muscle damage (order creatine kinase and urine myoglobin)
  - Resuscitation: requires more IVF to prevent acute renal failure from rhabdomyolysis
  - Heart damage and arrhythmias (order EKG/telemetry)
- Consider transfer to a burn center

TREATMENT
- ABCs, may need intubation
- Large bore IV, pain control, tetanus
- Elevate burned limbs, serial pulse checks
- Resuscitate IV fluids
  - Parkland formula for 20% TBSA or more
- Prophylactic antibiotics are *never* indicated
- Escharotomy for circumferential burns to prevent compartment syndrome
- Debridement and skin grafting (third- and fourth-degree burns)

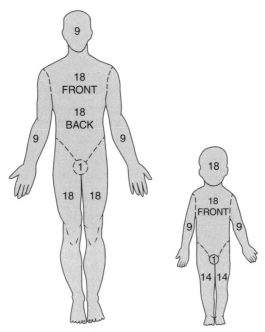

FIGURE 5.1. The "rule of nines" roughly estimates the TBSA burned. (From Roberts JR, Hedges JR, ed. *Hedges' Clinical Procedures in Emergency Medicine.* 6th ed. Philadelphia, PA: Saunders/Elsevier; 2013. Figure 38.5 MD consult.)

- Small burns
  - First degree: A and D or antibiotic ointment
  - Second degree: antibiotic ointment and nonadherent petroleum dressing
  - Silver sulfadiazine for deep second- and third-degree burns

● HYPERTHERMIA AND HYPOTHERMIA

Heat Stroke

BASICS
- Life-threatening
- Loss of thermoregulation leads to multisystem organ failure
- Mortality 21% to 63%

ETIOLOGY
- Chronically ill, elderly, alcoholics, athletes
- Strenuous exertion in high heat and humidity
- Risk factors
  - Lack of acclimatization
  - Dehydration
  - Obesity
  - Poor physical fitness

SIGNS AND SYMPTOMS
- Core temperature >104° to 106°F measured rectally
- Anhidrosis, dehydration

- Neurologic changes
- May be hemodynamically unstable

TREATMENT
- ABCs, supportive care, rapid cooling, including rectal temperature
- Monitor for complications: rhabdomyolysis, renal failure, disseminated intravascular coagulation
- Cooling with mist, fans, ice water immersion, ice packs on neck, groin, axillae
  - Severe cases consider peritoneal lavage and cardiopulmonary bypass
- Use benzodiazepines for shivering
- No role for acetaminophen
- Admission

Frostbite

BASICS
- Freezing injury and tissue destruction

SIGNS AND SYMPTOMS
- Numbness
- White, waxy skin
- Distal areas at greatest risk: fingers, toes, ears, nose, and penis
- Black eschar if severe

TREATMENT
- Remove wet clothing, insulate and immobilize affected area
- Avoid friction massage
- Tetanus, pain control, limb elevation, topical aloe vera
- Consider aspirating clear blisters
- Rapid thaw of tissue by immersion in water temperature 40° to 42°C/104° to 108°F

Hypothermia

BASICS
- Core temperature <35°C/95°F

SIGNS AND SYMPTOMS
- Mild (90° to 95°F/32° to 35°C)
  - Shivering, poor judgment, loss of fine motor skills, tachycardia
- Moderate (86° to 90°F/30° to 32°C)
  - Shivering stops, dysrhythmias, bradycardia, dilated pupils
- Severe (<86°F/<30°C)
  - Hypotension, coma, unresponsive

DIAGNOSTICS
- History and rectal temperature measured <35°C
- ECG: may have Osborne or "J" wave (Figure 5.2)

TREATMENT
- ABCs, stabilize patient
- Rewarm
  - Passive: insulation, warm blankets
  - Active external: warm blankets, warm water immersion, Bair Hugger
  - Active internal: heated IVF, heated humidified O_2, peritoneal lavage, hemodialysis, cardio-pulmonary bypass
  - Active rewarming for moderate to severe hypothermia (<32.2°C)

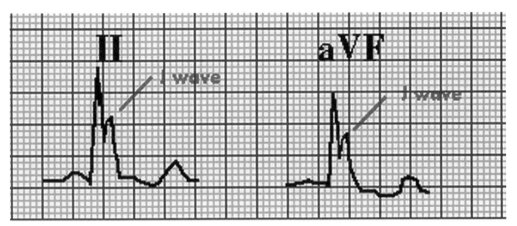

FIGURE 5.2. J waves or Osborn waves may be seen in hypothermia. (From Prutkin JM. ECG tutorial: miscellaneous diagnoses. In: Post TW, ed. *UpToDate*. Waltham, MA: UpToDate; 2014. Graphic 80836 Version 2.0.)

- Mainstay treatment for cardiac dysrhythmias is rewarming and advanced cardiac life support protocol
- Should rewarm patient before pronouncing dead

INHALATION OF CO

BASICS
- Binds to hemoglobin, which impairs O_2 transport and utilization
- CO is responsible for most common cause of death due to poisoning in US
  - Home generators, vehicle exhaust, fires

SIGNS AND SYMPTOMS
- Headache (most common), malaise, nausea, vomiting, dizziness, diarrhea, occasional cherry-red skin
- Severe: seizure, syncope, myocardial infarction, arrhythmias, pulmonary edema, acidosis

DIAGNOSIS
- History and carboxyhemoglobin (HbCO)
  - Normal: nonsmoker (0% to 3%), smoker (10% to 15%)
- Pulse oximetry and arterial blood gas cannot screen for exposure

TREATMENT
- High-flow O_2 non-rebreather
- Consider hyperbaric oxygen chamber and intubation if: Loss of consciousness (LOC), AMS, end-organ damage, **pregnant**

NOTES

Head, Ear, Eye, Nose, and Throat Disorders—5%

Tara Itrich, Noelia Kvaternik, Benjamin L. Miller, Kristen Vella Gray, and Fred Won

CROUP, EPIGLOTTITIS, PEDIATRIC UPPER RESPIRATORY INFECTION, AND PERTUSSIS

Croup

BASICS
- Laryngotracheobronchitis
- Peak incidence late fall/early winter
- Children 3 months to 3 years old most common

ETIOLOGY
- Parainfluenza 1 is most common
- Swelling leads to varying degrees of obstruction
- Spasmodic croup less common and associated with asthma and allergies

SIGNS AND SYMPTOMS
- **Barking seal-like cough**, hoarse voice, inspiratory stridor, respiratory distress
- Retractions, grunting, fatigue
- Prodrome 1 to 2 days, peak symptoms 2 to 3 days, resolution 5 to 7 days

DIAGNOSTICS
- Clinical, consider x-rays
- **Steeple sign** on lateral neck x-ray indicative of subglottic narrowing

TREATMENT
- Nebulized racemic epinephrine in severe cases
- Glucocorticoids
- Cool mist unproven

Epiglottitis

BASICS
- A life-threatening inflammatory condition of the epiglottis and surrounding soft tissue

ETIOLOGY
- Acute bacterial infection, usually *Haemophilus influenzae* type B (HIB)

SIGNS AND SYMPTOMS
- Sore throat, high fever, rapid onset, inspiratory stridor, dysphagia, drooling
- **Tripod posture**
- **"Muffled, hot potato voice"**

DIAGNOSTICS
- Clinical
- Lateral soft tissue neck film, "**thumb sign**"

TREATMENT
- Antibiotics (Ceftriaxone or Unasyn)
- Early airway management, preferably in OR

Pediatric Upper Respiratory Infection

BASICS
- Children get 6 to 8 colds per year

ETIOLOGY
- Most infections viral
- Children in day care get more colds

SIGNS AND SYMPTOMS
- Mucopurulent rhinitis is common
- Cough and nasal discharge may last 2 weeks
- Low-grade fever

TREATMENT
- No antibiotics
- Education for parents is key
- Fluids, acetaminophen, ibuprofen, nasal saline, humidifier
- Avoid over-the-counter cold preparations in kids
- Consider pertussis or mycoplasma pneumonia if cough lasts more than 2 weeks

Pertussis

BASICS
- Highly contagious
- Lower respiratory tract infection

ETIOLOGY
- Bordetella pertussis

SIGNS AND SYMPTOMS
- Persistent cough
- Rhinorrhea, low-grade fevers, conjunctival injection

DIAGNOSTICS
- Pertussis kit, including nasal pharyngeal swabs

TREATMENT
- Droplet precautions
- Macrolides, albuterol as needed
- Admit patients <1 year old

● EPISTAXIS AND NASAL FOREIGN BODY

Epistaxis

BASICS
- Ninety percent of bleeds occur at **Kiesselbach plexus** (anterior nasal septum)
- Ten percent posterior bleeds occur at sphenopalatine artery

ETIOLOGY
- Number one cause in children is trauma
- Infection, foreign body, cocaine, hypertension (HTN)
- Patients on anticoagulants

SIGNS AND SYMPTOMS
- Anterior
  - Usually unilateral
  - Do not feel blood in posterior pharynx
  - Bright red blood
- Posterior
  - Severe
  - Cannot visualize site of bleeding
  - Patient has blood in posterior pharynx and/or both nares
  - Blood is dark red

DIAGNOSTICS
- Complete blood count and coags if severe bleeding

TREATMENT
- Direct pressure
- Vasoconstrictors such as Afrin, oxymetazoline
- Chemical, electrical, thermal cautery
- Nasal packing
- Posterior bleeds require balloon device, ENT consult, and admission

Nasal Foreign Body

BASICS
- Most common in children
- Beads, buttons, toy parts
- Usually unilateral

DIAGNOSTICS
- History and physical exam

TREATMENT
- Mechanical removal if visible
  - Suction or forceps
  - Positive pressure ventilation with parent blowing air into child's mouth while blocking opposite nostril
- ENT referral if unable to remove

● EXTERNAL, MIDDLE, AND INNER EAR DISORDERS

Otitis Externa

BASICS
- Infection of the external ear, external canal, or external surface of tympanic membrane (TM)
- Necrotizing otitis externa: starts in ear canal and progresses through periauricular tissue toward base of skull
- Common in moist environments

ETIOLOGY
- Most common pathogen: *Pseudomonas aeruginosa* and *Staphylococcus aureus*

SIGNS AND SYMPTOMS
- Fullness and itching of ear
- Drainage, swelling, and erythema of canal

DIAGNOSTICS
- Clinical, visual inspection
- Pain with motion of pinna/tragus
- CT/MRI if suspecting bony involvement

TREATMENT
- Cleanse ear canal and keep dry
- Polymyxin-neomycin-hydrocortisone (Cortisporin) ear drops
- **Ofloxacin drops (drug of choice for perforated TMs)**
- Consider wick placement

Acute Otitis Media

BASICS
- Viral or bacterial infection of the middle ear
- Most commonly occurs in children less than 10 years of age

ETIOLOGY
- Most common pathogens: *Streptococcus pneumoniae* 50%, *H. influenzae* 20%, and *Moraxella catarrhalis* 10%
- Dysfunction of Eustachian tube leads to retention of secretions

SIGN AND SYMPTOMS
- Unilateral ear pain and fullness
- Decreased hearing
- Poor feeding or irritability in infants
- Bulging and erythematous TM
- Loss of light reflex and limited mobility of TM (most sensitive)

DIAGNOSTICS
- Clinical, visual inspection

TREATMENT
- Analgesia, typically self resolves without antibiotics
- If severe or less than 6 months of age, use Amoxicillin

Acute Mastoiditis

BASICS
- Inflammation, infection, or destruction of the mastoid air cells caused by acute purulent otitis media

ETIOLOGY
- Distribution of organisms can differ from those of otitis media

SIGNS AND SYMPTOMS
- Swelling, erythema, tenderness, and fluctuance over the mastoid process
- Ear pain, mild to moderate hearing loss, fever, headache

DIAGNOSTICS
- Mastoid plain films can reveal opacification of the mastoid air cells
- CT better at showing destruction of air cells as well as abscess formation
- MRI if suspecting brain involvement that cannot be confirmed by CT

TREATMENT
- Third-generation cephalosporins are preferred as better penetration into central nervous system
- ENT consult for consideration of surgical drainage

HEARING LOSS
BASICS
- Can involve the external ear, middle ear, or TM
- **Conductive**
  - Results from causes that limit amount of external sound from gaining access to inner ear, such as cerumen impaction, fluid
- **Sensorineural**
  - Results from disorders of inner ear, cochlea, CN VIII

DIAGNOSTICS
- History and physical exam
- **Rinne test**: air conduction (AC) is greater than bone conduction (BC). Abnormal test of BC >AC suggests conductive hearing loss
- **Weber test**: sound heard equally on both sides. If lateralizes to "good" side, suggests sensorineural loss. If lateralizes to "bad" side, suggests conductive hearing loss

TREATMENT
- Hearing aids, cochlear implants
- Auditory, speech-language training
- Removal of cerumen if impacted

OCULAR DISORDERS
General approach to the eye exam includes assessment of visual acuity, extraocular muscles, visual fields, pupils (reactivity, symmetry, shape), conjunctivae, cornea, anterior chamber, iris, orbital rim, lens, vitreous, retina

Chemical Burn
BASICS
- Chemical exposure to the eye can cause permanent damage
- Extent of damage depends on substance

ETIOLOGY
- Most occur at work or from home-cleaning products
- Alkali substance, acidic substance, irritants

SIGNS AND SYMPTOMS
- Redness, irritation, burning

DIAGNOSTICS
- Clinical findings
- Check pH:
  - Substances with pH values <7 are acids, >7 are alkaline (more dangerous)

TREATMENT
- Most are treated with liters of normal saline irrigation. ± Morgan lens, until pH becomes a neutral 7
- Irrigation contraindications: dry lime, phenol, hydrochloric acid, sulfuric acid, metals (K and Na)
- Emergent ophthalmology consult, further treatment based on acid or base
- Usual recommendation includes analgesic eye drops and ophthalmic fluoroquinolone

Open Globe

BASICS
- *Never* add drops or pressure!

ETIOLOGY
- Trauma

SIGNS AND SYMPTOMS
- Distortion of eye, loss of vision, displaced lens, traumatic hyphema, hemorrhagic swelling of the conjunctivae, shallow or deep anterior chamber

DIAGNOSTICS
- Clinical findings
- **Seidel test**: screening tool used to asses for corneal injury. After application of fluorescence, asses for aqueous fluid "stream" across cornea
- Consider CT

TREATMENT
- Emergent Ophthalmology consult given risk of vision loss
- Place rigid shield over, but not touching the globe
- Pain medication to avoid Valsalva and grimacing
- IV Antibiotics: cephalosporin, if there is soil then clindamycin
- Surgery

Traumatic Hyphema

BASICS
- Blood in anterior chamber
- Rule out an open globe first!
- Elevated intraocular pressure (IOP) occurs in 30% (>21 mm Hg), can develop up to 1 week posttrauma

ETIOLOGY
- Trauma most common
- Hemophilia, sickle cell disease
- Cancer

SIGNS AND SYMPTOMS
- Photophobia, decreased visual acuity, anisocoria

DIAGNOSIS
- Blood in the anterior chamber
- Slit lamp for microhyphema

TREATMENT
- Elevate head of bed >30 degrees, eye shield, pain control, avoid blood thinners/nonsteroidal anti-inflammatory drugs
- Ophthalmology consult
  - If increased IOP—start dilation drops (atropine), steroid drops (prednisolone), topical antibiotics, acetazolamide
  - Consider surgery

Corneal Abrasions

BASICS
- Defect on cornea

ETIOLOGY
- Caused by injury or foreign body

SIGNS AND SYMPTOMS
- Pain, tearing, foreign body sensation, photophobia, decreased visual acuity

DIAGNOSTICS
- Slit lamp: fluorescein uptake on cobalt blue light

TREATMENT
- Remove foreign body by irrigation, cotton swab, or needle tip
- Use of automated burr to remove rust ring
- No contact lenses or patching
- Antibiotic ointment or drops (erythromycin, Cipro)
- Pain control
- Ophthalmology follow-up
- Usually improves in 24 to 48 hours

Retinal Detachment

BASICS
- Emergent condition where the retina pulls away from the blood supply
- Usually occurs weeks to months after trauma, within 6 months

ETIOLOGY
- Trauma, age, diabetes, inflammatory disorders

SIGNS AND SYMPTOMS
- Floaters, flashing lights
- Curtain/shade in a visual field

DIAGNOSTICS
- Visual field deficit and dilated pupil on ophthalmoscopic exam

TREATMENT
- Ophthalmology consult
- Surgery

Iritis

BASICS
- Inflammatory process of the iris and anterior chamber

ETIOLOGY
- Infection
- Immune reaction
- Systemic disorders

SIGNS AND SYMPTOMS
- Unilateral, painful, red eye
- Photophobia, blurry vision

DIAGNOSTICS
- Slit lamp

TREATMENT
- Ophthalmology referral
- Pain control
- Steroids

Central Retinal Artery Occlusion

BASICS
- Form of ischemic stroke involving the central retinal artery, which supplies the inner retina and surface of the optic nerve

ETIOLOGY
- Most commonly caused by cholesterol embolus causing profound vision loss
- The incidence is very low; population at risk is those at risk for other types of vasculopathy (HTN, diabetes mellitus, smoking)

SIGNS AND SYMPTOMS
- Acute, **painless monocular loss of vision**

DIAGNOSTICS
- Clinical history
- Fundoscopic exam shows cherry-red spot at the fovea
- Retinal angiography performed by an ophthalmologist is the diagnostic gold standard

TREATMENT
- Conservative therapy includes ocular massage, which may dislodge clots
- Emergent ophthalmic consult is a must
- Consider acetazolamide, thrombolytics, and reducing IOP

Blepharitis

BASICS
- Inflammation of eyelid

ETIOLOGY
- May be caused by *S. aureus*

SIGNS AND SYMPTOMS
- Crusting, itching of eyelids
- "Sand in eye when blink"

DIAGNOSTICS
- Clinical, visual inspection

TREATMENT
- Careful washing of lids
- Warm compresses

Periorbital and Orbital Cellulitis

BASICS
- Periorbital
  - Involves the anterior structures, that is, lids, and does not involve the orbit or deeper structures
- Orbital
  - Involves the structures of the orbit such as muscles and fat and is therefore much more serious
  - Can lead to intracranial extension, abscess formation, thrombosis and central retinal artery occlusion

ETIOLOGY
- The paranasal sinuses are the main source of infection in orbital
- Strep species, *S. aureus* and anaerobes

SIGNS AND SYMPTOMS
- Unilateral eye pain, erythema, swelling
- They are distinguishable by **pain with extraocular muscle**

DIAGNOSTICS
- CT imaging if orbital cellulitis is suspected

TREATMENT
- Periorbital can be treated outpatient with Augmentin
- Orbital is treated with broad-spectrum IV antibiotics, ophthalmology consult, admission

Acute Angle Closure Glaucoma

BASICS
- Glaucoma is an optic neuropathy, which leads to visual field/peripheral vision loss, usually associated with increased IOP
- Two types: open angle and closed angle
  - Ninety percent of glaucoma is open angle and is painless and progressive
  - Ten percent of glaucoma is closed angle

ETIOLOGY
- Sudden closing or narrowing of the anterior angle (normally, this angle provides for proper flow/drainage of aqueous humor) causes an outflow obstruction of aqueous humor, leading to a sudden, rapid rise in IOP and damage to the optic nerve
- Risk factors include age >45, female, hyperopia, certain medications (anticholinergics, over-the-counter decongestants)

SIGNS AND SYMPTOMS
- Severe eye pain, decreased vision, headache, halo effect around lights, and vomiting
- Conjunctiva may be injected and the pupil mid-dilated (4 to 6 mm) and poorly reactive to light

DIAGNOSTICS
- Evaluation should include visual acuity, pupil evaluation, and IOP >21

TREATMENT
- Timolol and pilocarpine eye drops
- Emergent ophthalmic consult who will consider systemic medications such as acetazolamide and mannitol
- **This is a true ophthalmic emergency**

● ORAL AND DENTAL EMERGENCIES

Dental Abscess

ETIOLOGY
- Decay of tooth beyond enamel into the pulp
- Polymicrobial

SIGNS AND SYMPTOMS
- Severe dental pain
- Swelling, fever
- Fluctuance
- Lymphadenopathy

DIAGNOSTICS
- Usually based on exam
- Consider CT if concerned infection extends into deeper space

TREATMENT
- Antibiotics
- Incision and drainage if possible
- Referral to dentist

Dental Fracture

See Table 6.1
- For tooth avulsions:
  - Store tooth in milk, saline
  - A delay more than 2 hours affects prognosis

Ludwig Angina

BASICS
- Life-threatening infection of the floor of the mouth
- Rapidly spreading gangrenous cellulitis, necrotizing fasciitis of submaxillary, sublingual, submandibular spaces
- Most deaths due to respiratory obstruction

ETIOLOGY
- Usually from bacterial odontogenic infections, poor dental hygiene
- Most commonly caused by mouth anaerobe *Bacteroides*
- Also *Streptococcus viridans, Staphylococcus aureus, Staphylococcus epidermidis*

SIGNS AND SYMPTOMS
- Submandibular pain
- Tongue elevation, protrusion, swollen neck
- Trismus, odynophagia, fever
- Patient prefer sitting or sniffing position
- **Hard, "woody,"** painful submandibular area

DIAGNOSTICS
- Head and neck CT

TABLE 6.1. **Dental Fracture Classification**			
Type	**Definition**	**Symptoms**	**Treatment**
Ellis I	Enamel	Painless	Dental
Ellis II	Enamel + dentin	Painful	Calcium hydroxide/dental foil Consult dentist in 24 h
Ellis III	Pulp	Bleeding, red line or dot	Dental consult Treat in 48 h

TREATMENT
- ABCs, supportive care
- Emergent ENT consult for surgical drainage/excision
  - IV antibiotics: penicillin, Flagyl, or clindamycin
  - Admit to ICU for airway monitoring

● PERITONSILLAR AND RETROPHARYNGEAL ABSCESS
Peritonsillar Abscess
BASICS
- Most common deep infection of the head and neck
- Can lead to jugular vein thrombosis (Lemierre disease)

ETIOLOGY
- Direct bacterial invasion into peritonsillar space
- Polymicrobial

SIGNS AND SYMPTOMS
- Unilateral sore throat, fever, lymphadenopathy
- Unilateral peritonsillar bulge on soft palate
- Uvular deviation away from affected side

DIAGNOSTICS
- Clinical, visual inspection
- Consider CT neck

TREATMENT
- ABCs, IV fluid
- Antibiotics against oral flora: Unasyn, Clinda
- Steroids for inflammation
- Incision and drainage
- ENT consult

Retropharyngeal Abscess
BASICS
- Infection of the retropharyngeal space
  - Anterior to prevertebral space, posterior to pharyngeal mucosa

ETIOLOGY
- Often preceded by bacterial or viral upper respiratory infections
- Many are idiopathic

SIGNS AND SYMPTOMS
- Fever, dysphagia, stridor
- Hyperextension of neck
- Neck swelling, drooling
- Toxic appearing

DIAGNOSTICS
- CT neck with contrast

TREATMENT
- ABCs, IV fluids, antibiotics
- ENT consult and drainage preformed in OR

● SINUSITIS

BASICS
- Inflammation and/or infection of the paranasal sinuses
- Viral upper respiratory infection is the most common cause

ETIOLOGY
- Occurs when there is sinus drainage obstruction
- Caused by viruses, *S. pneumoniae, H. influenzae*

SIGNS AND SYMPTOMS
- Pain/pressure over sinuses
- Headache, fever
- Purulent nasal discharge
- Tenderness to palp or percussion over sinuses

DIAGNOSTICS
- Usually by clinical diagnosis
- CT if diagnosis is uncertain; if patient is immunocompromised or toxic appearing

TREATMENT
- Supportive with decongestants, antihistamines
- Antibiotics if suspecting bacterial cause
  - Amoxicillin or Augmentin are first-line choices

NOTES

NOTES

Hematologic Disorders—2%

Hana Dubsky, Patricia Gatcomb, and Michelle Higgins

● ANEMIAS

Iron-Deficiency Anemia

BASICS

- Microcytic anemia
- Occurs in infants, adults, and elderly

ETIOLOGY

- **Most common cause in women of childbearing age is menstruation**
- Most common cause in men is gastrointestinal bleed (GIB)
- Poor nutritional intake

SIGNS AND SYMPTOMS

- Glossitis, cheilitis, pica, koilia, jaundice, enlarged spleen, pale mucosa, tachycardia
- Fatigue, weakness, palpitations

DIAGNOSTICS

- Hematocrit, serum iron level, total iron-binding capacity, ferritin

TREATMENT

- Oral iron supplements

Thalassemia

BASICS

- Microcytic anemia
- More common those of Mediterranean descent

ETIOLOGY

- Hereditary—autosomal recessive
- Dysfunction with synthesis of globin subunits of α- or β-hemoglobin

SIGNS AND SYMPTOMS

- Pale mucosa, jaundice, facial bone deformities, slow growth, enlarged spleen
- Fatigue, weakness

DIAGNOSTICS

- Hematocrit, peripheral smear shows target cells, hemoglobin electrophoresis

TREATMENT
- Packed red blood cell (PRBC) transfusion to ameliorate anemia
- Splenectomy, iron chelation, bone marrow transplant for severe cases
- No treatment necessary for α- or β-thalassemia minor

Lead Poisoning

BASICS
- Microcytic anemia
- Buildup of lead in bloodstream and tissues, usually over months or years
- Children under age 6 are especially vulnerable

ETIOLOGY
- Inhalation, ingestion, absorption of lead from dust or contaminated paint in soils or older buildings

SIGNS AND SYMPTOMS
- Developmental delay, irritability, weight loss, fatigue, abdominal pain, vomiting, constipation, hearing loss

DIAGNOSTICS
- Blood lead level >5 μg per dL is unsafe in children

TREATMENT
- Treatment at blood lead level >45 μg per dL
- Remove contamination, chelation therapy

Vitamins B$_{12}$ Deficiency

BASICS
- Macrocytic anemia
- Often seen in nutritionally compromised patients, alcoholics, older adults

ETIOLOGY
- Vitamin B$_{12}$ or intrinsic factor deficiency
- Patients with prior history of bariatric surgery cannot produce intrinsic factor

SIGNS AND SYMPTOMS
- Glossitis, diarrhea, weight loss
- **Distinguished from folate deficiency with neuro symptoms:** paresthesias, peripheral neuropathies, dementia, ataxia

DIAGNOSTICS
- B$_{12}$ level, folate level, methylmalonic acid, homocysteine levels

TREATMENT
- Monthly intramuscular injections of B$_{12}$
- Severe B$_{12}$ deficiency left untreated can cause *irreversible* dementia

Folate Deficiency

BASICS
- Macrocytic anemia
- Folate is found in liver, green vegetables, cereals, cheese
- Seen most commonly in alcoholics, nutritionally compromised patients

ETIOLOGY
- Nutritional deficiency of folate

SIGNS AND SYMPTOMS
- Pale mucosa and skin, glossitis
- Malaise, anorexia, poor growth, recurrent infection

DIAGNOSTICS
- Hematocrit, B_{12} level, folate level

TREATMENT
- 1 to 2 mg folic acid po daily

Aplastic Anemia

BASICS
- Nonmegaloblastic macrocytic anemia
- Acquired failure of the hematopoietic stem cells, results in pancytopenia

ETIOLOGY
- Due to damage to the pluripotent stem cell
- Common complication of parvovirus B19 infection

SIGNS AND SYMPTOMS
- Fatigue and cardiopulmonary compromise due to anemia
- Recurrent infections
- Increased menstrual flow

DIAGNOSTICS
- Hematocrit
- Profound hypocellularity on bone marrow biopsy

TREATMENT
- Remove the offending agent
- Bone marrow transplant, corticosteroids, growth factor

G6PD Deficiency

BASICS
- Hemolytic anemia
- More common in African American and Mediterranean descent

ETIOLOGY
- Due to an inability to regenerate reduced glutathione
- Hemolysis is precipitated by drugs, infection, fava beans

SIGNS AND SYMPTOMS
- Classic course is episodic stress or infection-induced hemolytic anemia: jaundice, dark urine

DIAGNOSTICS
- Hematocrit, "blister cells" on peripheral smear, elevated indirect bilirubin, lactate dehydrogenase, low haptoglobin, nicotinamide adenine dinucleotide phosphate formation on G6PD assay

TREATMENT
- Treatment is supportive—PRBCs, vigorous hydration to protect the kidneys
- Avoid offending agents

Sickle Cell Disease

BASICS
- Hemolytic anemia characterized by sickled RBCs
- More common in African Americans

ETIOLOGY

- Hereditary—autosomal recessive
- Amino acid substitution of β-globin chain of Hgb
- Sickling shortens RBC survival time, causes microvascular obstruction, ischemia, infarction
- Sickling is accentuated by hypoxia, acidosis, fever, dehydration, infection

SIGNS AND SYMPTOMS

- Acute: precipitated by infection, dehydration, hypoxia, parvovirus B
  - Bone pain, abdominal pain, priapism, stroke
  - **Acute chest syndrome:**
    - ○ Fever, cough, chest pain, shortness of breath
    - ○ Chest x-ray may show pulmonary infiltrates
    - ○ Major cause of mortality
- Chronic:
  - Jaundice, biliary gallstones, splenomegaly, pretibial ulcers, dactylitis

DIAGNOSTICS

- Most diagnoses are made with newborn screening tests
- Hematocrit, hemoglobin electrophoresis, peripheral smear, retic count
- If suspect acute chest consider chest x-ray

TREATMENT

- Acute: intravenous fluids (IVFs), oxygen, opioids, transfusions
- Chronic: hydroxyurea maintenance therapy, splenectomy

● COAGULATION DISORDERS

BASICS

- Coagulation pathway (Figure 7.1)

Bleeding on Anticoagulants

BASICS

- Types of anticoagulation
  - Coumadin (vitamin K antagonists)—inhibits activation of vitamin K-dependent clotting factors: II (prothrombin), VII, IX, X; antithrombotic effect primarily due to reduction in prothrombin
  - Unfractionated heparin: activates antithrombin III—blocks thrombin
  - Low molecular weight heparin (Lovenox): does not require partial thromboplastin time monitoring, has more predictable plasma level
  - Inhibitors of factor Xa (fondaparinux): inhibits Xa via antithrombin activation
  - Direct factor Xa inhibitors: (rivaroxaban)

ETIOLOGY

- Increase risk of bleeding through inhibition of coagulation pathway

SIGNS AND SYMPTOMS

- Minor versus major bleeding can cause hemodynamic instability
- GIB, epistaxis, intracranial hemorrhage (ICH)

DIAGNOSTICS

- Laboratory testing including prothrombin time/international normalized ratio

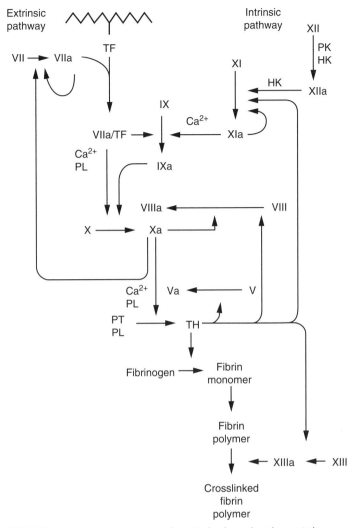

FIGURE 7.1. Coagulation cascade. HK, high-molecular-weight kininogen; PK, prekallikrein; PL, phospholipid; PT, prothrombin; TF, Tissue Factor; TH, thrombin. (From Leung LK. Overview of hemostasis. In: Post TW, ed. *UpToDate*. Waltham, MA: UpToDate; 2014. Graphic 69920 Version 1.0. Adapted from Ferguson et al, Eur Heart J 1998; Suppl 19:8.)

TREATMENT
- ABCs (airway, breathing, circulation), supportive, IVFs,
- Consider transfusions
- Patients with major bleeding use reversal agents depending on type of anticoagulant:
  - Coumadin:
    - Vitamin K 10 mg IV slowly
    - Profile nine with fresh frozen plasma (FFP)
    - Kcentra (four factor prothrombin complex concentrate)
  - Fragmin, heparin, or Lovenox recent use can be reversed with Protamine

Hemophilia

BASICS
- X-linked deficiency
- Two types:
  - **Hemophilia A:**
    - Reduced or lack of clotting factor VIII
    - Most common
  - **Hemophilia B:**
    - Reduced or lack of clotting factor IX
    - Christmas disease

SIGNS AND SYMPTOMS
- Signs of hemorrhage: epistaxis, GIB, hematuria, ICH, hemarthrosis
- Tachycardic, hypotensive, orthostatic
- Signs of infectious process

DIAGNOSTICS
- Clinical suspicion if unprovoked or excessive bleeding
- Complete blood count (CBC), coagulation studies

TREATMENT
- ABCs, supportive
- Control acute hemorrhage with aggressive hemostatic techniques and replacement of factors
- Consider transfusion

Von Willebrand Disease

BASICS
- **Most common hereditary bleeding disorder**

ETIOLOGY
- Deficiency of von Willebrand factor, which is important component in the blood clotting process

SIGNS AND SYMPTOMS
- Bleeding episodes may be mild from epistaxis and hemarthropathies to heavy menses, to severe and potentially life-threatening ICH

DIAGNOSTICS
- CBC, coagulation studies, ristocetin cofactor activity, and concentration of von Willebrand factor antigen

TREATMENT
- Desmopressin (DDAVP) and transfusion von Willebrand factor-containing factor VIII concentrates, FFP; consult hematology

Thrombocytopenia

BASICS
- Low platelets caused by many different disease processes (Table 7.1)

NEUTROPENIA

BASICS
- Granulocyte disorder characterized by abnormally low neutrophil count
- Common in patients undergoing chemotherapy

TABLE 7.1.	Sepsis, Leukemia, Hereditary Syndromes	
Disease	**Basics**	**Treatment**
Disseminated intravascular coagulation (DIC)	➤ Seen in cancer, sepsis, trauma ➤ Activation of clotting cascade causes clots → ischemia ➤ Up to 50% of patients will die	➤ ABCs, supportive ➤ Treat underlying cause
Heparin induced thrombocytopenia (HIT)	➤ Type 1: exposure to heparin, a nonimmune disorder, due to a direct effect of heparin on platelet activation ➤ Type 2: immune-mediated; occurs 4–10 d after exposure ➤ May see DVT, PE, MI, CVA	➤ ABCs, supportive ➤ Discontinue drug
Hemolytic uremic syndrome (HUS)	➤ Seen in children ➤ **Caused by *E. coli*** ➤ Causes bloody diarrhea, renal failure ➤ Hemolytic anemia	➤ ABCs, supportive ➤ Consider dialysis
Idiopathic thrombocytopenic purpura (ITP)	➤ Autoimmune condition ➤ In children, it is acute and self-limiting ➤ In adults, it is chronic ➤ Bruised, petechiae, gum bleeding	➤ Supportive ➤ Steroids ➤ Possible splenectomy
Thrombotic thrombocytopenic purpura (TTP)	➤ Idiopathic, cancer, HIV ➤ **Classic pentad:** hemolytic anemia, renal failure, fever, thrombocytopenia, neuro diseases	➤ ABCs, supportive ➤ Plasma exchange ➤ High mortality

DVT, deep venous thrombosis; PE, pulmonary embolism; MI, myocardial infarction; CVA, costovertebral angle.

- Types:
  - Mild—1,000 to 1,500 white blood cell (WBC) per mm^3
  - Moderate—500 to 999 WBC per mm^3
  - Severe—0 to 499 WBC per mm^3
- **Absolute neutrophil count (ANC)** = WBC count multiplied by total percentage of neutrophils (segs plus bands)

ETIOLOGY
- Cancers that affect the bone marrow directly (e.g., leukemia, lymphoma)
- Chemotherapy and radiation, which can damage defense mechanisms and integrity of mucous membranes
- Other causes include benign ethnic neutropenia, drug-induced neutropenia, nutritional deficiencies, collagen/vascular disorders, infections, and hematologic conditions

SIGNS AND SYMPTOMS
- May be asymptomatic
- Fever, cough, altered mental status, chills, myalgia

DIAGNOSTICS
- CBC with diff
- Febrile neutropenia = fever + neutropenia (<500 neutrophils/mm^3)

TREATMENT
- ABCs, IVFs, supportive
- Antibiotics

● TRANSFUSION AND BLOOD COMPONENT THERAPY

BASICS
- Restores volume and oxygen carrying capacity, improves clotting
- Decision to transfuse is based on transfusion triggers, clinical symptoms, rate of ongoing blood loss, cardiac function, need for operative intervention

DIAGNOSTICS
- ABO-Rh, antibody screen, crossmatch, prothrombin time/partial thromboplastin time, international normalized ratio, fibrinogen levels

TREATMENT
- **Whole blood**
  - High levels of K, NH_3, H_2
  - Low levels of clotting factors
  - Its use is now fairly obsolete
- **PRBCs**
  - Primarily used to improve oxygen delivery to the tissues
  - **One unit raises Hct by 3% and Hgb by 1 g per dL**
- **Washed PRBC**
  - Washing removes all but traces of plasma, leukocytes, platelets
- **Irradiated RBCs**
  - Gamma radiated to kill lymphocytes
  - Used for immunocompromised, lymphoma, stem cell/marrow transplants
- **Leukoreduced PRBC**
  - 99.9% of white cells are filtered out
  - Reduced risk of cytomegalovirus, Epstein–Barr virus, human T-lymphotropic virus, febrile reactions
  - Used for immunocompromised
- **Platelets**
  - Primarily used to reduce, minimize, or prevent bleeding
  - Indications: thrombocytopenia, active bleeding, need for surgical intervention
  - Usually transfuse when platelets <10,000/μL
- **Cryoprecipitate antihemophilic factor (CRYO)**
  - Contains factor VIII, fibrinogen, fibronectin, von Willebrand factor, factor XIII
  - Used primarily for correction of inherited and acquired coagulopathies
- **FFP**
  - Replaces coagulation factors
  - Indications: liver disease, urgent reversal of warfarin therapy, disseminated intravascular coagulation (DIC), thrombotic thrombocytopenic purpura (TTP), dilutional coagulopathy, congenital factor deficiencies
  - Use 1 unit FFP for every 4 to 5 units PRBCs transfused

Transfusion Reaction

BASICS
- A serious complication that occurs after transfusion
- Always monitor patients for adverse reactions when giving a transfusion

ETIOLOGY
- Antibodies in the patient's blood can attack the donor blood if the two are not compatible

SIGNS AND SYMPTOMS
- Urticaria, hypotension, fever, tachycardia, hemoglobinuria and microvascular bleeding

DIAGNOSTICS
- Clinical findings
- Laboratory testing

TREATMENT
- ABCs, supportive, stop transfusion
- Treat allergic reaction symptoms with antihistamines

NOTES

Immune System Disorders—2%

Hannah S. Dodd and Nicole Kostarellas

● ALLERGIC REACTIONS

BASICS
- IgE-mediated hypersensitivity that releases mediators from mast cells, may cause a vascular inflammatory response

ETIOLOGY
- Idiopathic, food, drug, contact allergies

SIGNS AND SYMPTOMS
- Urticaria, rhinitis, conjunctivitis, bronchospasm, angioedema, laryngeal edema, hypotension, nausea, vomiting, diarrhea, abdominal pain
- Contact dermatitis: may start with red, dry, scaly skin, then develops to small vesicular lesions that are oozing and crusted

DIAGNOSTICS
- Clinical exam findings
- Skin allergy testing
- Skin/scrape biopsy

TREATMENT
- Antihistamine (diphenhydramine or hydroxyzine) and corticosteroids (prednisone) depending on severity may need a longer taper. May additionally take H2 blockers (Pepcid) if there is a concern for food allergy
- Contact dermatitis: remove allergen. Wash with water! May need additional topical or oral steroids. Consider antihistamine for pruritus
- Follow up with an allergist, make a food journal, avoid extremities of temperature, fragranced soaps, and lotions
- Please refer to anaphylaxis for more severe allergy treatment

● ANAPHYLACTIC REACTION

Anaphylaxis

BASICS
- Defined as severe hypersensitivity reaction characterized by multisystem involvement (at least two or more body systems), which may include hypotension or airway compromise

ETIOLOGY
- Foods, medications, insect bites, and exercise can cause an IgE antibody response, which leads to mast cell and basophil immune mediators, leading to anaphylaxis

SIGNS AND SYMPTOMS
- Vasodilatation, shock, respiratory distress
- Bronchospasm, laryngeal edema
- Gastrointestinal and uterine muscle contraction
- Flushing, pruritus, urticaria
- Angioedema

DIAGNOSTICS
- History and clinical presentation

TREATMENT
- ABCs, supportive
- Maintain the airway!
- Adults: **Epinephrine 1:1,000 intramuscular 0.3 to 0.5 mg**
- Children: 0.01 mg per kg (no more than 0.3 mg)
- Can repeat this every 10 to 15 minutes depending on severity and can start an Epi drip at 1 to 4 µg per minute
- Racemic Epi for bronchospasm
- Antihistamines:
  - Adults: Benadryl 50 mg IV every 6 hours
  - Children: Benadryl 1 mg per kg every 6 hours
- H2-Receptor antagonists:
  - Adults: Ranitidine 40 mg IV
  - Children: Ranitidine 0.5 mg per kg IV
- Steroids:
  - Adults: methylprednisolone 125 mg IV
  - Children 1 to 2 mg per kg IV (max 125 mg)
- Inhaled β-agonist nebulization: albuterol, albuterol & ipratropium
- Intubation may be needed to protect the airway
- Hypotension treatment with intravenous fluids and additional pressors
- When safe for discharge to home, remember to give a prescription for EpiPen, allergist follow-up, and recommend a medical alert tag/ID

Accidental Epi-Pen Injection

BASICS
- Especially in extremities
- Unwanted vasoconstriction with risk of tissue compromise

TREATMENT
- Pain management, gentle massage, warm compresses
- **Phentolamine Mesilate**: short-acting α-blocker injection to affected area
- Dilute 1.5 mg of phentolamine 10 mg per mL amp in 1 mL lidocaine 2% and inject into site until reperfusion and skin becomes pink again

● HEREDITARY ANGIOEDEMA

BASICS
- Rare autosomal dominant disorder which causes systemic swelling of the body

ETIOLOGY
- Complement pathway deficiency
- Caused by a low level or improper function of a protein called the C1 inhibitor
- Dental procedures, sickness (including colds and the flu), minor trauma, and surgery may trigger attacks

SIGNS AND SYMPTOMS
- Swelling
- Abdominal cramping
- Upper respiratory reaction
- Usually no hives or itching

DIAGNOSTICS
- Serum testing during an attack

TREATMENT
- C1 inhibitor concentrate
- Antihistamines do not work well
- Epinephrine should be used in life-threatening reactions

NOTES

Musculoskeletal Disorders—5%

Nicole Dwyer and Ashley A. Hughes

● BACK PAIN
Cauda Equina

BASICS
- Compression of lumbar and sacral nerve

ETIOLOGY
- Most commonly from tumor or disc herniation

SIGNS AND SYMPTOMS
- Back pain
- Bowel or bladder dysfunction (urinary retention, overflow incontinence, loss of bowel or bladder control)
- Saddle paresthesias
- Leg weakness

DIAGNOSTICS
- MRI

TREATMENT
- Pain control
- Urgent surgical decompression

Cord Compression

BASICS
- Condition that causes pressure on the spinal cord
- Early recognition is key to improved outcomes

ETIOLOGY
- Common complication of malignancy, usually from metastatic tumor
- Also caused by arthritis, trauma, infection
- Thoracic spine (60%), lumbar spine (30%), cervical spine (10%)

SIGNS AND SYMPTOMS
- Back pain is first symptom
- Motor weakness, followed by gait disorders, then paralysis
- Sensory symptoms less common
- Bowel and/or bladder dysfunction

DIAGNOSTICS
- MRI of entire spine imaging of choice
- CT plus myelogram for those with contraindication to MRI

TREATMENT
- Pain control, steroids, surgical decompression, or radiation
- Preserving or improving neurological function

Epidural Abscess

BASICS
- Abscess anywhere along spinal cord which can compress

ETIOLOGY
- Most common pathogen *Staphylococcus aureus*
- Risk factors include intravenous drug abuse (IVDA), vertebral osteomyelitis, bacteremia, recent spinal/epidural anesthesia or procedure/surgery, diabetes mellitus, HIV, trauma

SIGNS AND SYMPTOMS
- **Classic triad: fever, spinal pain, extremity weakness**

DIAGNOSTICS
- MRI test of choice for diagnosis followed by CT with IV contrast
- Blood cultures
- CT-guided aspiration for culture

TREATMENT
- Surgery and long-term antibiotics

Herniated Disc

BASICS
- Most commonly occurs at L4 to L5
- Most common cause of chronic low back pain

SIGNS AND SYMPTOMS
- Back pain, radiating down leg
- Limited spine flexion
- Decreased reflexes

DIAGNOSTICS
- Straight leg raise
- Outpatient MRI

TREATMENT
- Conservative
  - Nonsteroidal anti-inflammatory drugs (NSAIDs), muscle relaxants, physical therapy
- Consider surgical referral

Spinal Stenosis

BASICS
- Narrowing of spinal canal, nerve root canals, or intervertebral foramina
- Causes nerve root entrapment

ETIOLOGY
- Congenital, herniated discs, tumors, injury

SIGNS AND SYMPTOMS
- Back pain, pain and tingling in legs, pain in calf/lower leg with ambulation and resolving with rest
- Pain relieved with sitting/spine flexion

DIAGNOSTICS
- Plain x-ray can show degeneration
- MRI to assess nerve root entrapment and to rule out malignancy

TREATMENT
- Conservative management with NSAIDs
- Physical therapy, epidural steroid injections
- Surgery can improve symptoms and functionality after conservative measures fail
- Urgent treatment required where there are neuro deficits

INFLAMMATORY AND INFECTIOUS DISORDERS OF JOINTS AND BONES

Gout

See Table 9.1

BASICS
- Painful inflammatory arthritis usually involving a single joint

ETIOLOGY
- Uric acid forms crystals that build up in the joints
- Risk factors: trauma, diet, dehydration, alcohol ingestion, medications, chronic kidney disease

SIGNS AND SYMPTOMS
- Severe pain, redness, swelling, warmth over 24 hours
- Podagra: inflammation of first metatarsophalangeal, most common

DIAGNOSTICS
- Uric acid levels have no significant value
- Joint aspiration reveals **negatively birefringent crystals**

TREATMENT
- NSAIDs are first-line therapy (Indomethacin)
- Colchicine often aborts flairs if taken as soon as symptoms begin, dose often limited by gastro-intestinal side effects
- Allopurinol used for chronic prevention
- Steroids may be given intra-articularly or orally

TABLE 9.1.	**Gout**			
Type	**Etiology**	**Location**	**Diagnostics**	**Treatment**
Gout	Uric acid crystals	Smaller joints, 1st MTP most common	Negatively birefringent crystals	NSAIDs, colchicine
Pseudogout	Calcium pyrophosphate crystals	Larger joints, knee most common	Positively birefringent crystals	NSAIDs

MTP, metatarsophalangeal.

Septic Arthritis

BASICS
- Infection of joint
- Risk factors: immunocompromised, intravenous drug abuse, recent joint surgery

ETIOLOGY
- **S. aureus is most common**, followed by *Streptococcus*

SIGNS AND SYMPTOMS
- Single swollen painful joint
- Swelling, tenderness, localized warmth
- Fevers
- Pain with range of motion of joint
- Knee most common joint, followed by hip

DIAGNOSTICS
- Arthrocentesis
  - Fluid usually purulent with white blood cell (WBC) 50,000 to 150,000
  - Cellulitis is contraindicated
- Erythrocyte sedimentation rate and C-reactive protein elevated

TREATMENT
- IV antibiotics, pain control
- OR for washout

Disseminated Gonococcal Infections

BASICS
- Three times more common in women
- Most common form of septic arthritis

ETIOLOGY
- Bacteremic spread of *Neisseria gonorrhoeae*

SIGNS AND SYMPTOMS
- Swollen, tender, erythematous joint
- May have cervicitis, maculopapular rash, or Fitz-Hugh–Curtis syndrome
- May have tenosynovitis

DIAGNOSTICS
- Synovial fluid cultures often negative
- Obtain genital cultures for GC

TREATMENT
- Pain control, supportive care
- IV antibiotics: Ceftriaxone or Quinolone
- Ortho consult, admit, consider OR

Osteomyelitis

BASICS
- Infection localized to bone

ETIOLOGY
- *S. aureus* is the most common organism

SIGNS AND SYMPTOMS
- Pain at site, fever, may have redness, swelling at site
- Subacute disease with symptoms over weeks

DIAGNOSTICS
- Erythrocyte sedimentation rate, C-reactive protein, complete blood count
- Radiologic imaging may show bone destruction and gas
- MRI
- Aspiration, bone biopsy to determine pathogen and if diagnosis uncertain

TREATMENT
- Debridement and antibiotics
- If hardware from an orthopedic procedure in place may require long-term suppressive therapy

Lyme Disease
BASICS
- Patients with untreated early Lyme can develop arthritis
- Infectious arthritis with an inflammatory synovial response, late form of Lyme disease

ETIOLOGY
- *Borrelia burgdorferi*

SIGNS AND SYMPTOMS
- Acute **monoarthritis** with knee most common
- Weeks or months after rash, fever, and arthralgias
- Often not occurring with fever

DIAGNOSTICS
- Knee aspirate with lower WBC counts (10,000 to 25,000)

TREATMENT
- Doxycycline 100 mg twice a day for 28 days

● OVERUSE INJURIES
Carpal Tunnel Syndrome
BASICS
- Overuse injury of the hand and wrist, leading to numbness in hand and fingers
- Occurs more often in women than in men

ETIOLOGY
- Occurs when the medial nerve gets compressed in the carpal tunnel, causing symptoms
- Carpal tunnel can be hereditary or hormonal changes in pregnancy

SIGNS AND SYMPTOMS
- Numbness in the palm or fingers, typically thumb, index, and middle finger (median nerve distribution)
- Occurs more frequently with holding objects and driving, and at night

DIAGNOSTICS
- **Phalen test**: hand tingling after full wrist flexion for 60 seconds
- **Tinel sign**: hand tingling after tapping on median nerve
- Electromyography (EMG) to assess for median nerve function

TREATMENT

- Nonsurgical management includes bracing or splinting to keep the wrist in neutral position, NSAIDs, and corticosteroid injections
- Treat pregnancy-related carpal tunnel as it resolves after delivery
- Definitive treatment is surgery
  - Transverse carpal ligament is cut in order to make more room for the medial nerve and the flexor tendons

Dequervain Tenosynovitis

BASICS

- Overuse injury of the wrist
- Pain over the thumb side of the wrist

ETIOLOGY

- Occurs when the tendons at the base of the thumb become inflamed
- Caused by lifting babies/toddlers, giving rise to the name "mommy's thumb"

SIGNS AND SYMPTOMS

- Pain with lifting objects or twisting motions of the wrist
- Sensation of a "snap" that occurs with thumb movement
- **Finkelstein test**: pain over the first extensor tendon with fist made over a flexed thumb and wrist ulnar deviated

DIAGNOSTICS

- Clinical diagnosis

TREATMENT

- Splinting, activity modification
- NSAIDs, corticosteroid injection
- Surgery to release the inflamed tendon in cases that are severe or refractory to conservative management

Rotator Cuff Tendonitis

BASICS

- Shoulder pain that is typically due to repetitive motion activities
- Rotator cuff pain can be due to shoulder impingement, tendonitis, or bursitis
- **Muscles include:**
  - **Supraspinatus**
  - **Infraspinatus**
  - **Teres minor**
  - **Subscapularis**

ETIOLOGY

- Overhead activities such as swimming, weight lifting, painting, and construction can lead to rotator cuff tendonitis

SIGNS AND SYMPTOMS

- Pain with shoulder range of motion
- With more severe cases, there can be arm weakness

DIAGNOSTICS

- Shoulder MRI to identify which soft tissue structures in the shoulder are affected

TREATMENT
- Nonsurgical management: shoulder rest, NSAIDs, corticosteroid injection, physical therapy
- Surgical management: Can be either arthroscopic or open shoulder surgery to make more space for the rotator cuff

Medial Epicondylitis

BASICS
- Pain over the medial aspect of the elbow and can be any of the following tendons:
  - Pronator teres, flexor carpi radialis, flexor carpi ulnaris, flexor digitorum superficialis, and palmaris longus
- Also known as "golfer elbow"

ETIOLOGY
- Due to activities that overuse the flexor tendons of the elbow
- Golfing, baseball, and lifting heavy suitcases

SIGNS AND SYMPTOMS
- Burning pain over the medial epicondyle of the elbow where the insertion of tendons occur
- Weakness in the arm of the affected side

DIAGNOSTICS
- Primarily a clinical diagnosis
- EMG or MRI may be used to rule out other causes of elbow pain

TREATMENT
- Nonsurgical management: rest, NSAIDs, corticosteroid injection, and physical therapy
- Surgical management: reserved only for pain and weakness that is refractory to conservative management for 6 to 12 months

Lateral Epicondylitis

BASICS
- Pain over the lateral aspect of the elbow
- Also known as "tennis elbow"
- Pain typically due to inflammation of the extensor carpi radialis brevis tendon

ETIOLOGY
- Due to activities that overuse the tendon such as tennis and racquet sports

SIGNS AND SYMPTOMS
- Burning pain over the lateral epicondyle with elbow extension
- Weakness in the arm of the affected side

DIAGNOSTICS
- Primarily a clinical diagnosis
- EMG or MRI may be used to rule out other causes of elbow pain

TREATMENT
- Nonsurgical management: rest, NSAIDs, corticosteroid injection, and physical therapy
- Surgical management: reserved only for pain and weakness that is refractory to conservative management for 6 to 12 months

Olecranon Bursitis

BASICS
- Inflammation of the olecranon bursa, which leads to pain in the elbow

ETIOLOGY
■ Direct trauma to the elbow or prolonged pressure on the elbow

SIGNS AND SYMPTOMS
■ Initial symptom is painless swelling over the olecranon process
■ As swelling increases, the bursa becomes more irritated and pain develops
■ Bursa can become infected
  • When infected, the bursa is red, warm, and hot to touch

DIAGNOSTICS
■ Clinical diagnosis
■ If bursa appears infected, an aspiration of the contents of the bursa should be done to exclude infection

TREATMENT
■ Noninfected bursa: elbow pads and NSAIDs initially. If no response to treatment, then may aspirate for symptomatic relief
■ Infected bursa: antibiotics and if persistent infection despite antibiotics, then surgical removal of bursa

Osgood–Schlatter Disease

BASICS
■ Overuse injury of the knee, which occurs primarily in adolescents
■ Inflammation of the patellar tendon, causing knee pain

ETIOLOGY
■ Adolescents participating in sports are most at risk

SIGNS AND SYMPTOMS
■ Knee pain and swelling
■ Tenderness over the patellar tendon
■ Pain with activity

DIAGNOSTICS
■ Primarily clinical diagnosis
■ Knee x-rays may reveal irregular ossification fragment of the tibial tubercle
■ Normal x-rays do not exclude this diagnosis

TREATMENT
■ RICE therapy, self-limiting disease
■ May last throughout the adolescent growth spurt

NOTES

NOTES

Nervous System Disorders—5%

10

Sabrina E. Serino, Patricia Gatcomb, Nicole Kostarellas, Noelia Kvaternik, and AJ Maselli

BELL'S PALSY

BASICS
- Unilateral (sometimes bilateral) **motor dysfunction of cranial nerve (CN) VII**

ETIOLOGY
- Associated with pregnancy, diabetes mellitus, trauma, infection, neoplasm, Lyme disease, herpes simplex virus

SIGNS AND SYMPTOMS
- Abrupt onset of symptoms
- Unilateral face paralysis of forehead and lower face
  - Cannot close eye, raise eyebrow, smile on affected side
  - **Central lesions (i.e., stroke) spare the forehead**
- May include pain in ipsilateral ear, hyperacusis, impaired taste, lacrimation

DIAGNOSTICS
- Clinical exam finding
- Consider head CT or MRI if risk factors for CVA or symptoms atypical

TREATMENT
- Most resolve spontaneously
- Treat with oral prednisone
- Consider acyclovir

CORD SYNDROMES

Transection (Segmental) Syndrome

- Loss of all sensation, weakness below affected level
- Bladder dysfunction
- Trauma, hemorrhage, abscess, transverse myelitis, metastatic lesions

Dorsal Syndrome

- Bilateral symptoms, including corticospinal tracts, central autonomic tracts to bladder
- Gait ataxia, weakness, muscle flaccidity hyperreflexia

Anterior Cord Syndrome

- Ventral two-third of spinal cord, includes corticospinal tracts, spinothalamic tracts, descending autonomic tracts to bladder control
- Muscle weakness and reflex changes, urinary incontinence

Central Cord Syndrome

- Focal to level of injury, do not ascend or descend
- Loss of pain and temperature
- Syringomyelia, tumor

Brown-Séquard Syndrome

- Aka hemi cord
- Lateral hemisection injury (trauma, bullet, stabbing) that affects the ipsilateral part of your body
- Weakness, loss of proprioception, pain, temperature, and vibration

Pure Motor syndrome

- Only weakness no sensory changes
- Upper motor neuronal injury = hyperreflexia, extensor plantar responses
- Lower motor neuron injury = muscle atrophy and fasciculations
- Chronic myelopathies

Conus Medullaris Syndrome

- Lesions at L2
- Early and significant urine/bowel incontinence
- Saddle anesthesia (S3 to S5)
- Tumors, disc herniation, fracture

● DEMENTIA

BASICS

- Chronic and progressive decline of function that interferes with independence and daily function
- Nonreversible
- Alzheimer disease is most common

ETIOLOGY

- Reduced cerebral production of choline acetyl transferase, which leads to a decrease in acetylcholine synthesis and impaired function

SIGNS AND SYMPTOMS

- Impairment in learning, reasoning, memory, handling complex tasks, spatial ability and orientation, language, learning and retaining new information
- Aphasia, apraxia, agnosia, impaired executive function

DIAGNOSTICS

- History and physical exam
- History from family members is particularly beneficial
- Screening for B_{12} deficiency and thyroid disorders
- Cognitive testing
- Mini-mental status exam
- Structural imaging with MRI or CT to rule out other etiologies

TREATMENT

- Symptomatic: treatment of behavioral disturbances, environmental manipulations to support function, and counseling
- Cholinesterase inhibitors, such as tacrine, rivastigmine, galantamine
- Memantine for moderate to severe Alzheimer dementia

DELERIUM

BASICS
- Acute, rapid, transient disturbance of consciousness

ETIOLOGY
- Fluid and electrolyte disorders, infections, drug or alcohol toxicity or withdrawal, metabolic disorders, low perfusion states, postoperative states

SIGNS AND SYMPTOMS
- Decreased ability to focus and change in level of awareness
- Sleep impairment, hallucinations, distractible
- Emotional disturbances, such as fear, depression, euphoria

DIAGNOSIS
- History and physical exam, mental status exam
- Lab testing and imaging to identify underlying etiology

TREATMENT
- Correct underlying medical disorder
- Antipsychotics for impulsive, violent, or unpredictable patients

GUILLAIN–BARRÉ SYNDROME

BASICS
- Acute immune-mediated polyneuropathy, progressing over about 2 weeks

ETIOLOGY
- Exact cause is unknown
- Sixty percent caused by a preceding infection

SIGNS AND SYMPTOMS
- Progressive, symmetric muscle weakness, usually **ascending**
- Weakness can be mild to nearly complete paralysis of all extremities, facial, respiratory, and bulbar muscles
- Decreased DTRs, respiratory muscle weakness and depression, back and extremity pain, paresthesias

DIAGNOSIS
- Cerebrospinal fluid from **lumbar puncture (LP) reveals elevated protein** with normal WBC
- Electromyography and nerve conduction studies

TREATMENT
- Plasmapheresis
- IV immunoglobulin

HEADACHE AND MIGRAINE
Life-Threatening

- Subdural, epidural, subarachnoid
  - See specific section
- Infections (meningitis, encephalitis, brain abscess)
  - See specific section
- Vascular:
  - Malignant hypertension (HTN), vertebral dissection (associated with exertion, chiropractor), thrombosis, cerebral aneurysm

- Temporal arteritis:
  - Unilateral frontotemporal severe headache (HA), tender to palpation of temporal artery
  - Diagnosis: erythrocyte sedimentation rate >50
  - Treatment: prednisone

Red Flags

- Age >50, rapid onset, severe intensity, no prior HA, fever, trauma, vision changes, immunosuppression, HTN, neuro deficits, altered mental status (AMS)

Benign

- Tension
  - Band-like, aching (nonpulsatile), bilateral, lacking secondary symptoms (nausea, vomiting, photophobia)
  - No focal neuro deficits
  - Tenderness to posterior cervical and temporal muscles
  - Precipitated by stress, sleep deprivation, hunger, eyestrain, alcohol
  - Treatment: supportive, nonsteroidal anti-inflammatory drugs, Tylenol, muscle relaxants
- Cluster
  - Severe, burning/pulsating, **unilateral, periorbital HA** with associated ipsilateral lacrimation, conjunctival injection, nasal congestion, myosis, ptosis
  - Short duration occurring several times per day for weeks
  - Most commonly in male >30 years
  - Treatment: high-flow O_2, IM/intranasal triptans
- Migraine
  - Unilateral, severe, throbbing, associated photophobia, phonophobia, nausea, vomiting, aura (visual, auditory, smell)
  - Common in women near menses, family history
  - Treat with analgesia/antiemetics (Tylenol, nonsteroidal anti-inflammatory drugs, chlorpromazine, Reglan)
    - Adjust environment (quiet/dark room)
    - Caffeine
    - Triptans
    - Ergotamines (do not use ergotamine within 24 hours of triptan use due to vasoconstrictive effect)
  - Prophylaxis propanolol, amitriptyline, fluoxetine, Topamax, Neurontin, valproate

● MYASTHENIA GRAVIS

BASICS

- Autoimmune neuro muscular disorder characterized by muscle weakness

ETIOLOGY

- Antibodies block acetylcholine receptor in the postsynaptic membrane
- Onset in the second and third decades (females predominantly) or sixth to eighth decade (males)

SIGNS AND SYMPTOMS

- Features fluctuating muscle weakness and fatigue, tends to be worse later in the day and with repetitive activity
- Diplopia, ptosis, dysarthria, dysphagia, loss of facial muscles, "loss of smile"
- Respiratory muscle weakness is most serious, can cause respiratory failure, or "myasthenic crisis"

DIAGNOSTICS

- Clinical diagnosis by history and physical

- **Tensilon test:** administering an anticholinesterase drug which will temporarily relieve muscle weakness
- Serologic test for antibodies
- Electromyography to detect impaired muscle to nerve transmission
- CT or MRI to rule out thymoma (present in 10% to 15% of patients with MG)

TREATMENT
- Symptom control by anticholinesterase drugs such as neostigmine or pyridostigmine
- Steroids and immunosuppressive drugs such as prednisone and tacrolimus to suppress production of antibodies

● PERIPHERAL NEUROPATHY

BASICS
- Damage to the peripheral nervous system
- May affect sensation, movement, organ function

ETIOLOGY
- Metabolic (diabetes, hypothyroid, liver failure)
- Vitamin deficiency
- Medication (chemotherapy)
- Traumatic injury
- Excessive alcohol consumption
- Immune system disease or infection (Guillain–Barré, lupus, leprosy, multiple sclerosis, Lyme disease)
- Shingles

SIGNS AND SYMPTOMS
- Gradual onset of numbness and tingling in hands and feet
- Burning, sharp, electric-like pain
- Extreme sensitivity to touch and heat intolerance
- Muscle weakness if motor nerves are affected
- Ankle jerk reflex is classically absent in peripheral neuropathy

DIAGNOSTICS
- History and physical, including neurologic exam
- Lab testing: CT, MRI, LP to exclude other causes
- Electromyography

TREATMENT
- There is no cure
- Depends on the cause and is focused on treating symptoms
- Antiseizure medications, including Gabapentin (Figure 10.1)

● SEIZURE AND STATUS EPILEPTICUS

Seizure

BASICS
- Partial:
  - Simple
    - ○ Consciousness preserved
    - ○ Isolated limb jerking or "Jacksonian march"—motor symptoms that start in one part of body and march down the rest

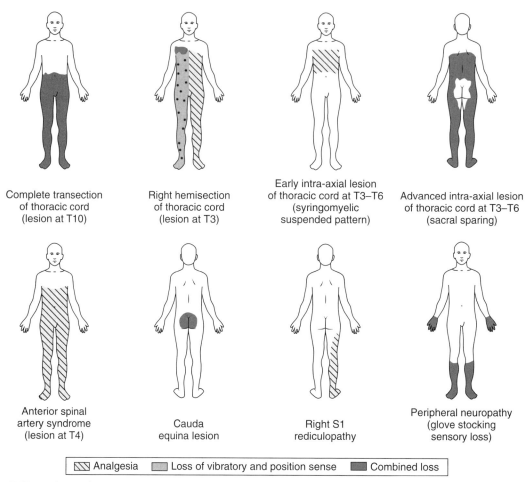

FIGURE 10.1. Characteristic sensory disturbances found in various spinal cord lesions in comparison with peripheral neuropathy. (From Daroff RB, Fenichel GM, Jankovic J, Mazziotta JC, eds. *Bradley's Neurology in Clinical Practice.* 6th ed. Philadelphia, PA: Saunders Elsevier; 2012. Figure 24.2 MD Consult.)

- Complex
  - Altered consciousness
  - May be preceded by "aura" of auditory/sensory/gustatory/perceptive symptoms (i.e., smells, tastes, epigastric sensation, déjà vu, visual)
  - Automatisms: lip smacking/blinking
  - Commonly located in **temporal lobe**
- Secondarily generalized
  - A partial seizure that turns generalized
■ Generalized:
  - Absence (blank stare)
  - Myoclonic (sharp brief jerks)
  - Clonic (contract flexor muscles)
  - Tonic (extensor muscles)
  - Tonic-clonic (sudden loss of muscle tone)

ETIOLOGY
■ Idiopathic: usually onset in children, genetic

- Secondary: electrolyte change, hyperthyroid, cocaine, phencyclidine, alcohol withdrawal, meds, trauma, intracranial hemorrhage (ICH), ischemic stroke, vasculitis, arteriovenous malformation (AVM), meningitis, abscess, tumors, Alzheimer's

SIGNS AND SYMPTOMS
- Asymmetric posturing, tongue laceration, incontinence, myoclonic jerks, loss of consciousness, increased heart rate and BP, prodrome of aura
- Postictal state: confusion, fever, lethargy, HA, **Todd paralysis** (weakness on one side of body that resolves within 48 hours)

DIAGNOSTICS
- Lab testing to look for toxic, metabolic, or infectious causes
- Consider head CT if first-time seizure
- EEG

TREATMENT
- Correct underlying provoking factor
- Generally outpatient management with instructions to avoid swimming and driving
- Check level of any antiseizure medications and adjust appropriately
- **If pregnant and there is evidence of eclampsia: magnesium sulfate IV**

Status Epilepticus

BASICS
- Life-threatening emergency
- Continuous or intermittent seizures for more than 5 minutes **without recovery** of consciousness

TREATMENT
- ABCs (airway, breathing, circulation), supportive, protect airway as there is a risk of aspiration and hypoxia
- Benzodiazepines (Ativan), followed by phenytoin, and consider phenobarbital for refractory seizures
- Neurology consult for admission

● SUBARACHNOID, EPIDURAL, AND SUBDURAL HEMORRHAGE
Subarachnoid Hemorrhage (SAH)

BASICS
- Bleeding into subarachnoid space, which is the space between the arachnoid membrane and pia mater

ETIOLOGY
- Head trauma is the most common cause
- Rupture of berry aneurysm versus AVM (~10%, typically congenital, men > women)
- Risk factors: HTN, smoke, hyperlipidemia (HLD), polycystic ovarian syndrome (PCOS), trauma

SIGNS AND SYMPTOMS
- **Sudden onset, worst HA of life**
- Nausea, vomiting, AMS
- Confusion, nuchal rigidity

DIAGNOSTICS
- CT before LP (xanthochromia) to rule out ICH or elevated intracranial pressure
- CT may have findings of hyperdensity within subarachnoid space, prominent in the sulci or cerebral peduncles

TREATMENT
- ABCs, supportive, blood pressure control
- Neurosurgical evaluation

Epidural Hematoma (EDH)

BASICS
- Bleeding between the dura and skull

ETIOLOGY
- The middle meningeal artery is most common
- Usually from direct trauma over the temporoparietal region

SIGNS AND SYMPTOMS
- **Lucid period**
- Blown pupil on exam

DIAGNOSIS
- CT: biconvex density adjacent to skull, does not cross suture lines

TREATMENT
- ABCs, supportive
- Burr hole drainage

Subdural Hematoma (SDH)

BASICS
- Tearing of veins between the brain and dura

ETIOLOGY
- Occurs with acceleration-deceleration
- Risk factors include brain atrophy (elderly, alcoholics)

SIGNS AND SYMPTOMS
- Slow, progressive HA
- AMS
- Neuro deficits

DIAGNOSIS
- CT: concave density adjacent to the skull, crosses suture lines

TREATMENT
- ABCs, supportive
- Surgical drain versus observation

● TRANSIENT ISCHEMIC ATTACK, STROKE, AND CEREBRAL ANEURYSM

Transient Ischemic Attack

BASICS
- Sudden onset of focal neuro deficit lasting few minutes to hours, **resolving completely within 24 hours**

ETIOLOGY
- Emboli is the most common cause; most common source is carotid or vertebrobasilar circulations
- Afib, mitral valve disease, infective endocarditis, polycythemia, sickle cell disease

SIGNS AND SYMPTOMS
- *Carotid circulation*: contralateral arm/leg weakness or sensory loss, aphasia, monocular vision loss (amaurosis fugax)
- *Vertebrobasilar circulation*: diplopia, vertigo, perioral numbness, blurring of vision, dysarthria

DIAGNOSTICS
- Arteriography is definitive, but MRI can exclude small cerebral hemorrhage
- EKG, echo (murmur, patent foramen ovale, vegetation), Holter (arrhythmia), carotid ultrasound (stenosis, clot)
- Labs including complete blood count, glucose, cholesterol, coags
- **ABCD2 score:**
  - Assesses risk of stroke at 2, 7, and 90 days from transient ischemic attack (TIA)
  - 0 to 3 low risk, 4 to 5 moderate, 6 to 7 high risk
  - **A**ge >60 (1 point)
  - **B**lood pressure: systolic blood pressure>140 or diastolic blood pressure >90 (1 point)
  - **C**linical features: isolated speech disturbance (1 point), unilateral weakness (2 point)
  - **D**uration of symptoms: <60 minute (1 point), >60 minute (2 point)
  - **D**iabetes (1 point)

TREATMENT
- Neurology consult and consider admission
- Antiplatelets (aspirin or Plavix)
- Carotid thromboendarterectomy if severe stenosis

Stroke

BASICS
- Lack of blood flow to the brain, causing neurologic deficit

ETIOLOGY
- Ischemic
  - Most common, 80%
  - Types: thrombotic, embolic, hypoperfusion
  - Risk factors: HTN, hyperlipidemia, Afib, diabetes mellitus, smoking, hypercoagulable, prior stroke, family history
- Hemorrhagic
  - Less common, 20%
  - ICH, SAH
  - Risk factors: HTN, male, liver disease, alcohol use, brain tumor, coagulopathies, anticoagulant meds

SIGNS AND SYMPTOMS
- Middle cerebral artery
  - Most common
  - Contralateral weakness, sensory loss in face, arm, and leg, homonymous hemianopsia, aphasia (dominant hemisphere), apraxia/neglect (nondominant hemisphere)
- Anterior cerebral artery
  - Contralateral weakness in legs, urinary incontinence, confusion, personality changes
- Posterior cerebral artery
  - Subtle to minimal signs and symptoms, including dizziness, nausea
  - Ocular and visual abnormalities, **CN III palsy**
- Vertebrobasilar
  - Vertigo, nausea, vomiting, ataxia, diplopia, sensory symptoms in **ipsilateral face and contralateral limbs**

- Cerebellum
  - Nausea, vomiting, central vertigo, diplopia, lack of hemisensory, and hemiparesis deficit
- Lacunar
  - Contralateral pure motor or pure sensory deficit, or ipsilateral ataxia, clumsy hand

DIAGNOSTICS
- Labs: CT, MRI/MRA, EKG, ECHO, carotid ultrasound

TREATMENT
- ABCs, supportive, blood pressure monitoring
- Ischemic:
  - Tissue plasminogen activator if symptom onset <3 to 4.5 hour
    - Contraindications:
      - Recent major surgery or trauma
      - Uncontrolled blood pressure (>185/110)
      - Seizure at stroke onset
      - Head trauma or stroke in past 3 months
      - MI in previous 3 months
      - Gastrointestinal bleeding in past 21 days
      - Known ICH
      - Arterial puncture at noncompressible site in past 7 days
      - Intracranial neoplasm
      - AVM or aneurysm
      - Heparin use within 48 hours
      - PLT <100 K, glucose <50, INR >1.7
  - Carotid thromboendarterectomy if severe stenosis
  - Anticoagulation if cardioembolic, antiplatelets if noncardioembolic
- Hemorrhagic:
  - ABCs, supportive treatment, BP control
  - Mannitol, steroids for edema
  - Neurosurgery consult for consideration of clipping and/or coiling
- **NIHSS** used to objectively quantify the impairment caused by a stroke and determine thrombolytic need

Cerebral Aneurysms

BASICS
- Most are located in the anterior circle of Willis
- Aneurysm may leak or rupture, causing SAH
- Classified by size and type: saccular, lateral, fusiform

ETIOLOGY
- Weak or thin spot on blood vessel in the brain which balloons and fills with blood
- More common with connective tissue diseases, may be congenital
- Trauma, high BP, infection, tumors, atherosclerosis and smoking are risk factors

SIGNS AND SYMPTOMS
- Small unchanging aneurysms are usually asymptomatic
- If ruptured, sudden and severe "thunderclap" HA, diplopia, nausea, vomiting, stiff neck, loss of consciousness
- Photophobia, ptosis, AMS, seizures

DIAGNOSTICS
- Head CT to look for intracerebral bleeding

- If CT is negative and high index of suspicion persists, LP with cerebrospinal fluid analysis
- Cerebral angiography is gold standard of diagnosis

TREATMENT
- Outpatient follow-up for small asymptomatic aneurysms
- If ruptured:
  - Neurosurgery consultation
  - Antiepileptics (Dilantin or Keppra)
  - Antihypertensives (Nicardipine to decrease arterial vasospasm)
  - Reverse coagulopathy with vitamin K or fresh frozen plasma

VERTIGO

BASICS
- Sensation of movement (room spinning)

ETIOLOGY
- *Peripheral*: most common causes are benign paroxysmal positional vertigo (BPPV), labyrinthitis, and Meniere disease (triad of vertigo, hearing loss, and tinnitus)
- *Central:* most common causes are vertebrobasilar TIA, brainstem infarction or hemorrhage, cerebellar infarction or hemorrhage

SIGNS AND SYMPTOMS
- Peripheral
  - Usually positional, worse with eyes closed and movement, nausea, vomiting
  - Nystagmus is usually horizontal. Fast phase beats in the direction of unaffected side
  - Transient gait impairment, may feel a sense of falling over, usually able to ambulate if head position is not changing
- Central
  - Usually not alleviated by rest, persistent (may be recurrent if recurrent TIAs)
  - Nystagmus: may be horizontal or vertical. Fast phase may change direction with gaze from side to side
  - May be unable to ambulate, may feel a sensation of falling over to either side
  - Exhibit abnormality in cerebellar function testing (dysmetria), numbness or weakness in the face or extremities, dysphagia, abnormality of vision or speech, respiratory depression/ failure

DIAGNOSTICS
- Clinical exam findings and detailed history
- **HINTS:** Can reliably distinguish peripheral cause from central
  - Head impulse testing
    - Tests vestibulo-ocular reflex
    - Have patient fix his or her eyes on provider's nose
    - Move his or her head in the horizontal plane to the left and right
      - If reflex is intact, his or her eyes will stay fixed on nose
      - If reflex is abnormal, eyes will move with their head and will not stay fixed on nose
    - It is reassuring if the reflex is abnormal
  - Nystagmus
    - Benign nystagmus only beats in one direction no matter which direction his or her eyes look
    - Abnormal nystagmus beats in every direction their eyes look
      - If patient looks left, you will see left-beating nystagmus
      - If looks right, you will see right-beating nystagmus

- Test of skew
  - ○ Vertical dysconjugate gaze is concerning
  - ○ Alternating cover test
    - – Have patient look at nose with his or her eyes and then cover one eye
    - – When rapidly uncovering the eye, look to see if the eye quickly moves to realign
- Consider CT/CTA, MRI/MRA if concerned for central process

TREATMENT
- Peripheral: H2 blockers (meclizine) or benzodiazepines (diazepam)
- Central: stroke management (thrombolytics, anticoagulation, embolectomy, reversal of anticoagulation, surgical coiling, BP control, and airway management)

NOTES

NOTES

Obstetrics and Gynecology—5%

11

Heather R. Becker, MacKenzie Bohlen,
Hannah S. Dodd, and Noelia Kvaternik

● ECTOPIC PREGNANCY

BASICS
- Pregnancy located outside the uterus
  - Fallopian tube ectopic (outer one-third most common)
  - Cervical and extrauterine ectopic (rare)

ETIOLOGY
- Conditions that block the fallopian tube
  - History of sexually transmitted disease
  - Past ectopic
  - Past abdominal surgeries
  - Endometriosis
  - Intrauterine device or tubal ligation reversal
- Increased risk with age >35, smoking, and fertility treatments

SIGNS AND SYMPTOMS
- Pelvic pain (sudden, sharp, diffuse, or local)
- Vaginal bleeding, spotting
- Low back pain, shoulder pain
- Weakness, dizziness, syncope
- Tachycardic, hypotensive if ruptured

DIAGNOSTICS
- Pelvic ultrasound, consider ultrasound bedside *fast* exam if concern for rupture
- Lab tests: β-hCG (human chorionic gonadotropin), complete blood count (CBC), type and screen, comprehensive metabolic panel

TREATMENT
- ABCs (airway, breathing, circulation), supportive, IVFs, transfuse when necessary
- Immediate obstetric/gynecologic (OB/GYN) consultation for consideration of:
  - Removal of the abnormal pregnancy
  - Salpingectomy
  - Methotrexate

● ENDOMETRITIS

BASICS
- Inflammation of the endometrium
- Can be acute or chronic

ETIOLOGY
- Caused by anaerobes and aerobes from genital tract
- *Chlamydia trachomatis* and *Neisseria gonorrhoeae* are uncommon causes
- Instrumentation, cesarean delivery, prolonged labor, multiple cervical exams, abortion

SIGNS AND SYMPTOMS
- Postpartum fever, tachycardia, midline lower abdominal pain, uterine tenderness, malaise, purulent discharge

DIAGNOSTICS
- History and clinical exam findings

TREATMENT
- Supportive, IVFs, pain control, antibiotics for anaerobic coverage

● MASTITIS

BASICS
- Inflammation of breast tissue that may or not be associated with infection
- Primarily women of childbearing age
- Most common in first-time nursing mothers

ETIOLOGY
- Can be classified into three major categories:
  - *Infectious*
    - Lactational mastitis is most common
    - Associated with abscesses; cellulitis is rare
    - Common pathogens are *Staphylococcus aureus* (MRSA is most common), less frequently *Streptococcus pyogenes, E. coli,* or *Bacteroides*
  - *Noninfectious*
    - Postirradiation mastitis, periductal mastitis, superficial thrombophlebitis of the breast, duct ectasia
  - *Malignancy associated*
    - Large tumors can cause secondary infection as tissue becomes necrotic

SIGNS AND SYMPTOMS
- Severe soreness, hardness, redness, heat, swelling of breast, generalized chills and fever

DIAGNOSTICS
- History and clinical exam findings
- Consider ultrasound for abscess

TREATMENT
- Antibiotics can be used for infectious and noninfectious causes:
  - Outpatient: dicloxacillin or cephalexin or clindamycin
  - If at risk for MRSA: Bactrim or clindamycin
  - Severe infection requiring admission: vancomycin
- Pain control, increased fluid intake, ice
- Continue nursing or pumping on infected breast and make sure to empty breast completely
- If symptoms persist with antibiotics, consider abscess or malignancy

● MISCARRIAGES

BASICS
- A pregnancy that has failed prior to 20 weeks gestation
- **Complete abortion:** passage of all products of conception (POC)

- **Incomplete abortion:** partial passage of POC
- **Inevitable abortion:** POC have not passed, but cervical os is open with vaginal bleeding
- **Threatened abortion:** vaginal bleeding without POC passage and closed cervical os
- **Missed abortion:** death of embryo or fetus without passage of POC

ETIOLOGY
- Chromosomal abnormalities, advanced maternal age, congenital abnormalities, trauma, hypothyroidism, medications, or substance abuse

SIGNS AND SYMPTOMS
- Vaginal bleeding, abdominal cramping

DIAGNOSTICS
- Lab testing including: CBC, β-hCG, Rh
- Pelvic ultrasound which can be performed outpatient if known intrauterine pregnancy

TREATMENT
- Hemodynamic monitoring for blood loss
- Rhogam for Rh-negative patients
- Consider OB/GYN consultation for possible D+C if patient is hemodynamically unstable

● OVARIAN MASS, OVARIAN CYST, AND OVARIAN TORSION
Ovarian Masses

BASICS
- Common, ranging from small physiologic cysts to large masses causing ovarian torsion and necrosis, to malignancy

ETIOLOGY
- Typically benign, but are defined as pathologic if >2.5 cm
- Women of all ages are at risk
- Most common in reproductive years

SIGNS AND SYMPTOMS
- Often asymptomatic, mild to moderate pelvic and abdominal pain, dyspareunia
- Abdominal and/or pelvic tenderness, adnexal tenderness

DIAGNOSTICS
- Ultrasound
- Labs including hCG to rule out ectopic, CBC if concern for hemorrhagic cyst (Table 11.1)

TREATMENT
- Control pain, outpatient follow-up for repeat ultrasound

TABLE 11.1.	Ultrasound Characteristics of Ovarian Masses
Benign Cysts	**Malignant**
➤ Thin-walled	➤ Solid
➤ Fluid-filled	➤ Internal septations
➤ ±Small free fluid in pelvis	➤ Internal echos
➤ ±Hemorrhage	➤ Daughter cysts
	➤ Thickened walls
	➤ Large free fluid in pelvis/ascites

- Most will resolve within 1 to 3 months
- If malignancy suspected, refer to gynecology oncologist for laboratory testing and possible surgical exploration

Ruptured/Hemorrhagic Ovarian Cyst

BASICS
- A rupture of a follicular cyst can be asymptomatic, mild transient pain, or significant pain
- In severe cases, intraperitoneal hemorrhage can occur

ETIOLOGY
- Occurs to women of reproductive years
- Exact etiology is unknown though can occur in trauma

SIGNS AND SYMPTOMS
- Severe, unilateral pelvic pain mid-menstrual cycle immediately following sexual intercourse, or with pelvic exam (can occur at other times of cycle or without sexual intercourse)
- Abdominal and/or pelvic tenderness, adnexal tenderness; can have tachycardia and hypotension if significant blood loss

DIAGNOSTICS
- Ultrasound
- Serum β-hCG, hemoglobin /hematocrit (platelet count, prothrombin time (PT), partial thromboplastin time (PTT) if on antiplatelet or warfarin therapy or history of coagulopathy)

TREATMENT
- Hemodynamically stable:
  - Control pain with po or IV pain medications
  - Consider serial hematocrit and observation if ongoing pain or anemia
- Hemodynamically unstable:
  - NPO, two large-bore IV, type and screen, pain control
  - Surgery indicated only for brisk blood flow to ovary and continued bleeding

Ovarian Torsion

BASICS
- Twisting or rotation of the ovary, which can lead to occlusion of the ovary's blood supply
- Three percent of all GYN emergencies
- Prompt diagnosis is imperative to preserve function of ovary

ETIOLOGY
- Most often occurs when a mass or functional cyst is present on ovary
- Twisting of both ovary and fallopian tube on vascular pedicle → venous/lymphatic destruction → congestion and edema → ischemia and necrosis → infarction
- Risk increases with size of mass until mass is so large that it becomes fixed in the pelvis

SIGNS AND SYMPTOMS
- Sudden onset of unilateral, severe, sharp pelvic pain, often with vomiting, generally occurs midcycle
- Low-grade fever; abdominal, pelvic, and adnexal tenderness

DIAGNOSTICS
- Detailed history and clinical exam findings with an ovarian cyst
- Labs including: serum β-hCG to rule out ectopic pregnancy; CBC, basic metabolic panel (BMP), type and screen
- Urgent pelvic ultrasound with doppler, can be misleading due to dual blood supply of ovary

TREATMENT
- ABCs, supportive, IV fluids, pain control
- Consult GYN for emergent laparoscopy
  - **Even if blood flow is normal on ultrasound**
  - Laparoscopy is gold standard to confirm torsion and assess viability of ovary

PELVIC INFLAMMATORY DISEASE

BASICS
- Inflammation of pelvic organs, which can lead to infertility in women

ETIOLOGY
- Bacteria, usually gonorrhea and *Chlamydia*, from the vagina or cervix travels into the uterus, fallopian tubes, ovaries, pelvis or the upper reproductive tract
- Risk factors include:
  - Sexual partner with gonorrhea or *Chlamydia*
  - Multiple sexual partners
  - Past history of any sexually transmitted infection/pelvic inflammatory disease (PID)
  - Recent insertion of an intrauterine device
  - Sexual activity during adolescence/young age
  - Age <25 years
  - Unprotected sex

SIGNS AND SYMPTOMS
- Pelvic and lower abdominal pain
- Vaginal discharge
- Fevers and chills
- Postcoital bleeding
- Painful sexual intercourse
- Tubo-ovarian abscess (TOA): unilateral adnexal tenderness, systemic symptoms

DIAGNOSTICS
- PID: pelvic exam with findings of vaginal discharge, cervical motion tenderness (chandelier sign)
- TOA: pelvic ultrasound
- Cultures may show *N. gonorrhoeae* or *C. trachomatis*

TREATMENT
- *Centers for Disease Control and Prevention recommended regimen* for outpatient treatment
  - Ceftriaxone 250 mg intramuscular in a single dose *plus* doxycycline 100 mg orally twice a day for 14 days with or without metronidazole 500 mg orally twice a day for 14 days
- Consider inpatient therapies if patient pregnant, unable to tolerate orals, or TOA
  - Cefotetan or cefoxitin plus doxycycline
  - Clindamycin plus gentamicin

PLACENTAL ABRUPTION AND PLACENTAL PREVIA

Placental Abruption

BASICS
- Premature separation of placenta from uterine wall
- Significant cause of maternal and perinatal morbidity

ETIOLOGY
- Chronic placental disease, abnormalities in early implantation, blunt abdominal trauma or rapid uterine decompression, uterine abnormalities, cocaine use, smoking

■ Risk factors: hypertension (HTN), preeclampsia, advanced maternal age, thrombophilia, prior spontaneous abortion, prior abruption, smoking, cocaine use, trauma, chorioamnionitis

SIGNS AND SYMPTOMS
■ **Painful,** vaginal bleeding (dark and scant to large-volume bright red blood)
■ Uterine tenderness, increased uterine tone, fetal distress; if severe, can lead to disseminated intravascular coagulation

DIAGNOSTICS
■ CBC, BMP, liver function test (LFT), PT, PTT, and type and screen, disseminated intravascular coagulation panel as indicated
■ Ultrasound: often not useful as high rate of false negative results
■ Any woman with small bleeding from placental separation is at risk of severe abruption

TREATMENT
■ ABCs, supportive, place on left side, IV fluids, consider transfusion, Rhogam
■ Urgent GYN consultation for further management and delivery

Placenta Previa

BASICS
■ Implantation of placenta over cervical os

ETIOLOGY
■ Risk factors: previous placenta previa, previous C-section or intrauterine surgical procedure, multiple gestation, multiparity, advanced maternal age, infertility treatment, previous abortion, smoking, cocaine use, male fetus

SIGNS AND SYMPTOMS
■ **Painless, bright red vaginal bleeding** after 20 weeks gestation
■ Defer full speculum exam to OB/GYN

DIAGNOSTICS
■ Prompt pelvic ultrasound to evaluate placental location
■ Labs including: CBC, BMP, LFT, PT, PTT, fibrinogen level, type and screen, Rh

TREATMENT
■ Most women require conservative care after first episode if no severe bleeding
■ ABCs, supportive, place on left side, IV fluids, consider transfusion, Rhogam
■ Urgent GYN consultation for further management and delivery
■ Emergent delivery for fetal distress, maternal hemorrhage refractory to treatment, significant bleeding after 34 weeks
  • **Cesarean section is method of choice**

● PREECLAMPSIA, ECLAMPSIA, AND HELLP

BASICS
■ A syndrome of HTN (>140/90), proteinuria, and edema after 20 weeks gestation
■ **Eclampsia includes above plus seizure**
  • Generally seen in third trimester or up to 10 days postpartum

ETIOLOGY
■ Exact cause is unknown
■ Risk factors include:
  • Young or advanced maternal age

- History of HTN
- Diabetes, kidney disease
- Multiple gestation
- Hydatidiform mole

SIGNS AND SYMPTOMS
- Hypertension, peripheral edema, headache, visual changes, papilledema
- Eclampsia includes seizures

DIAGNOSTICS
- Physical exam including attention to blood pressure, lower extremities
- Labs including urine to evaluate for proteinuria

TREATMENT
- Treatment is blood pressure control with hydralazine
- Consult GYN for further management and fetal and maternal monitoring
- Eclampsia:
  - Left lateral decubitus position to increase blood flow to uterus
  - **Seizure treatment:**
    - **Magnesium sulfate**
    - If refractory, use Phenytoin or diazepam
  - Definitive treatment is *delivery of fetus*

● HELLP

BASICS
- Severe, clinical variant of preeclampsia
  - **H**emolysis
  - **E**levated **l**iver enzymes
  - **L**ow **p**latelets

ETIOLOGY
- Exact cause is unknown
- Risk factors include:
  - Maternal age >35
  - Multiparity
  - White race
  - History of poor pregnancy outcomes

SIGNS AND SYMPTOMS
- Abdominal pain (usually epigastric or right upper quadrant), nausea, vomiting, malaise

DIAGNOSTICS
- Labs including: urinalysis, CBC with smear, BMP, LFT, PT, PTT, 24-hour urine
- Hemolytic anemia with schistocytes
- Platelet count <150,000
- Aspirate aminotransferase >70 IU per L
- Total bilirubin >1.2 mg per dL

TREATMENT
- Definitive treatment is urgent delivery, but can be timed based on safety and severity of maternal illness
- Treat HTN and seizure prophylaxis

● VULVOVAGINITIS

Bacterial Vaginosis (BV)

BASICS
- Not sexually transmitted infection
- Associated with multiple sex partners, vaginal lactobacilli, douching

ETIOLOGY
- Overgrowth of anaerobic microorganisms primarily: *Gardnerella vaginalis*

SIGNS AND SYMPTOMS
- Vaginal irritation, pain, pruritus, white, thick malodorous discharge

DIAGNOSTICS
- **Wet mount**
- pH 5.0 to 5.5, clue cells, fishy odor with KOH (whiff test)

TREATMENT
- Metronidazole 500 mg po bid ×7 days (or)
- MetroGel PV (or)
- Clindamycin cream PV
- Treat pregnant women *only* if symptomatic

Trichomoniasis

BASICS
- Sexually transmitted infection
- Men/women commonly asymptomatic

ETIOLOGY
- Protozoa: *Trichomonas vaginalis*

SIGNS AND SYMPTOMS
- Malodorous frothy yellow-green vaginal discharge dyspareunia, abdominal pain

DIAGNOSTICS
- **Wet mount**
- pH >4.5 and trichomonads

TREATMENT
- Metronidazole 2 g po single dose
- Metronidazole 500 mg bid ×7 days
- Treat all sexual partners

Vulvovaginal Candidiasis

BASICS
- Pregnancy, diabetes, antibiotics

ETIOLOGY
- Yeast/fungi: *Candida albicans*

SIGNS AND SYMPTOMS

■ Vulvar pruritus, white, curd-like vaginal discharge, erythema, dyspareunia, dysuria

DIAGNOSTICS

■ **Wet mount**
■ pH <4.5, pseudohyphae, culture (+) for *Candida*

TREATMENT

■ Fluconazole 150 mg po single dose (nonpregnant women only) (or)
■ Topical antifungal PV

NOTES

Psychobehavioral Disorders—3%

Rachel Frances, Carla Novaleski,
and Audrey Ranieri

ABUSE

Elder Abuse and Neglect

BASICS

- Neglect or failure of the individual responsible to provide needs and protection to a vulnerable person
- Considered elder abuse in patients >60 years old
- Failure to provide food, water, medicine, and clothing or financial exploitation
- Risk factors include advanced age, disability in self-care, low socioeconomic status, or institutional staffing shortages

SIGNS AND SYMPTOMS

- Suspicious pressure ulcers, skin tears, wounds, and burns
- Fractures, bruises
- Malnutrition and dehydration
- Signs of sexual abuse such as sores or bleeding genital/anal areas

DIAGNOSTICS

- Detailed history and clinical exam findings for signs of abuse
- Screening questions

TREATMENT

- Social work consultation
- Report reasonable suspicion to designated governmental resources

Sexual Abuse

BASICS

- Nonconsensual sexual mistreatment against a vulnerable individual
- Occurs at any age in domestic or institutional settings
- Typically by someone in a position of authority over the victim

SIGNS AND SYMPTOMS

- Sexually transmitted diseases or unplanned pregnancies
- Evidence of forced penetration into oral cavity, rectum, or female genitalia
- Trauma of the genitalia or anal area, including lesions, sores, or irritation
- Sexually abused children can be hypersexual or sexually permissive

DIAGNOSTICS
- Clinical exam findings, including genital, pelvic, and rectal exam
- Screening questions

TREATMENT
- Social work consultation
- Medical treatment for sexually transmitted infection and wounds
- Report reasonable suspicion to designated governmental resources

Intimate Partner Abuse (Spousal or Domestic Abuse)

BASICS
- Physical, psychological, or sexual harm is inflicted or threatened by a spouse or partner

SIGNS AND SYMPTOMS
- Inappropriate or distant affect
- Injuries similar to abused patient, including fractures, bruising, bleeding, or sores on genitals or anal area
- Inconsistent explanations, missed appointments

DIAGNOSTICS
- Detailed history and clinical exam findings
- Screening questions

TREATMENT
- Social support consultation
- Report reasonable suspicion to designated governmental resources

Child Abuse

BASICS
- Physical or psychological harm imposed upon a child
- Neglect or failure to provide protection and basic needs
- Includes Munchausen syndrome by proxy, abuse inflicted by a parent or guardian

SIGNS AND SYMPTOMS
- Suspicious injuries for which the mechanism is not adequately explained
- Bruises, **fractures (commonly spiral fractures),** and burns
- Retinal hemorrhages can be seen in shaken baby syndrome
- Psychological or psychiatric disturbances as a result of the abuse

DIAGNOSTICS
- Detailed history and clinical exam findings
- Screening questions

TREATMENT
- Social work consultation
- Report reasonable suspicion to designated governmental resources

● BEHAVIORAL AND PERSONALITY DISORDERS
Attention Deficit Disorder/Attention Deficit Hyperactivity Disorder

BASICS
- Impulsivity, inattentiveness, and/or hyperactivity causing impaired social function
- Typically diagnosed in childhood and can persist throughout adulthood

SIGNS AND SYMPTOMS
- Fails to follow instructions
- Poor concentration
- Difficulty organizing
- Easily distracted by outside stimuli
- Forgetful

DIAGNOSTICS
- Diagnosis requires hyperactivity, impulsivity, or inattentiveness
- Before age 7
- Demonstrates in two separate environmental settings

TREATMENT
- First line: methylphenidate, dextroamphetamine, or combination medications
- Noncontrolled substances, including antidepressant medications or some serotonin-norepinephrine reuptake inhibitors
- Behavioral therapy should be used in addition to pharmacotherapy

Disruptive Behavior Disorder

BASICS
- Childhood behavioral disorders
- Conduct disorder
  - Violates social norms and basic rights of other people, animals, or property
- Oppositional defiant disorder
  - Deliberately defies authority and rules
  - Purposely annoys or angers others

SIGNS AND SYMPTOMS
- Hostile, defiant, negative attitude, loses temper easily

TREATMENT
- Focused individual, group or family psychotherapy

Pervasive Developmental Disorder

BASICS
- Causes severe deficit in social interaction with impaired communication
- Autism, Asperger syndrome

SIGNS AND SYMPTOMS
- Methodical, repetitive, or stereotyped behavior
- Impaired social interaction
- Difficult communication or nonverbal
- Poor relationship development

TREATMENT
- Individual therapy according to needs

Personality Disorders

BASICS
- Characteristics that range across social, interpersonal, and environmental contexts
- Impair adaptation and function in social, occupational, and domestic settings (Table 12.1)

TABLE 12.1. **Personality Disorders**		
Cluster A "wild and mad"	**Cluster B "wild and bad"**	**Cluster C "whiny and sad"**
➤ **Paranoid personality disorder:** pervasive distrust of others, preoccupied with the suspicion that they are being exploited	➤ **Antisocial personality disorder:** impulsive, manipulative individual with disregard for laws or social norms and tends to lack empathy	➤ **Avoidant personality disorders:** social anxiety due to a fear of rejection, inferiority complex, and poor self-image
➤ **Schizoid personality disorder:** withdrawn, detached, and sometimes eccentric individual, tends to be quiet and does not desire close relationships	➤ **Borderline personality disorder:** volatile, unpredictable, and unstable individual with a poor self-image and fears abandonment	➤ **Dependent personality:** tends to be clingy, lacks self-confidence, and has difficulty making decisions
➤ **Schizotypal personality disorder:** similar to schizophrenia, individual demonstrates pervasive pattern of eccentric, superstitious behavior with magical thinking	➤ **Histrionic personality disorder:** dramatic, easily excitable, and sometimes seductive individual with attention seeking behavior, tends to exaggerate thoughts or feelings	➤ **Obsessive-compulsive personality disorders:** pervasive need for orderliness and rules, is inflexible and rigid
	➤ **Narcissistic personality disorder:** grandiose, with a superior self-image, tends to feel entitled or special and lacks empathy	➤ **Personality disorder NOS:** includes passive-aggressive, depressive, and sadomasochistic personality disorders

SIGNS AND SYMPTOMS
- See above chart for specific characteristics of each type of personality disorder

TREATMENT
- Tend to be unaware of their disorder and may not seek treatment
- Individual and group therapy with insight orientation
- Referral to psychiatric services
- Comorbidities include substance abuse, suicidal ideation, depression, anxiety, and functional impairment
- Medical therapy with antidepressant, antianxiety, and mood-stabilizing medications to treat associated symptoms

● BIPOLAR DISORDER
BASICS
- Prolonged depression with episodes of mania
- Females > males
- High suicide risk

SIGNS AND SYMPTOMS
- Mania
  - Decreased need for sleep
  - Pressured speech
  - Increased libido
  - Reckless behavior, excessive spending without regard
  - Grandiosity
  - Severe thought disturbances

DIAGNOSTICS
- Manic episode criteria
  - Greater than 1 week of elation, irritability, or expansiveness *plus* three mania symptoms

TREATMENT
- Drug and alcohol screen
- Assess for suicidal ideations
- Anxiolytics, benzodiazepines (lorazepam, clonazepam)
- Psych consult for consideration of hospital admission

DEPRESSION

BASICS
- Three types:
  - Major depression
  - Minor depression
  - Dysthymic disorder

ETIOLOGY
- Genetics
- Environmental, that is, major life event
- Disturbance in central nervous system 5-hydroxytryptamine levels and neuroendocrine abnormalities

SIGNS AND SYMPTOMS
- Depressed mood, diminished interest or pleasure in activities
- Weight change, sleep disturbances
- Psychomotor agitation or retardation, fatigue, feeling of worthlessness
- Thoughts of death or suicide
- Diminished ability to concentrate

DIAGNOSTICS
- Major depression: five depressive symptoms daily >2 weeks
- Minor depression: two depressive symptoms for >2 weeks
- Dysthymic disorder: mild depressive symptoms >2 years

TREATMENT
- Selective serotonin reuptake inhibitors (SSRIs), serotonin-norepinephrine reuptake inhibitors, atypical antidepressants, MAOIs (do not combine with SSRI; serotonin syndrome risk), tricyclic antidepressant s (avoid in suicidal patients)
- Outpatient referral for consideration of psychotherapy, electroconvulsive therapy, light therapy
- If patient expresses suicidal ideations in the emergency department:
  - Must search and/or remove belongings
  - 1:1 sitter for safety monitoring
  - Place patient on section 12
  - Psychiatry consult to determine disposition

GRIEF REACTIONS

BASICS
- Powerful emotional stressor relating to the loss of someone close
- Grief reaction in response, causing emotional pain
- Anticipatory grief with the knowledge of impending loss
- Complicated bereavement is prolonged or persistent grief

SIGNS AND SYMPTOMS
- Feelings of shock, disbelief, numbness
- Overwhelming sadness, depression, anxiety

TREATMENT
- Self-limiting with resolution within 6 months
- Prolonged or complicated bereavement persists longer than 6 months

● PANIC AND ANXIETY DISORDER

Panic Disorder

BASICS
- Panic attack: acute episode of intense physical symptoms and fear, rapidly peaks in 10 minutes, resolves in ~20 minutes
- Panic disorder: recurrent panic attacks or fear of another attack
- Genetic, family history is common

ETIOLOGY
- Limbic system: release of norepinephrine and serotonin
- Risk factors:
  - Female
  - Family history
  - Illness
  - Drug abuse
  - History of recent major life event (<1 year)

SIGNS AND SYMPTOMS
- Cardiac: palpitations, tachycardia, chest pain
- Respiratory: shortness of breath, choking
- Neurologic: dizzy, tremor, faint, paresthesia, sweating, chills, flushing
- Gastrointestinal: nausea, abdominal pain
- Intense fear of myocardial infarction (MI) or death

DIAGNOSTICS
- Detailed history
- Labs: toxicology screen, complete blood count (CBC), basic metabolic panel, thyroid-stimulating hormone
- Consider EKG to rule out cardiac etiology

TREATMENT
- Patient education of symptoms
- High-potency benzodiazepines
  - Lorazepam: quick onset, long duration
  - Clonazepam: slow onset, long duration
  - Alprazolam: avoid if possible, risk of rebound anxiety
- Avoid low-potency benzodiazepines (diazepam, chlordiazepoxide)
- Panic disorder outpatient treatment
  - SSRI, clonazepam

Generalized Anxiety Disorder

BASICS
- Anxiety so intense and long lasting that it interferes with daily functioning
- Not focused on a particular objection or situation
- Lasts at least 6 months in duration

ETIOLOGY
- Previous life experiences
- Environmental factors, genetic component

SIGNS AND SYMPTOMS
- Excessive worry, restlessness, feeling on edge, easily fatigued, difficulty concentrating, irritability, muscle tension, sleep disturbance, increased heart rate (HR), diaphoresis, tachypnea, dry mouth

DIAGNOSTICS
- Consider labs, imaging to rule out physiologic or medical explanations behind signs and symptoms

TREATMENT
- Combination therapy: psychotherapy and psychopharmacology
- Stress reduction techniques
- Antidepressants (often SSRIs) for long-term therapy
- Benzodiazepines for short-term use

PSYCHOSIS

BASICS
- Gross impairment of reality
- Broad term to categorize a condition that can result from a variety of psychiatric and medical illnesses

ETIOLOGY
- Psychiatric disorders:
  - Schizophrenia
  - Schizoaffective disorder
  - Mood disorders
  - Delusional disorder
  - Post-traumatic stress disorder
- Medical conditions:
  - Delirium, stroke, malignancy, endocrine disease, autoimmune disorders, nutritional deficiencies, electrolyte imbalance, neurodevelopmental disorders, multiple sclerosis, Alzheimer disease, Parkinson disease
- Substance abuse:
  - Cannabis, cocaine, amphetamines, psychedelic drugs, alcohol, prescription medications

SIGNS AND SYMPTOMS
- Hallucinations and delusions
- Thought disorder: incoherence, thought blocking, clanging, echolalia, concreteness, poverty of speech, overinclusiveness

DIAGNOSTICS
- Labs and imaging must be performed to rule out psychosis as a secondary cause (toxicology, brain MRI, electrolyte levels, etc.)

TREATMENT
- Atypical antipsychotics: clozapine, olanzapine, risperidone, quetiapine, aripiprazole
- Psychotherapy

Neuroleptic Malignant Syndrome

BASICS
- Life-threatening neurologic reaction to antipsychotic medications

ETIOLOGY
- Most commonly from antipsychotic drugs
  - Haldol
  - Chlorpromazine
- Atypical psychotics:
  - Clozapine
  - Risperidone
  - Olanzapine
- Dopaminergic drugs:
  - Levodopa
  - Reglan

SIGNS AND SYMPTOMS
- Muscle cramps and tremors
- Fever
- Hypertension, tachycardia
- Alerted mental status

DIAGNOSTICS
- Detailed history, including medication list
- Labs including CBC, creatine kinase, myoglobin, LFTs

TREATMENT
- ABCs, IV fluids, supportive
- Discontinue antipsychotics
- Dantrolene: treats symptoms including muscle rigidity

● SUBSTANCE ABUSE AND OVERDOSE

BASICS
- Abuse: self-administration of psychoactive drugs in ways that deviate from a culture's social norms
- Dependence can be physical (addiction) or psychological
- Tolerance: increasingly larger drug doses are required to produce the same effect
- Withdrawal syndrome: symptoms associated with discontinuation of habit forming substance (Table 12.2)

TABLE 12.2. Most Commonly Used and Abused Drugs

Drug Category	Drug Examples	Main Effects	Adverse Effects	Withdrawal Symptoms	Treatment Options
Depressants	Alcohol, barbiturates	Relaxation, elation, lowered inhibitions, emotional volatility, slurred speech, drowsiness	Nausea, vomiting, cognitive changes, memory impairment, poor motor coordination, sexual dysfunction, depression, hypertension, liver and heart disease, addiction, death	Tremors, agitation, psychotic symptoms, seizures, delirium tremens	Benzodiazepines, IVF (vitamin, thiamine, and folate infused), disulfiram, acamprosate, naltrexone, topiramate, psychotherapy
Stimulants	Tobacco, nicotine, caffeine, amphetamines, cocaine, methamphetamine	Alertness, increased energy, euphoria, hallucinations, decreased appetite, increased metabolism, increased HR and BP	Anxiety, insomnia, paranoia, irritability, confusion, psychosis, tremors, nausea, sexual dysfunction, seizures, MI, stroke, weight loss	Headache, fatigue, anxiety, shakiness, cravings, dysphoria, irritability, hypersomnolence	Benzodiazepines, IVF, psychotherapy
Opiates	Heroin, opium, morphine, codeine	Drowsiness, analgesia, euphoria, impaired coordination, miosis	Dizziness, confusion, nausea, sedation, decreased respirations, constipation, exposure, death	Tachycardia, hypertension, diaphoresis, rhinorrhea, lacrimation, dilated pupils, tremor, chills, anorexia, abdominal cramps, and diarrhea	Naloxone + buprenorphine, methadone, clonidine, psychotherapy **Fast-acting reversal agent = Narcan**
Hallucinogens	LSD, mescaline, psilocybin	Hallucinations, euphoria, alerted perceptions, increased HR and BP, decreased appetite, mydriasis	Delusions, short-term memory loss, paranoia, insomnia, nightmares, panic attacks, diaphoresis, dizziness, weakness	Psychotic symptoms, anxiety, recurring hallucinations	Supportive, antipsychotics, benzodiazepines

(continued)

TABLE 12.2.	Most Commonly Used and Abused Drugs (*Continued*)				
Drug Category	Drug Examples	Main Effects	Adverse Effects	Withdrawal Symptoms	Treatment Options
Club drugs	MDMA, GHB, flunitrazepam	Increased energy, increased sex drive, euphoria, sedation, muscle relaxation	Visual hallucinations, nausea, headache, dry mouth, hyperactivity, trismus, arrhythmias, lowered inhibition, anxiety, perspiration, impaired memory, depression, dizziness, seizures, coma, hyperthermia	Muscle aches, fatigue, depression, poor concentration	IVF, benzodiazepines
Dissociative drugs	Ketamine, PCP, salvia, dextromethorphan	Out-of-body experience	Amnesia, nausea, anxiety, tremors, impaired motor function, respiratory depression, impulsiveness, paranoia, panic reactions	Persistent psychosis and hallucinations	Supportive
Prescription medications	Most common: CNS depressants (benzodiazepines), stimulants, opioid pain relievers	See main effects for depressants, stimulants, and opiates	See adverse effects for depressants, stimulants, and opiates	See withdrawal symptoms for depressants, stimulants, and opiates	See treatment options for depressants, stimulants, and opiates **Fast-acting reversal agent for benzodiazepines: flumazenil**

CNS, central nervous system; IVF, intravenous fluids; BP, blood pressure; LSD, lysergic acid diethylamide; MDMA, methylenedioxymethamphetamine; GHB, γ-hydroxybutyrate; PCP, phencyclidine.

NOTES

NOTES

Pulmonary Disorders—9%

Erin Bradley, Kelly Devine, Hannah S. Dodd,
Christie Lucente, and Kristen Vella Gray

BRONCHITIS, PNEUMONIA, LUNG ABSCESS, AND EMPYEMA

Bronchitis

BASICS
- Infection of the conducting airways of the lung (bronchial inflammation)

ETIOLOGY
- Generally viral (influenza, parainfluenza, respiratory syncytial virus [RSV])

SIGNS AND SYMPTOMS
- Cough, fever, sputum production, malaise, congestion

DIAGNOSTICS
- Chest x-ray if clinical concern for bacterial pneumonia (PNA)
- Clinical criteria:
  - Acute cough (2 weeks but up to 2 months)
  - No prior lung disease
  - Wheezes/rhonchi on lung exam
  - Bullous myringitis (may indicate mycoplasma PNA)

TREATMENT
- Supportive treatment
- Albuterol if wheezing
- Antitussive agents (robitussin, codeine, Tessalon Perles)
- No antibiotics for healthy individuals (unless pertussis or atypical PNA suspected)
- For acute exacerbations of chronic bronchitis, antibiotics are indicated (azithromycin, levofloxacin)
- **Clinical pearls:** up to 20% of patients with cough persisting for 2 to 3 weeks have pertussis

Pneumonia

BASICS
- Inflammation of the lung parenchyma characterized by consolidation of the affected area, including terminal airways, alveolar spaces, and interstitium
- Sixth leading cause of death in the United States

ETIOLOGY

■ Four categories:
  • Community-acquired
  • Hospital-acquired:
    ○ Occurs 48 hours after hospital admission
  • Health care–associated:
    ○ In patients who have been hospitalized within 90 days of the infection
    ○ Residing in a skilled nursing facility
  • IV antibiotics, chemotherapy, or wound care within 30 days
  • Ventilator-associated: occurs 48 hours after intubation
■ ***Streptococcus pneumoniae* is responsible for up to 90% of all bacterial PNA**
■ *E. coli, Pseudomonas aeruginosa, Klebsiella pneumoniae, Staphylococcus aureus, Haemophilus influenzae,* and group A streptococci account for majority of remaining 10%
■ *Legionella* and anaerobes (aspiration) are less frequent
■ Respiratory viruses, *Mycoplasma,* and *Chlamydia* are responsible for the majority of atypical PNA (Table 13.1)
■ Two main routes of infection
  • Inhalation of airborne pathogen
  • Aspiration of oropharyngeal flora
■ Less common routes: blood borne (sepsis), direct extension from infection adjacent to the lung

SIGNS AND SYMPTOMS

■ **Typical:**
  • Sudden onset of fever/chills/rigors, productive cough with purulent sputum, pleuritic chest pain
  • Bronchial breath sounds and crackles over affected area
  • Egophony, dullness to percussion, increased fremitus
■ **Atypical:**
  • Gradual onset of headache (HA), myalgias, fatigue, anorexia with a dry cough
  • Scattered rhonchi or fine crackles

DIAGNOSTICS

■ Chest x-ray
■ Sputum cultures, blood cultures when sepsis suspected or patient requires ICU level of care

TABLE 13.1. **Pathogens and Unique Features**	
Pathogen	**Unique Feature**
Pneumococcus	Abrupt; rusty brown sputum
Legionella species	Often involve GI symptoms and AMS
	Cruise ships; aerosolized water
Mycoplasma	Bullous myringitis
Chlamydia pneumoniae	College age, nonproductive cough
H. influenzae	More common among smokers and the elderly
Aspiration/anaerobes	Right lower lobe, ETOH or seizure history
S. aureus	Follows viral illness particularly measles
K. pneumoniae	Currant jelly sputum

GI, gastrointestinal.

TREATMENT

- Treatment of patients with high suspicion for PNA should be started empirically
- **Community-acquired pneumonia (CAP):**
  - Outpatient: po azithromycin, levofloxacin, doxycycline
  - Inpatient: IV fluoroquinolone as monotherapy or ceftriaxone + azithromycin
- **Health care–associated pneumonia (HCAP)/hospital-acquired pneumonia:**
  - Antipseudomonal cephalosporin (cefepime/ceftazidime) *or*
  - Antipseudomonal carbapenem (imipenem/meropenem) *or*
  - Piperacillin/tazobactam *plus* antipseudomonal fluoroquinolone (levofloxacin/ciprofloxacin)
  - Consider anti-MRSA agent (vancomycin, linezolid)
  - Consider double coverage for *Pseudomonas* in areas where multidrug-resistant (MDR) *Pseudomonas* common
- **Aspiration:** consider adding anaerobic coverage, including clindamycin, Augmentin
- **Admission versus discharge**
  - **HCAP:** must be admitted for IV antibiotics
  - **CAP:** admit when there is high suspicion for poor outcomes
  - **Pneumonia outcome research trial score:**
    - ○ Clinical prediction rule used to calculate the probability of morbidity and mortality among patients with CAP
    - ○ The presences of any of the following increases the score, thus increasing the likelihood of poor outcomes
    - ○ Risk class I (outpatient treatment), II to III (case by case basis), IV to V (require admission)
      - Age
      - Gender: males
      - Nursing home resident
      - Comorbidity: cerebrovascular, renal, liver disease, congestive heart failure (CHF), cancer
      - Physical exam: altered mental status, systolic blood pressure <90, temp <35 or ≥40 respiratory rate ≥30, heart rate (HR) ≥125
      - Labs: pH <7.35, PO_2 <60 or Sat <90, Na <130, hematocrit <30, glucose >250, blood urea nitrogen >30, pleural effusion
  - **Clinical pearl:** awareness of airborne pathogens related to bioterrorism is becoming increasingly relevant (Table 13.2)

Pulmonary Abscess and Necrotizing PNA

BASICS

- Occurs when necrotic lung tissue is released into adjacent airway structures, causing formation of cavities containing necrotic debris or fluid caused by microbial infection

TABLE 13.2. Airborne Pathogens

Pathogen	Signs/Symptoms	Treatment
Bacillus anthracis (infected spores)	Causes skin lesions and lung infections; 1st flu-like symptoms progress to respiratory failure and coma	Ciprofloxacin or doxycycline
Yersinia pestis (etiologic agent of the plague)	48–72 h incubation period; fever, rigors, HA, cough, malaise, cyanosis	Streptomycin or doxycycline
Francisella tularensis (etiologic agent of tularemia)	Fever, chills, drenching sweats, severe weakness	Streptomycin

ETIOLOGY

■ Commonly associated with aspiration PNA, periodontal disease, bacteremia, endocarditis, intravenous drug use (IVDU), and Lemierre syndrome (oropharyngeal infection complicated by septic thrombophlebitis of the internal jugular)

SIGNS AND SYMPTOMS

■ Fever, chills, cough, sputum production (foul smelling), malaise, anorexia, weight loss
■ Symptoms may be indolent over weeks or months

DIAGNOSTICS

■ Complete blood count, sputum culture, acid-fast bacillus stain (if tuberculosis (TB) suspected)
■ Chest x-ray or chest CT

TREATMENT

■ Admit, prolonged antibiotic treatment (4 to 6 weeks), physiotherapy with postural drainage
■ Antibiotics should always include anaerobic coverage
   • Clindamycin and Augmentin are both effective
■ Percutaneous catheter drainage or lobectomy for refractory cases

Empyema

BASICS

■ Parapneumonic effusion complicated by frank pus in the pleural space

ETIOLOGY

■ Caused by viral and bacterial PNA, trauma, hematogenous spread, and complications from surgery
■ Most common bacterial causes include *S. aureus*, *Klebsiella*, anaerobes, and mixed flora

SIGNS AND SYMPTOMS

■ Fever, chills, malaise, cough, chest pain, sputum production, weight loss

DIAGNOSTICS

■ Chest x-ray: pleural effusion (may appear loculated)
■ Chest CT: dense collection in the pleural space, often with gas locules
■ Thoracentesis: pleural fluid with elevated white blood cell, exudative pattern (in terms of lactate dehydrogenase, protein, and glucose)
   • Gram stain and culture positive for bacterial organisms

TREATMENT

■ Hospital admission, antibiotics (CAP/HCAP coverage), and chest tube placement (at least 28 Fr)
■ Thoracic surgery consultation for thoracoscopy/video-assisted thoracoscopic surgery

● CHRONIC OBSTRUCTIVE PULMONARY DISEASE, ASTHMA, BROCHIOLITIS

Chronic Obstructive Pulmonary Disease

BASICS

■ Characterized by chronic dyspnea and expiratory airflow obstruction
■ Fourth leading cause of death in the United States
■ Men more than women, predominantly over 40 years old
■ Characterized by airway inflammation, fibrosis, and mucous hypersecretion
■ Forced expiratory volume in 1 second (FEV1)/forced vital capacity (FVC): standard measure, FEV1 and its ratio to FVC

ETIOLOGY

- Smoking (most common), cystic fibrosis, α-1 antitrypsin deficiency, bronchiectasis and bullous lung diseases (rare), occupational exposures
- **Two main types**
  - **Chronic bronchitis**
    - Damage to endothelium → excessive mucous → airway obstruction → decreased ventilation and increased cardiac output → rapid circulation in a poorly ventilated lung → hypoxemia and polycythemia → hypercapnia and respiratory acidosis → pulmonary artery vasoconstriction and cor pulmonale
    - *"Blue bloaters"*: obesity, cyanosis, peripheral edema, wheezes/rhonchi
  - **Emphysema**
    - Destruction distal to the terminal bronchiole → gradual destruction of alveolar septa and of the capillary bed → decreased oxygenation → decreased cardiac output and hyperventilation → limited blood flow through a fairly well oxygenated lung → tissue hypoxia and pulmonary cachexia → muscle wasting and weight loss
    - *"Pink puffers"*: pink, thin, cachectic, pursed lip breathing, diminished breath sounds

SIGNS AND SYMPTOMS

- Chronic obstructive pulmonary disease (COPD) exacerbation: an acute increase in symptoms beyond normal day-to-day variation, usually from respiratory infection or environmental factors
  - Cough increases in frequency and severity
  - Sputum production increases in volume and/or changes character
  - Dyspnea on exertion, increased O_2 requirement

DIAGNOSTICS

- Oxygen saturation
- Arterial blood gas (ABG) in severe exacerbations
- Chest x-ray to assess for signs of PNA, pulmonary edema, pneumothorax (PTX)
- EKG

TREATMENT

- Continuous monitoring of oxygen saturation, cardiac monitoring
- **Pharmacotherapy**
  - **Oxygen:**
    - Goal saturation of 90% to 94% and PaO_2 of 60 to 70 mm Hg
  - **Inhaled β-agonist:**
    - Albuterol 2.5 mg diluted to 3 mL via nebulizer
  - **Inhaled anticholinergic agent:**
    - Ipratropium (often combined with albuterol—Duoneb)
  - **Systemic corticosteroid:**
    - Oral glucocorticoids, appear equally efficacious to IV
    - IV glucocorticoids used with severe exacerbations, those who respond poorly to oral glucocorticoids, or unable to take oral medications
    - Optimal dosing is unknown (e.g., methylprednisolone 60 to 125 mg IV or prednisone 30 to 60 mg po)
    - Five-day course often effective, although a taper may be necessary
  - **Antibiotics:**
    - Optimal regimen undetermined
    - Target likely pathogens (levofloxacin 750 mg IV/po or alternative)
    - Consider risks of *Pseudomonas* or local patterns of antibiotic resistance

- **Noninvasive positive pressure ventilation (NPPV)**
  - Moderate to severe exacerbations
  - Use only if tracheal intubation not immediately necessary and no other contraindications
  - Contraindications:
    - Impaired consciousness
    - Inability to clear secretions or protect airway
    - Facial deformity
    - High aspiration risk
  - Initial settings for bi-level NPPV: 8 cm H_2O inspiratory pressure (may increase up to 15 cm H_2O) and 3 cm H_2O expiratory pressure
- **Endotracheal intubation**
- **Criteria for hospitalization**
  - Inadequate improvement of symptoms with initial therapies
  - Worsening hypoxemia or hypercapnia
  - Mental status changes
  - Inadequate response to outpatient management
  - Acute respiratory acidosis

Asthma (Acute Exacerbation)

BASICS
- Obstructive lung disease characterized by airway narrowing, hyperreactivity, and airway inflammation

ETIOLOGY
- May occur at any age, but generally diagnosed in childhood
- May be precipitated by viral illness, environmental exposure, or exercise
- Has been associated with maternal cigarette smoking

SIGNS AND SYMPTOMS
- Wheezing, shortness of breath, cough, chest tightness

DIAGNOSTICS
- Clinical exam findings
  - Use of accessory muscles, diaphoresis, and inability to lie supine
- Pulse oximetry
- Peak flow
  - Normal values based on height, age, and gender
  - Peak flow <200 L per minute indicates severe obstruction
  - While useful, peak flow has not yet been shown to improve outcomes, predict need for admissions, or limit morbidity/mortality when used in the emergency department (ED)
- ABG: elevated or even normal $PaCO_2$ indicates severe airway narrowing
- Chest x-ray: obtain if at high risk for comorbidities or if suspect underlying bacterial infection

TREATMENTS
- Goal: rapid reversal of airflow obstruction and correction of hypoxemia and hypercapnia
- **Inhaled β-agonists**
  - Albuterol, levalbuterol
  - Standard regimens:
    - Nebulized: albuterol 2.5 to 5 mg every 20 minutes for three doses, then 2.5 to 10 mg every 1 to 4 hours as needed
    - Metered-dose inhaler joint with spacer: albuterol 4 puffs every 10 minutes, or 8 puffs every 20 minutes, for up to 4 hours, then every 1 to 4 hours as needed

- **Inhaled anticholinergics**
  - Ipratropium for severe airflow obstruction in those who fail to improve despite inhaled β-agonists, as well as patients with concomitant COPD
  - Standard regimens:
    - Nebulized: ipratropium 500 mcg every 20 minutes for three doses, then as needed
    - Metered-dose inhaler joint with spacer: ipratropium 8 puffs every 20 minutes, then as needed for up to 3 hours
- **Systemic glucocorticoids**
  - Moderate (peak expiratory flow <70% baseline) or severe exacerbation (peak expiratory flow <40% of baseline) or without significant improvement in peak flow with inhaled β-agonists
  - Peak serum levels achieved ~1 hour after administration; clinical benefit may not be apparent for up to 6 hours
  - Optimal dosing regimen unknown and based on expert opinion
  - Standard regimens:
    - PO and IV forms have identical efficacy and bioavailability
    - Impending or actual respiratory failure: methylprednisolone 60 to 125 mg IV initially
    - Prednisone 40 to 60 mg po per day in a single or divided dose
    - Pediatric asthma: prednisolone 1 to 2 mg per kg daily or divided dose
- Duration:
  - Based on resolution of symptoms and return of peak expiratory flow measurements to >70% of baseline
  - Generally 3 to 7 days, although taper should be considered in certain cases
- **Magnesium sulfate**
  - Exacerbation is life-threatening or remains severe (peak expiratory flow <40% of baseline) after 1 hour of intensive conventional therapy
  - Magnesium sulfate 2 g IV infused over 20 minutes
  - Contraindicated in renal insufficiency
- **Admission or observation**
  - Peak expiratory flow <40% predicted at time of disposition
  - For new onset asthma patients with peak expiratory flow 40% to 70% predicted
  - Multiple prior hospitalizations or ED visits for asthma, prior intubation
  - Failure of outpatient treatment with oral glucocorticoids

Bronchiolitis

BASICS
- Upper respiratory symptoms followed by lower respiratory infection with inflammation that results in wheezing and/or rales
- Clinical syndrome that occurs in children <2 years old (peak 2 to 6 months)
- Most common cause of respiratory distress/wheezing in infants
- More common in the fall and winter
- Clinical diagnosis, usually self-limited

ETIOLOGY
- Viruses → terminal bronchiolar epithelial cells → damage and inflammation in the small bronchi and bronchioles → edema, excessive mucus, and sloughed epithelium → obstruction of small airways and atelectasis
- **Most common: RSV, rhinovirus, parainfluenza**
  - Two or more viruses are detected in approximately one-third of children hospitalized
  - Adenovirus tends to cause more severe cases (bronchiolitis obliterans)
- **Risk factors for severe disease**
  - Prematurity (gestational age <37 weeks)
  - Age <12 weeks

- Chronic pulmonary disease, congenital and anatomic defects of the airways, congenital heart disease, and immunodeficiency
- Environmental risk factors: passive smoke inhalation, crowded household, daycare, concurrent birth siblings, older siblings, and high altitude

SIGNS AND SYMPTOMS
- Usually presents 3 to 6 days after symptom onset
- Preceded by 1 to 3 days of rhinorrhea and mild cough
- Fever (usually <38.4°C), cough, and mild respiratory distress
- Tachypnea, intercostal/subcostal retractions, and expiratory wheezing, prolonged expiratory phase and coarse/fine rales
- Mild hypoxemia
- Severe: respiratory distress, cyanosis with poor peripheral perfusion
- Wheezing may not be audible if airways are narrowed and when increased work of breathing results in exhaustion
- **Complications:** dehydration, apnea, respiratory failure, and hypercapnia

DIAGNOSTICS
- Clinical exam findings
- Radiographs: not routinely indicted, chest x-ray abnormalities are variable and nonspecific
- Laboratory studies: not necessary to make the diagnosis; however, may be necessary to assess the severity of illness
- Virology studies: not routinely performed

TREATMENT
- Supportive care: nasal/oral suctioning, supplemental O_2, IV fluids
- Bronchodilators and saline nebulizers are widely used, but data is mixed on their effectiveness
- **When to admit**
  - Persistent resting O_2 sat below 92% on room air
  - Persistent tachypnea, respiratory distress
  - Age younger than 3 months, prematurity, or significant comorbidities (congenital heart disease)
  - Inability to feed or maintain oral hydration

● INTERSTITIAL LUNG DISEASE

BASICS
- The term *interstitial* can be misleading since many disorders characterized as interstitial lung disease (ILD) involve pathology of the lung parenchyma as well as perivascular and lymphatic tissue

ETIOLOGY
- Occupational and environmental exposures
  - Asbestosis, silicosis, berylliosis, Coal worker's pneumoconiosis, (Farmer's lung)
- Drug-induced pulmonary toxicity (amiodarone, bleomycin, methotrexate)
- Radiation-induced lung injury
- Connective tissue disease related
  - Systemic lupus erythematosus, scleroderma, rheumatoid arthritis
- Idiopathic
  - Sarcoidosis, cryptogenic organizing PNA
  - Idiopathic pulmonary fibrosis
- Complete medical history can help identify the cause of suspected ILD
- High mortality

SIGNS AND SYMPTOMS

- Dyspnea, cough, pleuritic chest pain
- Lung exam: wheezes, rales, rhonchi, or may be normal
- Cardiac exam: usually normal or may suggest pulmonary hypertension (HTN) and cor pulmonale in advanced disease
- Extrapulmonary: clubbing, systemic arterial HTN, skin and eye changes, lymphadenopathy, pericarditis, hepatosplenomegaly, and muscle weakness
- ILD presenting with respiratory failure
  - Infection may unmask an underlying, previously undiagnosed ILD
  - Consider investigation into etiology of acute decompensation
    - Chest x-ray: infiltrates in the lower lung zones, ground-glass opacities, honeycombing in later stages
    - Consider chest CT, transthoracic echocardiogram, pulmonary artery catheterization, bronchoalveolar lavage, transbronchial biopsy, open lung biopsy
  - Acute ILD
    - Consider after other causes are excluded
      - Acute interstitial PNA
      - Acute exacerbation of interstitial pulmonary fibrosis
      - Cryptogenic organizing PNA

TREATMENT

- Antibiotics if underlying infection present
- Supplemental O_2
- Discontinue exposure to pulmonary irritants
- High-dose corticosteroids with or without immunosuppressive therapy

● PNEUMOTHORAX

BASICS

- Introduction of air into the pleural space
- **Types**
  - Primary PTX:
    - Absence of underlying lung disease
    - Risk factors: smoking, tall, thin stature, family history, Marfan syndrome
    - Usually in early 20s to 30s
  - Secondary PTX
    - Occurs with an underlying lung disease
    - Risk factors: COPD, cystic fibrosis, CA, necrotizing PNA
  - Traumatic PTX:
    - May occur with a hemothorax
    - Requires a 36 Fr chest tube
  - Tension PTX:
    - Hypotension, tracheal deviation, elevated jugular venous pressure
    - **Requires emergent needle decompression** followed by 24 to 36 Fr chest tube
    - Needle decompression with 14G angiocath into the second intercostal space at the midclavicular line

SIGNS AND SYMPTOMS

- Shortness of breath, tachypnea, tachycardia, hypoxia, decreased breath sounds, subcutaneous emphysema
- Tracheal deviation is a late finding
- Hemodynamic instability may indicate a tension PTX

DIAGNOSTICS
- Clinical exam findings
- Chest x-ray
- Ultrasound will show absence of lung sliding
- Chest CT scan

TREATMENT
- Small (<15% volume):
  - Observation, high-flow O_2 with non-rebreather facemask
  - Repeat chest x-ray
  - May resolve spontaneously
- Large (2 cm on upright posteroanterior chest x-ray equals a 50% PTX)
  - Chest tube insertion
  - Pigtail catheter placement
- Video-assisted thoracoscopic surgery pleurodesis:
  - Reserved for recurrent pneumothoraces and failure of lung to reexpand after chest tube placement

● PULMONARY EMBOLISM

BASICS
- Thrombi originating in the venous circulation of the right side of the heart

ETIOLOGY
- **Virchow triad:**
  - Venous stasis
  - Hypercoagulability
  - Vessel intimal injury
- General risk factors
  - Age
  - Immobilization longer than 3 days
  - Pregnancy and postpartum period
  - Major surgery in previous 4 weeks
  - Long plane or car trips (>4 hours) in previous 4 weeks
- Medical
  - Cancer, previous deep venous thrombosis (DVT), stroke, acute myocardial infarction, CHF, sepsis, nephrotic syndrome, ulcerative colitis, systemic lupus erythematosus, lupus anticoagulant
- Trauma
- Hematologic
  - Inherited disorders of coagulation/fibrinolysis
  - Antithrombin III deficiency, factor V Leiden, protein C and S deficiency
- Drugs/medications
  - IVDU
  - Oral contraceptives
  - Estrogens
- Pulmonary embolism (PE) develops in 50% to 60% of patient with lower extremity DVT: 50% of events are asymptomatic
- Hypoxemia results from vascular obstruction, leading to dead space ventilation, right to left shunting, and decreased cardiac output

SIGNS AND SYMPTOMS
- Dyspnea, pleuritic chest pain, cough, hemoptysis, palpitations, leg pain/swelling
- Tachypnea, tachycardia, rales, fourth heart sound

DIAGNOSTICS

- EKG: most common finding is sinus tachycardia
- S1Q3T3 on EKG is pathognomonic, but not common
- Chest x-ray:
  - Atelectasis, infiltrates, pleural effusions
  - Westermark sign: focal oligemia with prominent central pulmonary artery
  - **Hampton hump:** wedge-shaped opacity against the pleural surface from intraparenchymal hemorrhage/infarct
- Labs including: complete blood count, basic metabolic panel, prothrombin time/partial thromboplastin time, cardiac enzymes, B-type natriuretic peptide
  - D-dimer may be used to exclude PE in low to moderate risk groups
- Ventilation-to-perfusion (V/Q) scan
- **Helical CT arteriography is gold standard**
- Venous thrombosis studies (ultrasound)
- Pulmonary angiography
- Bedside echocardiogram: may see evidence of right ventricular (RV) strain
- *PE rule-out criteria (PERC) rule*
  - If age <50
  - HR <100
  - O$_2$ sat >94%
  - Without history of DVT
  - Recent trauma/surgery
  - Exogenous estrogen
  - Leg swelling
  - Hemoptysis
- *The Wells score:*
  - Clinically suspected DVT—3.0 points
  - Alternative diagnosis is less likely than PE—3.0 points
  - Tachycardia (heart rate >100)—1.5 points
  - Immobilization (≥3 days)/surgery in previous 4 weeks—1.5 points
  - History of DVT or PE—1.5 points
  - Hemoptysis—1.0 points
  - Malignancy (treatment within 6 months) or palliative—1.0 points
  - *Traditional interpretation*
    - Score >6.0—high
    - Score 2.0 to 6.0—moderate
    - Score <2.0—low
  - *Alternative interpretation*
    - Score >4—PE likely, consider diagnostic imaging
    - Score 4 or less—PE unlikely, consider D-dimer to rule out PE
- Massive PE: acute PE with sustained hypotension, pulselessness, or persistent bradycardia with signs of shock
- Submassive PE: acute PE without systemic hypotension but with either RV dysfunction or myocardial necrosis

TREATMENT

- Admit for anticoagulation and monitoring
- Classic anticoagulation regimen of unfractionated heparin (UFH) followed by warfarin to maintain the INR 2.0 to 3.0
- Factor Xa inhibitors or fondaparinux
- Thrombolytic therapy: indicated for massive PE and may be considered for submassive PE with significant RV dysfunction/myocardial injury

- Inferior vena caval filter
- Pulmonary embolectomy: reserved for patients with refractory shock who have an absolute contraindication to thrombolytic therapy

⬤ RESPIRATORY FAILURE

BASICS
- **Hypoxemic (type I):**
  - Arterial oxygen tension (PaO_2) <60 mm Hg with a normal or low arterial carbon dioxide tension ($PaCO_2$)
  - Most common form of respiratory failure
  - Common causes: COPD, PNA, pulmonary edema, pulmonary fibrosis, asthma, PTX, PE, pulmonary arterial HTN, cyanotic congenital heart disease, bronchiectasis, acute respiratory distress syndrome (ARDS), fat embolism, kyphoscoliosis, obesity
- **Hypercapnic (type II):**
  - $PaCO_2$ >50 mm Hg
  - Etiologies such as drug toxicities, neuromuscular disease, chest wall abnormalities, and severe airway disorders
  - COPD, severe asthma, drug toxicity, myasthenia gravis, polyneuropathy, poliomyelitis, porphyria, head and cervical spine injury, obesity, hypoventilation syndrome, pulmonary edema, ARDS, myxedema, tetanus
- **Acute versus chronic hypoxemic failure**
  - Cannot easily be determined through blood gas analysis
  - Look for clinical signs of chronic hypoxemia such as polycythemia or cor pulmonale
- Acute hypercapnic respiratory failure
  - Develops over minutes to hours
  - pH <7.3
- **Chronic hypercapnic respiratory failure**
  - Develops over days or more, giving time for renal compensation through an increase in bicarbonate
  - pH only slightly decreased

ETIOLOGY
- Result of a malfunction in:
  - Transfer of oxygen across the alveolus
  - Transport of oxygen to the tissues
  - Removal of carbon dioxide from blood into the alveolus and then into the environment
- **Hypoxemic respiratory failure**
  - Mechanisms
    - **V/Q mismatch**
      - Most common cause of hypoxemia
      - Hypoxemia can be corrected by administration of 100% O_2
      - Minute ventilation rate is increased
      - $PaCO_2$ generally not affected
    - **Shunt**
      - Deoxygenated blood bypasses ventilated alveoli and mixes with oxygenated blood
      - Persistent hypoxemia despite 100% O_2 inhalation
- **Hypercapnic respiratory failure**
  - Mechanism
    - Alveolar ventilation decreases due to a reduction in minute ventilation rate or an increase in the proportion of dead space ventilation
    - As ventilation decreases below 4 to 6 L per minute, $PaCO_2$ rises

SIGNS AND SYMPTOMS
- Dyspnea, altered mental status (AMS), diaphoresis, somnolence
- Tachypnea, tachycardia, accessory muscle use, wheezes/rales

DIAGNOSTICS
- ABG
- Chest x-ray
- EKG
- Consider echocardiogram, pulmonary function test, and/or right heart catheterization

TREATMENT
- ABCs, IV, monitor
- Stabilize patient's respiratory and hemodynamic status
- Correct patient's hypoxemia with high-flow O_2, 100% non-rebreather, NPPV, endotracheal intubation when indicated
- Identify and correct underlying pathophysiologic process
  - Broad-spectrum antibiotics if underlying infection suspected
  - β-Agonists for asthma/COPD
  - Nitrates/diuretics for CHF

● SLEEP APNEA

BASICS
- Pauses in breathing (apnea) during sleep, due to sleep-related changes in ventilatory control
- Breathing often resumes with choking or snorting sound

ETIOLOGY
- Risk factors
  - Obesity
  - Enlarged airway tissues/adenoids/tonsils
  - Men > women
  - Increased risk with age
- If untreated, associated with major health problems
  - HTN, myocardial infarction, costovertebral angle, diabetes mellitus, obesity, heart failure, arrhythmia
  - Work-related or car accidents
  - Increased mortality
  - Increased surgical complications

SIGNS AND SYMPTOMS
- Loud snoring, daytime sleepiness, morning HAs
- Poor memory and concentration, depression, sore throat on waking

DIAGNOSTICS
- History from patient, family, partner
- Exam for obesity, enlarged tonsils/uvula
- Sleep study

TREATMENT
- Weight loss, side sleeping, smoking cessation
- Avoid alcohol and sedating medication
- Continuous positive airway pressure
- Surgery (tonsillectomy, uvuloplasty)
- Obstructive sleep apnea has little bearing on emergency medicine

● TUBERCULOSIS

BASICS

- Airborne infection caused by a bacterium called *Mycobacterium tuberculosis*
- Usually involves the lungs, but can also have manifestations of the kidney, spine, and brain
- Transmission occurs via infectious droplets
- Most common cause of death from infectious disease (other than complications of HIV/AIDS)
- Risk factors include homelessness, HIV+, foreign-born, residents of shelters/prisons, IVDU
- **Primary TB**
  - Most frequently presents with new positive Mantoux test (purified protein derivative [PPD])
  - When symptomatic, most often presents with active pneumonitis or extrapulmonary symptoms
    - Ghon complex: calcified focus of infection with an associated lymph node
- **Reactivation TB**
  - Symptoms
    - Fever, night sweats, productive cough, hemoptysis, pleuritic chest pain, dyspnea
    - May present subacutely with cough, weight loss, fatigue, night sweats
  - Exam findings: rales, rhonchi, cervical lymphadenitis (scrofula)
  - Extrapulmonary symptoms develop in 15% of the cases of reactivation TB and include
    - Lymphadenitis (most common)
    - Pleural effusion
    - Pericarditis
    - Peritonitis
    - Meningitis
- **Miliary TB**
  - Multisystem involvement caused by massive hematogenous dissemination
    - Primarily affects children and the immunocompromised
    - Signs and symptoms include fever, cough, weight loss, lymphadenopathy, hypercalcemia
- **The HIV patient and TB**
  - Highly susceptible to TB and have atypical presentations (extrapulmonary TB is common)
  - Always consider TB in the HIV patient with respiratory complaints even if chest x-ray is normal
  - Likely to develop MDR-TB
- **MDR-TB**
  - Foreign-born persons accounted for 72% of MDR-TB in 2,000
  - Increase suspicion in patients with suboptimal medical care, homeless, HIV, and drug users

DIAGNOSTICS

- Chest x-ray: most useful diagnostic tool for active TB in the ED
  - Active primary TB: parenchymal infiltrates in any lung field, hilar and/or medial adenopathy can be seen with or without infiltrate
  - Reactivation TB: lesion in the upper lobes or superior segments of the lower lobes, cavitary lesions, scarring, atelectasis, and effusion may also be seen
  - Miliary TB: diffuse small nodular infiltrates (1 to 3 mm) in size
- **Clinical pearl**: cavitary lesion on chest x-ray is associated with higher rates of infectivity
- Chest CT: to evaluate lesions suspicious for TB seen on chest x-ray
- Sputum cultures: acid-fast staining of the sputum can detect mycobacteria in 60% of patients
  - Cultures sometimes positive even with negative acid-fast bacillus
  - Most hospitals require three negative sputum cultures to rule out definitively
  - Less sensitive in HIV population
- Extrapulmonary TB
  - Urine culture for renal TB
  - Cerebrospinal fluid for TB meningitis
  - MRI helpful in evaluating for TB involvement of brain or spine

- *Mantoux testing*
  - Intradermal tuberculin skin testing with PPD
  - Not useful in ED as results are read 48 to 72 hours after placement
  - HIV patients, the immunocompromised, and those with miliary TB often have false negative PPDs

TREATMENT

- Isolation, on droplet precautions
- When diagnosis is uncertain (i.e., infiltrate on chest x-ray in a patient with TB risk factors), avoid fluoroquinolones when treating empirically
  - Fluoroquinolones are associated with significant delays in treatment and resistant strains
  - **Initial therapy includes four drugs:**
    - Isoniazid
    - Rifampin
    - Pyrazinamide
    - Streptomycin or ethambutol
- Most patients remain on the above regimen for 2 months, and then isoniazid and rifampin for an additional 4 months
- Patients with a positive PPD and no active disease (latent TB) are treated with isoniazid for 6 to 9 months to prevent reactivation TB
- **When to admit the TB patient**
  - Indicated for clinical instability, diagnostic uncertainty, unreliable outpatient follow-up or compliance, active or high suspicion for MDR-TB
  - Standard of care in most EDs is isolation and admission, although outpatient protocols in stable patients exist

NOTES

Renal and Urogenital Disorders—3%

Noah Askman and Hannah S. Dodd

● ACUTE RENAL FAILURE

BASICS
- A rapid increase in blood urea nitrogen (BUN) and creatinine

ETIOLOGY
- Prerenal
  - Volume depletion, heart failure, liver failure, sepsis, burns, bilateral renal artery stenosis, drugs (nonsteroidal anti-inflammatory drugs, angiotensin-converting enzyme inhibitor)
- Postrenal
  - Obstruction (benign prostatic hyperplasia, calculi, tumors)
- Intrinsic
  - Renal ischemia
  - Nephrotoxin exposures
  - Acute tubular necrosis
    - ○ Most common
    - ○ Caused by renal ischemia secondary to trauma, sepsis, rhabdomyolysis (Table 14.1)

SIGNS AND SYMPTOMS
- Nausea, vomiting, oliguria
- Hyperkalemia
- Metabolic acidosis

DIAGNOSTICS
- Laboratory testing, including basic metabolic panel, urine electrolytes

TREATMENT
- IVFs
- Diuresis to prevent volume overload
- Monitor electrolytes

TABLE 14.1.	Acute Renal Failure Tests		
Test	**Prerenal**	**Postrenal**	**Renal**
Urine osmol	>500	<350	<350
Urine Na	<20	>40	>20
BUN/Cr	>20	>15	<15

- Dialysis if:
  - Critical electrolyte abnormalities
  - Unresponsive metabolic acidosis
  - Uremia
  - Toxic ingestion

● NEPHROLITHIASIS

BASICS

- A stone formed in the kidneys from dietary minerals

ETIOLOGY

- Eighty percent Ca (others:uric acid, struvite)
- Risk factors:
  - Previous stones
  - Male gender
  - Family history
  - History of gastric bypass
  - Medications (hydrochlorothiazide, allopurinol)
  - Diabetes
  - Gout
  - Dehydration

SIGNS AND SYMPTOMS

- Flank pain, can radiate to the groin
- Colicky, waxing, and waning pain
- Restless
- Hematuria (70% to 90%)
- Nausea, vomiting, urinary urgency, dysuria

DIAGNOSTICS

- Lab tests, including urinalysis, basic metabolic panel
- Imaging:
  - Noncontrast CT scan is test of choice
    - Ureterovesicular junction is most common site to see stones as it is the most narrow
  - Kidney, ureter, and bladder x-ray (can miss stones and does not show hydronephrosis)
  - Ultrasound

TREATMENT

- IV fluids, pain medication (nonsteroidal anti-inflammatory drugs and opiates)
- Urology consult for acute renal failure, urosepsis, unrelenting pain, stone >10 mm
- Stone passage: smaller, more distal stones more likely to pass (most <5 mm pass spontaneously, then the percentage drops proportionally to the increasing size of the stone)
- α-Blockers help facilitate the passage of the stone

● PARAPHIMOSIS AND PHIMOSIS

Paraphimosis

BASICS

- Inability to retract foreskin over glans (distally)

ETIOLOGY

- Uncircumcised males
- Failure to return foreskin after exam, cleaning, catheter

SIGNS AND SYMPTOMS
- Pain, edema with constricting skin around glans

DIAGNOSTICS
- Clinical exam findings

TREATMENT
- Manual reduction of the prepuce
  - Thumbs are placed on the glans, and the skin is rolled over the glans
- If unsuccessful, obtain urology consult for a dorsal slit
- Preventative interval circumcision

Phimosis

BASICS
- Inability to retract foreskin over glans (proximally)

ETIOLOGY
- Abnormal stricture of distal foreskin secondary to infections or inflammation

SIGNS AND SYMPTOMS
- Pain and inability to retract foreskin

DIAGNOSTICS
- Clinical exam findings

TREATMENT
- Manual retraction, then thorough cleaning and proper hygiene
- If unsuccessful, obtain urology consult

PRIAPRISM

BASICS
- Pathologic erection lasting >4 hours

ETIOLOGY
- Idiopathic, sickle cell disease, drugs (Viagra, hypertensives cocaine), spinal cord injury

SIGNS AND SYMPTOMS
- Erection can be painful
- End result can cause ischemia, necrosis, urinary retention, impotence

DIAGNOSTICS
- Clinical exam findings

TREATMENT
- **Phenylephrine and terbutaline injections**
- Needle aspiration of corpora cavernosa
- Ice packs, pressure dressing
- Recurrent episodes may require surgery

PYELONEPHRITIS, URINARY TRACT INFECTION, UROSEPSIS, PERINEPHRIC ABSCESS

Pyelonephritis

BASICS
- An inflammation and infection of the kidney
- Women more common than men

ETIOLOGY
- Most commonly caused by *E. coli*, followed by *Proteus, Klebsiella*
- The bacterial infection spreads up the urinary tract to the kidneys

SIGNS AND SYMPTOMS
- Dysuria, frequency, urgency, hematuria, fever, flank pain, vomiting
- Costovertebral angle (CVA) tenderness

DIAGNOSTICS
- Physical exam findings consisting of CVA tenderness, fever
- Urinalysis, urine culture
- Image if:
  - Persistent symptoms after 48 to 72 hours
  - Kidney stones or abscess suspected
  - Immunosuppression
- CT is the choice to assess for stone, gas-forming infections, hemorrhage, renal abscess

TREATMENT
- Based on prior culture data
- Cephalosporins or fluoroquinolones for 10 to 14 days
- Admit if:
  - Complicated/comorbidities
  - Patient not tolerating orals
  - Pregnant
  - Renal transplant, single kidney
  - Abscess

Urinary Tract Infection

BASICS
- Infection in any part of urinary system, most commonly bladder or urethra
- Affects women more than men

ETIOLOGY
- Common microbes: *E. coli, Proteus, Klebsiella, Enterobacter*

SIGNS AND SYMPTOMS
- Lower abdominal pain, dysuria, urinary frequency
- Foul-smelling urine

DIAGNOSTICS
- Urinalysis

TREATMENT
- Tailor to presumed microbes
- Antibiogram dependent, but often Bactrim and Keflex are first line
- Macrobid 100 mg bid for 5 days for pregnant patients
- Men must be treated for 14 days

Urosepsis

BASICS
- Severe illness that occurs when an infection starts in the urinary tract and spreads into the bloodstream
- Can be life-threatening if it is not treated immediately

ETIOLOGY

■ Caused by bacteria from urinary tract infections (UTIs) and pyelonephritis

■ Risk factors: elderly patients, HIV, transplant recipients, diabetics, and immunosuppressed patients

SIGNS AND SYMPTOMS

■ Fever, weakness, hypotension, flank pain

DIAGNOSTICS

■ Urinalysis, urine culture

■ Lab testing, including complete blood count, lactate, blood cultures

■ Consider imaging, including ultrasound, chest x-ray

TREATMENT

■ ABCs, supportive

■ IV fluids, antibiotics

■ Consider ICU admission if patient persistently hypotensive, hypoxic, on pressors

Perinephric Abscess

BASICS

■ Abscess in perinephric space

ETIOLOGY

■ Usually from obstructed pyelonephritis

■ Risk factors: stones, diabetes mellitus, bacteremia

SIGNS AND SYMPTOMS

■ Symptoms similar to severe pyelonephritis

■ Few symptoms in the elderly, neuropathy, diabetes mellitus, alcoholics

DIAGNOSTICS

■ Must have high clinical suspicion

■ Urinalysis may be normal if no communication with the collecting system

■ Ultrasound or CT scan

TREATMENT

■ IV antibiotics for 2 to 3 weeks, drainage, and relief of any urologic obstruction

■ Renal abscess >5 cm = percutaneous drainage and antibiotics

■ Renal abscess <5 cm = antibiotics initially and if no response can consider drainage

■ Perinephric abscess should be drained for diagnostic and therapeutic options

● SEXUALLY TRANSMITTED INFECTIONS

Genital Herpes

ETIOLOGY

■ Transmitted from sexual intercourse, usually herpes simplex virus type 2

SIGNS AND SYMPTOMS

■ Prodrome of hyperesthesia, parasthesia, or itching in area of peritoneum or genitals prior to outbreak

■ Occasional flu-like symptoms, inguinal lymphadenopathy, and fever

■ Exquisitely tender vesicles on erythematous base

DIAGNOSTICS

■ Clinical exam findings

■ Tzanck smear

TREATMENT
- Vesicles are self-limiting and last 1 to 2 weeks
- **Oral antiviral therapy (acyclovir, or valacyclovir) can shorten the outbreak**
- Advise patient that the virus can be transmitted even when there are no symptoms

Syphilis

ETIOLOGY
- *Treponema pallidum*

SIGNS AND SYMPTOMS
- Primary syphilis:
  - Usually with a chancre, a painless ulcer
- Secondary syphilis:
  - Various cutaneous lesions which are usually pink papules or macules often seen on palms and soles
  - Sore throat and fever
- Tertiary syphilis:
  - Neurology manifestations

DIAGNOSTICS
- Clinical exam findings
- Polymerase chain reaction

TREATMENT
- Primary and secondary should be **treated with benzathine penicillin G** 2.4 million units by intramuscular (IM) injection

Chlamydia and Gonorrhea

ETIOLOGY
- *Chlamydia trachomatis*
- *Neisseria gonorrhoeae*

SIGNS AND SYMPTOMS
- Men: asymptomatic or present with dysuria
- Females: dysuria, vaginal discharge, pelvic pain, cervicitis

DIAGNOSTICS
- Direct swab or collect urine/urethral swab

TREATMENT
- *Chlamydia*:
  - Azithromycin 1,000 mg po or doxycycline 100 mg po bid for 7 days
- Gonorrhea
  - Ceftriaxone 250 mg IM
  - If penicillin or cephalosporin allergy, may give double dose of azithromycin

Genital Warts

ETIOLOGY
- Human papillomavirus

SIGNS AND SYMPTOMS
- Fleshy warts appearing like cauliflower on the external genitalia

TREATMENT
- Freeze or remove the warts
- Immunization for preexposure prophylaxis

● TESTICULAR PAIN

Testicle Torsion

BASICS
- A surgical emergency that may result in the loss of the affected testicle if not treated promptly

ETIOLOGY
- Twisting of the spermatic cord constricts blood supply, which if left untreated can cause testicle necrosis
- More common in children and young adults

SIGNS AND SYMPTOMS
- Acute onset of pain and scrotal swelling
- Occasional nausea and vomiting
- The involved testis may be swollen or have a palpable torsed section

DIAGNOSTICS
- Ultrasound to evaluate blood flow

TREATMENT
- Occasional attempt at emergent manual reduction and emergent urologic consultation for surgical intervention

Orchitis

BASICS
- Inflammation of the testicles

ETIOLOGY
- Usually secondary to viral illness, **mumps**, or sexually transmitted infection

SIGNS AND SYMPTOMS
- Pain and swelling of the testicle

DIAGNOSTICS
- Ultrasound helpful to distinguish it from other pathology

TREATMENT
- Symptomatic treatment
- Treat the underlying etiology if suspected infectious cause

Epididymitis

BASICS
- Inflammation of the epididymis

ETIOLOGY
- Epididymal swelling caused by infection, trauma, or idiopathic
- Common causes: *C. trachomatis* and gonorrhea in young men who are sexually active; *E. coli*, *Pseudomonas*, and *Enterobacter* species in older men

SIGNS AND SYMPTOMS
- Gradual onset of unilateral pain and swelling over a few hours
- Epididymis and scrotum can be swollen and tender
- May also have signs of UTI, but not consistent

DIAGNOSTICS
- Urinalysis
- Ultrasound

TREATMENT
- If age <35:
  - Treat for both *C. trachomatis* and gonorrhea with ceftriaxone 250 mg IM and doxycycline 100 mg bid
- If age >35:
  - Assume enteric pathogen and treat with Cipro for 10 days
- Pain control and close urology follow-up

Fournier Gangrene

BASICS
- Necrotizing fasciitis of perineal, genital, or perianal regions

ETIOLOGY
- Polymicrobial
- High rate of mortality
- Most patients have diabetes

SIGNS AND SYMPTOMS
- Edema, erythema tenderness in groin and genitals
- Necrosis, crepitus of skin and subcutaneous tissue

DIAGNOSTICS
- Clinical exam findings
- Labs for leukocytosis
- X-ray or CT scan may show subcutaneous gas

TREATMENT
- ABCs, supportive, IV fluid, antibiotics
- Surgery and/or urology consult for consideration of surgical debridement

NOTES

NOTES

Systemic Infectious Disorders—6%

15

Matthew Brochu, Nicole Kostarellas, and Noelia Kvaternik

● CENTRAL NERVOUS SYSTEM INFECTIONS

Bacterial Meningitis

BASICS
- An acute inflammation and infection of the meninges which surround the brain and spinal cord

ETIOLOGY
- Children: **group B streptococci** and *E. coli*, *Streptococcus pneumoniae*, *Neisseria meningitidis*, Hib
- Adults: *S. pneumoniae*, *N. meningitidis*, group B streptococci

SIGNS AND SYMPTOMS
- Fevers, headache, nausea, vomiting, meningismus, altered mental status (AMS)
- *Kernig sign*:
  - Pain or resistance with passive knee extension with hip flexion
- *Brudzinski sign*:
  - Passive flexion of neck causes hip flexion

DIAGNOSTICS
- Consider head CT if neurologic deficits
- Lumbar puncture (LP)
  - Elevated white blood cell (WBC), protein
  - Decreased glucose in cerebrospinal fluid (CSF)
  - Often xanthochromia present

TREATMENT
- ABCs (airway, breathing, circulation), intravenous fluids, supplemental oxygen
- Seizure treatment as needed, consider steroids
- Mannitol 1 g per kg IV for increased intracranial pressure (ICP)
- Antibiotics:
  - Infants to 3 months: ampicillin 200 mg per kg and cefotaxime or ceftriaxone 100 mg per kg
  - Three months and older: cefotaxime or ceftriaxone 100 mg per kg and vancomycin 15 mg per kg
  - Adults 18 to 50 years old: ceftriaxone 2 g IV Q12 and vancomycin or rifampin if *S. pneumoniae* resistance
  - Adults older than 50 years old: consider coverage for gram negative: ceftriaxone 2 g IV Q12 and ampicillin 2 g IV Q4 plus vancomycin or rifampin if *S. pneumoniae* resistance
- Prophylaxis is considered for those in close contact

Viral Meningitis

BASICS
- Inflammation of meninges
- Less severe than bacterial meningitis, also called aseptic meningitis
- It can be severe or fatal depending on the virus causing the infection, the person's age, or if immunocompromised

ETIOLOGY
- **Enterovirus** is most common
- Epstein–Barr virus (EBV), herpes simplex viruses (HSVs), and Varicella zoster virus (VZV)
- Influenza, measles

SIGNS AND SYMPTOMS
- Headache, fever, stiff neck, photophobia

DIAGNOSTICS
- LP for CSF: WBC low to 1,000, low to normal protein, normal to high glucose
- HSV considered if AMS, or history of HSV virus

TREATMENT
- ABCs, IV fluids
- Consider antivirals (acyclovir)
- Fungal is considered for immunocompromised patients and those immunosuppressed from recent surgery, prednisone use
  - *Cryptococcus* is the most common
  - Fungal treatment is amphotericin B, flucytosine, and fluconazole

Encephalitis

BASICS
- Inflammation of brain parenchyma with inflammation of meninges or spinal cord

ETIOLOGY
- Most commonly caused by viral infection:
  - Herpes (HSV, VZV, cytomegalovirus [CMV])
  - Arboviruses (eastern equine encephalitis [EEE], West Nile virus)
  - Enteroviruses
- Less likely caused by bacterial or fungal pathogens
- Hematogenous versus neuronal spread to central nervous system (CNS), less often spreads through respiratory or gastrointestinal (GI) routes, blood transfusion, or organ transplantation

SIGNS AND SYMPTOMS
- Fever, headache, AMS
- Neurologic or psychiatric symptoms, cognitive deficits, focal neurologic deficits, or seizure

DIAGNOSTICS
- ABCs, supportive, IV fluids
- Head CT prior to LP
- MRI more sensitive and preferred imaging modality if high suspicion
- Head CT often normal but may show diffuse cerebral edema or focal edema
- If HSV encephalitis: parenchymal hemorrhages in frontal and/or temporal lobes with CSF normal or similar to that seen with viral infections causing aseptic meningitis

TREATMENT
- Empiric treatment with ceftriaxone, vancomycin, acyclovir, dexamethasone, after cultures but no need to wait for CT and LP
- Admit due to high mortality

Brain Abscess

BASICS
- Infection in brain tissue coming from local source

ETIOLOGY
- Usually polymicrobial
- Most common causes: *Staphylococcus aureus*, aerobic, and anaerobic streptococci
- **One-third of cases are due to sinus, otic, or odontogenic**
- Ten percent are due to direct implantation by neurosurgery or trauma

SIGNS AND SYMPTOMS
- Headache, fever, AMS, or neurologic deficit
- Seizures, increased ICP (confusion, vomiting, somnolence)

DIAGNOSTICS
- CT scan with contrast
- MRI is highly sensitive

TREATMENT
- ABCs, supportive, IV fluids
- Broad-spectrum antibiotics, including cefotaxime and Flagyl
- Neurology, neurosurgery, and ID consult
- Possible surgery needed

● FOOD AND WATER-BORNE ILLNESS

Infectious Diarrhea

BASICS
- Acute gastroenteritis is a common illness that is due to a variety of bacterial, viral, parasitic, and toxin-mediated causes
- Infection is spread easily through fecal–oral contamination and through person-to-person contact
- Main stay of disease prevention is hand hygiene

ETIOLOGY
- Ingestion of pathogen that leads to the development of acute diarrhea (Table 15.1)

TABLE 15.1.	**Causes of Acute Infectious Diarrhea**	
	Nonbloody	**Bloody**
Viral	Norovirus, rotavirus, adenovirus, astrovirus	
Bacterial	*E. coli, Shigella, Salmonella, Yersinia, Campylobacter*	*E. coli* O157:H7, *Shigella, Salmonella, Yersinia*
Parasitic	*G. lamblia, Cryptosporidium, Cyclospora*	*E. histolytica*
Toxin	*Clostridium difficile, S. aureus, Clostridium perfringens, Bacillus cereus*	

SIGNS AND SYMPTOMS

- Diarrhea may be bloody or nonbloody
- May be associated with vomiting
- Abdominal pain
- Fevers and chills

DIAGNOSTICS

- Stool studies for immunocompromised individuals, those at high risk for spread of infection (nursing home resident, health care worker, day care worker, food handler)
- *Clostridium difficile* toxin assay if suspecting *C. difficile*
- If healthy individual with nonbloody diarrhea and low risk for spread, no diagnostic stool studies are needed

TREATMENT

- Supportive therapy
- Geared toward specific pathogen responsible for infection

Norovirus (Norwalk Virus)

BASICS

- **Most common cause of acute gastroenteritis in the United States**
- People can become infected with norovirus many times in their lives
- Easily and rapidly spread virus
- Virus spread rapidly in nursing homes, day care facilities, and cruise ships
- Outbreaks common in the United States from November to April

ETIOLOGY

- Virus spread through ingestion of food contaminated by norovirus
- Fecal–oral route

SIGNS AND SYMPTOMS

- Fever
- Abdominal pain
- Nausea and vomiting
- Nonbloody diarrhea

DIAGNOSTICS

- Clinical diagnosis

TREATMENT

- Supportive care
- Infants, young children, and the elderly more likely to become dehydrated
- Treat with IV fluids for dehydration

Rotavirus

BASICS

- Viral cause of acute gastroenteritis
- Children affected more often
- Infection more likely to occur in December through June
- Symptoms appear about 2 days after exposure to rotavirus

ETIOLOGY

- Spread through fecal–oral route

SIGNS AND SYMPTOMS
- Fever
- Abdominal pain
- Nausea and vomiting
- Watery diarrhea

DIAGNOSTICS
- Clinical diagnosis

TREATMENT
- Supportive care
- Infants, young children, and the elderly more likely to become dehydrated
- Treat with IV fluids for dehydration

E. coli 0157:H7
BASICS
- Many types of *E. coli* bacteria normally live in the human intestines
- Certain types have the ability to cause severe diarrhea
- *E. coli* O157:H7 causes illness by producing a **Shiga toxin**

ETIOLOGY
- Infection occurs primarily through the fecal–oral route or consumption of unclean drinking water

SIGNS AND SYMPTOMS
- Low-grade fever
- Abdominal pain
- Bloody diarrhea

DIAGNOSTICS
- Stool studies for Shiga toxin

TREATMENT
- Supportive therapy
- No antibiotics or antidiarrheal agents as this will increase the risk for hemolytic uremic syndrome (HUS)

Campylobacter jejuni
BASICS
- Bacterial cause of acute diarrhea

ETIOLOGY
- Infection occurs through consumption of contaminated meat, poultry, or raw milk
- Symptoms can occur 2 to 5 days after exposure to the pathogen

SIGNS AND SYMPTOMS
- Fever
- Abdominal pain
- Nonbloody or bloody diarrhea
- Nausea and vomiting

DIAGNOSTICS
- Stool studies

TREATMENT
- Supportive care
- Symptoms can last for 10 days
- Ciprofloxacin or azithromycin for immunosuppressed individuals or severe cases

Salmonella

BASICS
- Bacterial cause of acute diarrhea
- Causes illness 12 to 72 hours after exposure
- Illness lasts about 4 to 7 days
- *Salmonella typhi* can lead to bacteremia and typhoid fever

ETIOLOGY
- Ingestion of undercooked foods such as chicken or eggs

SIGNS AND SYMPTOMS
- Fever
- Crampy abdominal pain
- Nausea, vomiting
- Watery diarrhea
- Diarrhea may be bloody
- About 30% of people develop reactive arthritis weeks to months after diarrhea resolves

DIAGNOSTICS
- Stool studies

TREATMENT
- Supportive care
- Consider antibiotics (Cipro) for outpatient management
- Salmonella bacteremia is treated with ciprofloxacin IV or ceftriaxone IV

Shigella

BASICS
- *Shigella dysenteriae* is responsible pathogen for worldwide deadly epidemics
- *Shigella* is a gram-negative bacteria similar to *E. coli*
- Symptoms begin 1 to 2 days after exposure to bacteria
- Illness lasts 5 to 7 days

ETIOLOGY
- Fecal–oral route of transmission
- Ingestion of food contaminated by person infected with *Shigella*
- Ingestion of water contaminated by person infected with *Shigella*

SIGNS AND SYMPTOMS
- Fever
- Abdominal pain
- Bloody diarrhea
- **Reiter syndrome** (arthritis, eye irritation, and painful urination) may occur in some individuals after *Shigella* infection

DIAGNOSTICS
- Stool studies for *Shigella*

TREATMENT
- Supportive care
- Antibiotic treatment for severe cases with ciprofloxacin, Bactrim, or azithromycin
- Avoid antidiarrheal medications

Yersinia

BASICS
- Acute diarrhea caused by *Yersinia enterocolitica*
- Symptoms develop 4 to 7 days after exposure
- Illness lasts 1 to 3 weeks

ETIOLOGY
- Consumption of undercooked or raw pork products
- Drinking unpasteurized milk or contaminated water supplies
- Direct person-to-person transmission due to poor hand hygiene

SIGNS AND SYMPTOMS
- Fever
- Abdominal pain; pain typically in right lower quadrant
- Bloody diarrhea
- Symptoms can mimic appendicitis
- Erythema nodosum can develop after infection and will self-resolve
- Around 2% to 3% risk of development of reactive arthritis that occurs after diarrhea resolves and this is also self-limiting

DIAGNOSTICS
- Stool studies for *Y. enterocolitica*

TREATMENT
- Supportive care for mild cases
- Ciprofloxacin, levofloxacin, or Bactrim for severe cases

Giardia lamblia

BASICS
- Microscopic parasite that causes diarrheal infection
- Most common intestinal parasitic infection causing human illness in the United States
- Symptoms begin 1 to 3 weeks after infection

ETIOLOGY
- Primarily causes infection through the ingestion of contaminated drinking water
- Often seen in campers who drink from streams and lakes

SIGNS AND SYMPTOMS
- Abdominal cramping
- Abdominal bloating
- Excessive flatulence
- Diarrhea
- Greasy stools

DIAGNOSTICS
- Stool studies to look for *Giardia*

TREATMENT
- Supportive therapy
- Metronidazole or tinidazole

Entamoeba histolytica

BASICS
- Ameba that is responsible for GI infection as well as extra intestinal infections
- Occurs more often in tropical countries and places with poor sanitation

ETIOLOGY
- Ingestion of dormant cysts from fecally contaminated water causes infection

SIGNS AND SYMPTOMS
- Stomach cramping
- Bloating
- Flatulence
- Diarrhea with intermittent constipation

DIAGNOSTICS
- Stool studies for *Entamoeba*

TREATMENT
- Supportive therapy
- Metronidazole plus paromomycin or iodoquinol

Cyclosporiasis

BASICS
- Parasite that causes acute diarrhea

ETIOLOGY
- Ingestion of oocysts from fecally contaminated water
- Ingestion of contaminated fruits and vegetables
- Illness may take 1 to 2 weeks to appear after ingestion of contaminated water

SIGNS AND SYMPTOMS
- Watery diarrhea
- Fatigue, weight loss
- Abdominal cramping and bloating
- Flatulence
- Decreased appetite

DIAGNOSTICS
- Stool studies to look for *Cyclospora*

TREATMENT
- Supportive care
- Bactrim

Cryptosporidium

BASICS
- Microscopic parasite responsible for acute diarrheal illness
- Symptoms begin about 7 days after infection
- Illness lasts 1 to 2 weeks

ETIOLOGY
- Illness caused by drinking fecally contaminated water supplies
- Can also become infected through contaminated soil or food

SIGNS AND SYMPTOMS
- Fever
- Abdominal pain
- Nausea and vomiting
- Diarrhea

DIAGNOSTICS
- Stool studies to look for *Cryptosporidium*

TREATMENT
- Supportive care
- Nitazoxanide

Staphylococcus aureus

BASICS
- *S. aureus* is a bacteria commonly found on the skin of individuals
- It does not cause GI illness unless the bacteria is ingested
- Symptoms begin as quickly as 1 to 6 hours after ingestion of bacteria

ETIOLOGY
- Primary route of transmission is through food contamination by food handlers with *S. aureus* on their hands
- Typical foods are unpasteurized milk and cheeses, sliced meats, and pastries
- Cooking food will not kill bacteria or toxin and prevent infection

SIGNS AND SYMPTOMS
- Abdominal cramping
- Nausea and vomiting
- Nonbloody diarrhea

DIAGNOSTICS
- Clinical diagnosis

TREATMENT
- Supportive care
- Self-limiting disease
- Antibiotics not indicated

C. difficile

BASICS
- Bacteria that causes colitis infection, which can be severe and prolonged
- Very young and elderly at risk for severe complications
- Complications include toxic megacolon, pseudomembranous colitis, and sepsis

ETIOLOGY
- Inappropriate or prolonged use of antibiotics can lead to change in gut flora, causing over proliferation of *C. difficile*
- Can be spread through hand contamination via health care workers or individuals with *C. difficile* infection

SIGNS AND SYMPTOMS

- Fever
- Abdominal pain
- Nausea and vomiting
- Watery diarrhea
- Weight loss

DIAGNOSTICS

- Test for *C. difficile* toxin

TREATMENT

- Supportive care
- Metronidazole for mild to moderate disease
- **Metronidazole IV and vancomycin po for severe complicated disease**

● HUMAN IMMUNODECIENCY VIRUS (HIV)

BASICS

- Blood-borne virus transmitted via semen, vaginal secretions, blood products, or transplacental transmission

ETIOLOGY

- Infection with HIV-1 or HIV-2 virus results in immune deficiency by depletion of helper T-cells (CD4)

SIGNS AND SYMPTOMS

- Acute seroconversion:
  - Flu-like symptoms: fever, malaise, rash, lymphadenopathy
- Asymptomatic phase:
  - May last for up to 10 years
  - **When the CD4 count falls to 500, patients more susceptible to opportunistic infections**
- Symptomatic HIV infection:
  - Fever, weight loss, night sweats, malaise

TREATMENT

- Multiple regimens of highly active antiretroviral therapy (HAART) available

MANIFESTATIONS

- Cutaneous manifestations:
  - Multiple skin disorders are associated with HIV
  - **Kaposi sarcoma:**
    - AIDS defining illness
    - Manifests as macular, papular, nodular, palpable lesions, sometimes with mucosal, pulmonary, and GI involvement
    - Brown, pink, red, or violaceous
  - Bacterial infections:
    - Cellulitis, abscess, folliculitis, bullous impetigo
    - Mycobacterial infections: *Mycobacterium avium-intracellulare* complex (MAC) infections present as disseminated rash with plaques, pustules, and ulcers
  - Syphilis:
    - Common coinfection with HIV
    - Primary syphilis presents with painless chancre
    - Secondary syphilis: disseminated mucocutaneous rash, involving palms and soles
  - Viral infections:
    - Herpes simplex and herpes zoster
    - EBV: oral hairy leukoplakia

- CMV: perineal ulcers
- Molluscum contagiosum
- Human papillomavirus: condyloma accuminata
- Fungal infections:
  - Candidal infections common
- Neurologic manifestations:
  - Toxoplasmosis:
    - **Leading cause of CNS disease in patients with AIDS**
    - Infection by parasite *Toxoplasma gondii*
    - Can occur in patients with CD4 <200, but patients <50 at greatest risk
    - Signs and symptoms:
      - Headache, fever, focal neurologic symptoms, AMS
    - Diagnostics:
      - Serum anti-*T. gondii* IgG/IgM, polymerase chain reaction (PCR) of CSF
      - CT/MRI: MRI more sensitive than CT. Single or multiple hypodense lesions that may be ring-enhancing
    - Treatment:
      - Pyrimethamine + folinic acid + sulfadiazine, or intravenous Bactrim
  - HIV-associated dementia:
    - End stages of the disease
    - Involves decreased cognitive function, memory impairment, decreased inhibition
  - *Cryptococcus*:
    - **Most common fungal CNS infection**
    - AIDS defining illness
    - Patients with CD4 <100 at risk
    - Signs and symptoms:
      - Headache, fever, malaise, stiff neck, AMS
    - Diagnostics:
      - CT, MRI (better test)
      - May see cryptococcal pseudocysts on CT
      - MRI may show meningeal enhancement or mass lesion (cryptococcoma)
      - CSF: CSF antigen, CSF culture (almost 100% positive)
    - Treatment:
      - Intravenous amphotericin B plus flucytosine for 2 weeks followed by po fluconazole × 2 weeks
  - HSV encephalitis:
    - Mortality is six times higher in immunocompromised patients
    - Signs and symptoms:
      - Fever, headache, vomiting, AMS
    - Diagnostics:
      - CSF viral culture, CSF PCR
    - Treatment:
      - IV acyclovir
      - Role of steroids remains unclear
  - Tuberculosis meningitis:
    - Mortality is high
    - Signs and symptoms:
      - Fever, headache, vision change, AMS, focal neuro deficits
      - Myelopathy/ascending paralysis in spinal meningitis
    - Diagnostics:
      - Hyponatremia secondary to syndrome of inappropriate secretion of antidiuretic hormone (SIADH) common

     – Purified protein derivative (PPD) of limited utility
     – CSF with elevated protein
     – CT/MRI: may show hydrocephalus, infarcts, edema, and tuberculoma
   ○ Treatment:
     – Early antibiotics improve mortality
     – Isoniazid + rifampin + pyrazinamide
■ Ophthalmologic manifestations:
  • CMV retinitis:
   ○ Slowly progressive
   ○ Suspect in patients with CD4 <50
  • Signs and symptoms:
   ○ Floaters, decreased visual acuity
   ○ Sclera/conjunctiva noninjected
  • Diagnostics
   ○ Visual acuity
   ○ Dilated slit lamp exam
   ○ Exam with "cheese pizza" appearance
   ○ Lesions typically peripheral
  • Treatment:
   ○ Consult ophthalmology and ID
   ○ Most important treatment is optimizing HAART
■ Pulmonary manifestations:
  • *Pneumocystis jiroveci* (formerly phencyclidine):
   ○ **Most common opportunistic infection in patients with HIV**
  • Signs and symptoms:
   ○ Fever, exertional dyspnea, nonproductive cough, chills, weight loss
  • Diagnostics:
   ○ Lactate dehydrogenase elevation, serum quantitative PCR, serum β-D-glucan
   ○ Sputum induction with inhaled hypertonic saline
   ○ Chest x-ray: **diffuse bilateral perihilar infiltrates**
  • Treatment
   ○ Bactrim or clindamycin plus primaquine
   ○ Consider corticosteroids
  • Histoplasmosis:
   ○ Fungal infection endemic to Ohio, Mississippi, and Missouri River Valleys
   ○ Signs and symptoms
     – Cough, fever, myalgia, arthralgia, dyspnea, chest pain
   ○ Diagnostics:
     – Pancytopenia in acute, progressive disseminated histoplasmosis
     – Sputum cultures, blood cultures, antibody titers, serum and urine antigen
     – Chest x-ray: can see hilar lymphadenopathy or patchy infiltrates
   ○ Treatment:
     – Mild cases: oral itraconazole 6 to 12 weeks
     – Severe cases: intravenous amphotericin B
     – May require surgical resection of pulmonary cavitary lesions if failed medical management

● INFECTIOUS MONONUCLEOSIS

BASICS

■ Infectious, viral disease, also called the kissing disease

ETIOLOGY
- Caused by EBV
- Transmitted by saliva

SIGNS AND SYMPTOMS
- Fever
- Sore throat
- Splenomegaly
- Lymphadenopathy
- Fatigue, malaise

DIAGNOSTICS
- Leukocytosis with atypical lymphocytes in the peripheral blood smear
- **Monospot test showing heterophil antibodies**

TREATMENT
- Self-limiting
- Symptomatic treatment
- Avoid contact sports to prevent splenic injuries

● PARASITIC INFECTIONS

Ascariasis
ETIOLOGY
- *Ascaris lumbricoides*
- Larvae hatch from ingested eggs and migrate to the lungs
- More common in children in underdeveloped countries due to exposure to feces

SIGNS AND SYMPTOMS
- Fever, cough, shortness of breath, hemoptysis, and eosinophilia

DIAGNOSTICS
- Stool studies

TREATMENT
- Albendazole or mebendazole as a single dose

Hookworm
ETIOLOGY
- Necator Americanus
- Prevalent in the Southern United States
- Eggs excreted in human feces → become filariform larvae → larvae penetrate skin of humans walking barefoot

SIGNS AND SYMPTOMS
- Cough, fever, abdominal pain, weight loss, guaiac positive stools, eosinophilia
- Marked by chronic anemia, as the worms feed on blood

DIAGNOSTICS
- Stool studies

TREATMENT
- Albendazole or mebendazole as a single dose

Pinworm

ETIOLOGY
- Enterobius vermicularis, white nematode
- Generally a pediatric condition
- Eggs hatch within the ileum and colon. Females then migrate to perianal region

SIGNS AND SYMPTOMS
- Anal pruritus or mild pain, generally worse at night or early morning
- White female pinworms visible on exam of the perianal region

DIAGNOSTICS
- **Cellophane tape test:**
  - Apply cellophane tape to the unwashed perianal region in the morning and apply to a slide
- Larvae and eggs can be seen on microscopy
- Stool for ova and parasites may also be positive for pinworm

TREATMENT
- Mebendazole
- Treat the entire family, or risk recurrence

Threadworm

ETIOLOGY
- *Strongyloides stercoralis*
- More common in the Southeastern United States and Appalachia
- Infestation of the small intestine
- Parasite penetrates skin (usually through the feet or via fecal–oral contact)
- Migrate to lungs via lymphatic system → up the trachea where they are swallowed and enter the GI tract
- Immunocompromised hosts can develop disseminated *Strongyloides*, leading to invasion of all tissues (CNS, heart, urinary tract)

SIGNS AND SYMPTOMS
- Causes erythematous rash with petechial hemorrhages (cutaneous larval migrans—very distinct)
- Cough, hemoptysis, abdominal pain, weight loss, bloody diarrhea

DIAGNOSTICS
- Stool for ova and parasite

TREATMENT
- Thiabendazole and ivermectin

Trichinellosis/Trichinosis

ETIOLOGY
- Nematodal infection of genus *Trichinella*
- Transmitted by ingestion of infected pork, beef, and walrus meat
- Larvae penetrate intestinal wall, enter the lymphatic system, and invade striated muscle cells

SIGNS AND SYMPTOMS
- Nausea, vomiting, diarrhea, urticaria, myalgia, periorbital edema, splinter hemorrhages, and headache
- Cardioneurologic syndrome: encephalopathy, neurologic deficits, myocardial injury (infarction, myocarditis, congestive heart failure)

DIAGNOSTICS

- Labs including complete blood count (CBC) with eosinophilia, creatine kinase, UA for myoglobinuria, parasite specific indirect IgG, muscle biopsy

TREATMENT

- Mebendazole and albendazole, which are only helpful during intestinal phase
- Prednisone/hydrocortisone for anti-inflammatory effects, decreased immunologic response to larvae

Schistosomiasis

ETIOLOGY

- Blood flukes of the genus *Schistosoma*
- Snails act as hosts
- More common in Africa, Caribbean, and Middle East
- Larvae released by infected snails; penetrates the skin through contact with infected water, resulting in maculopapular rash; invades the venous system

SIGNS AND SYMPTOMS

- Acute schistosomiasis (Katayama fever):
  - Fever, myalgia, cough, headache
- Chronic schistosomiasis
  - Intestinal: diarrhea, portal hypertension, and esophageal varices
  - Urogenital: dysuria, frequency, hematuria
  - Cardiopulmonary: cough, dyspnea, cor pulmonale
  - CNS: headache, seizures, transverse myelitis

DIAGNOSTICS

- Labs including CBC and basic metabolic panel
- Schistosoma may be isolated from urine, blood, and stool

TREATMENT

- Praziquantel and corticosteroids for acute schistosomiasis

Whipworm

ETIOLOGY

- *Trichuris trichiura*
- Parasite found in rural areas of the United States
- Spread by fecal–oral route
- Eggs hatch in the small bowel and immature worms migrate to the colon, imbedding half their bodies in the intestinal mucosa

SIGNS AND SYMPTOMS

- Anorexia, abdominal pain, diarrhea, fever, weight loss
- Colitis and rectal prolapse in children

DIAGNOSTICS

- Microcytic hypochromic anemia, stool for O&P

TREATMENT

- Mebendazole, albendazole

Tapeworm

ETIOLOGY

- *Taenia solium*—pork tapeworm
- Central America and Middle East

- Ingestion of undercooked pork
- Taenia saginata: beef tapeworm

SIGNS AND SYMPTOMS
- Abdominal pain, anorexia, nausea, constipation
- Most common complication is appendicitis
- Larval cysts within the brain may cause seizure, headache, or psychiatric disturbance

DIAGNOSTICS
- CBC with eosinophilia. Stool for O&P. Head CT may reveal cysts and granulomata, or edema consistent with dead worms

TREATMENT
- Praziquantel, Niclosamide
- Decadron in the event of increased ICP
- Ocular, ventricular, and spinal lesions may require surgical management

Giardiasis
BASICS
- Flagellate protozoan *G. lamblia*
- Most common parasitic intestinal infection in the United States
- Endemic in regions with poor sanitation

ETIOLOGY
- Cysts ingested via contaminated water → develop into trophozoites, which colonize the duodenum and jejunum

SIGNS AND SYMPTOMS
- Watery diarrhea, flatus, abdominal cramping, nausea, weight loss

DIAGNOSTICS
- Stool antigen testing

TREATMENT
- Metronidazole, tinidazole

Amebiasis
BASICS
- Amebic dysentery
- Protozoan *E. histolytica*
- Endemic in developing countries with poor sanitation

ETIOLOGY
- Ingestion of cysts from contaminated water/soil/hands from food handlers
- Trophozoites inhabit the colon, causing mucosal destruction and ulceration

SIGNS AND SYMPTOMS
- Bloody diarrhea, fever, abdominal pain, nausea, anorexia
- Complications: liver, lung, brain abscesses, pericarditis, toxic megacolon, ameboma

DIAGNOSTICS
- **CBC generally *without* eosinophilia**, liver function test elevation
- Stool for ova and parasite, culture, and antigen
- Serum IgG
- Colonoscopy: scraping of ulcers may reveal trophozoites

TREATMENT
- Metronidazole

Trypanosomiasis

BASICS
- Protozoan parasite *Trypanosoma cruzi* causes Chagas disease
- More common in the Southwestern United States and South America

ETIOLOGY
- Humans come into contact with feces from infected blood-sucking insects
- After entry into the skin, they invade the bloodstream and lymphatics

SIGNS AND SYMPTOMS
- Acute phase:
  - Chagoma (inflammatory lesion where *T. cruzi* enters the skin)
  - Fever, headache, anorexia, conjunctivitis
  - Resolves in 3 to 8 weeks
- Chronic phase:
  - GI complications: megacolon (abdominal pain and constipation), megaesophagus (dysphagia, chest pain)
  - Cardiac: cardiomyopathy, atrioventricular block, thromboembolism

DIAGNOSTICS
- Thick and thin smear, enzyme-linked immunosorbent assay

TREATMENT
- Benznidazole or nifurtimox for the acute phase
- Antiparasitic treatment not given to those with GI and cardiac complications from chronic infection

Cholera

BASICS
- Common, bacterial infection by *Vibrio cholerae*
- Found in developing countries, specifically sub-Saharan Africa

ETIOLOGY
- Water-borne, also through fecal–oral spread and person-to-person contact

SIGNS AND SYMPTOMS
- Watery diarrhea, vomiting, dehydration

DIAGNOSTICS
- Serum PCR, examination of stool under dark field microscopy, stool culture

TREATMENT
- Aggressive rehydration and maintenance
- Ciprofloxacin, erythromycin, doxycycline, and Bactrim

● RABIES

BASICS
- Disease of mammals only
- Once symptomatic: **nearly 100% mortality**
- High-risk animals:
  - Raccoons, skunks, foxes, coyotes
    - Assume rabid and always vaccinate

- Bats
  - Very high risk
  - Vaccinate for any other bite/scratch/saliva exposure or if patient wakes up with bat in bedroom
- Other mammals
  - Domestic cats and dogs
    - Confirm vaccination status of animal
    - Most are low risk
      - Unknown rabies vaccine
      - Observe animal for 10 days OR
      - Vaccinate after consulting with Department of Public Health (DPH)
  - Livestock, small rodents generally low risk

SIGNS AND SYMPTOMS
- Similar to the flu including general weakness, fever, headache
- Late stages: delirium, abnormal behavior, hallucinations
- The acute period of disease typically ends after 2 to 10 days

TREATMENT
- If signs of clinical disease: ABCs, supportive, the disease is nearly always fatal
- If animal bite and/or exposure:
  - Clean wounds
  - Vaccinate
    - Human rabies immune globulin (HRIG) 20 IU per kg on day 0
      - Infiltrate full dose around wound if possible
    - **Rabies vaccine 1.0 mL IM days 0, 3, 7, and 14**
      - Do not inject in same site as HRIG

● SEPSIS

BASICS
- *Bacterial sepsis* is a clinical term used to describe symptomatic bacteremia, with or without organ dysfunction
- Defined as the presence of infection in conjunction with **systemic inflammatory response syndrome (SIRS):**
  - Body temp $< 36°C$ (96.8°F) or $> 38°C$ (100.4°F)
  - Heart rate >90
  - Tachypnea: respiratory rate >20 or arterial partial pressure of CO_2 <32 mm Hg
  - Leukocytes $<4,000$ cells per mm^3 or $>12,000$ cells per mm^3, or presence of $>10\%$ bands
- Patients with diabetes mellitus, systemic lupus erythematosus, ETOH abuse, and chronic steroid use at higher risk

ETIOLOGY
- Infectious versus noninfectious
- Noninfectious include adrenal insufficiency, pulmonary embolism, aortic aneurysm/dissection, cardiac tamponade, anaphylaxis, drug overdose

DEFINITIONS
- Sepsis
  - SIRS plus documented infection
  - Goals in the ED: early identification of sepsis with early administration of appropriate empiric antimicrobial therapy and surgical intervention are critical

- Severe sepsis
  - Sepsis-related organ dysfunction or signs of hypoperfusion (lactate >2 mmol/L, oliguria, AMS, hypoxia, elevated liver function tests)
  - Hypotension: systolic blood pressure <90 or mean arterial pressure <60
- Septic shock
  - Severe sepsis with persistent hypotension refractory to fluid bolus
- MODS: multiple organ dysfunction syndrome
  - More than one major system failure, associated with >50% mortality

DIAGNOSTICS
- Laboratory studies, including blood cultures and lactic acid, arterial blood gas/venous blood gas, urinalysis, and culture
- Chest x-ray

TREATMENT
- ABCs, IV fluids, supportive, transfusion if needed (if hematocrit <30)
- Initiate appropriate broad-spectrum antibiotics, goal within 3 hours of arrival in the ED
- Blood cultures prior to antibiotics
- Early goal-directed therapy
  - Antibiotics generally institution specific
  - Consider Methicillin-resistant *S. aureus*, *Pseudomonas* coverage, especially if recently hospitalized (health care–associated pneumonia—2-day hospital admission in the last 90 days)
    - ○ If hypotensive, give fluid bolus 20 to 40 mL per kg
    - ○ If persistently hypotensive despite fluid bolus, initiate vasopressors via central line

● TETANUS

BASICS
- A serious bacterial infection affecting nervous system
- Also called "lock jaw"

ETIOLOGY
- Bacteria *Clostridium tetani*
- Found in soil, dust, and animal feces
- Bacteria produces a toxin (tetanospasmin) which impairs motor neurons

SIGNS AND SYMPTOMS
- Muscle spasms
- Difficulty breathing
- Fever, hypertension, diaphoresis

DIAGNOSTICS
- Clinical exam findings

TREATMENT
- ABCs, supportive
- **Vaccine**
  - Tetanus vaccine nearly 100% effective after three doses
  - Immunity declines after 5 to 10 years, booster recommended every 10 years
  - Combined vaccine with diphtheria
  - **Recommended for all pregnant women** (third trimester preferred)

●TICK-BORNE AND VECTOR-BORNE ILLNESSES

Tick removal: Grab the head with forceps and gently pull away from the skin

Lyme Disease

BASICS
- Most common tick-borne disease

ETIOLOGY
- Spirochete *Borrelia burgdorferi*
- Transmitted by deer tick, genus Ixodes nymph stage
- Highest incidence in the Northeast
- Tick must be attached >24 hours

SIGNS AND SYMPTOMS
- Early localized:
  - **Erythema chronicus migrans**
  - Annular (target) lesions
  - May include systemic symptoms: fever, chills, headache, malaise
  - Symptoms occur 3 to 32 days after tick bite
- Early disseminated:
  - Longer than 4 weeks
  - Neuro: headache, meningitis, facial nerve palsy, radiculoneuropathy
  - Cardiac: atrioventricular block, all types
- Late:
  - Migratory polyoligoarthritis involving large joints (knee, shoulder, elbow), encephalitis

DIAGNOSTICS
- Clinical exam findings
- Serology: Lyme titer/antibody (not reliable)
- CSF studies

TREATMENT
- Stage I:
  - **Doxycycline 100 mg bid for 21 days**
  - Children and pregnant women: Amoxicillin, penicillin, or erythromycin
- Stage II:
  - Ceftriaxone 1 g Q12H × 10 to 14 days
- Stage III:
  - Arthritis treatment doxycycline for 28 days
  - Encephalitis requires IV treatment
- Posttreatment Lyme disease syndrome:
  - 10% to 20% of people previously diagnosed with Lyme develop chronic fatigue, myalgia, and arthralgia
  - No evidence that patients who receive prolonged course of antibiotics for this do better than those who receive placebo

Babesiosis

ETIOLOGY
- *Babesia:* protozoal parasite that causes a malaria-like syndrome
- Same tick vector as Lyme
- Coinfection with Lyme is possible
- More common in asplenic patients

SIGNS AND SYMPTOMS
- Fever, malaise, anorexia, fatigue, headache
- Exam: unremarkable, splenomegaly noted in 40% of patients

DIAGNOSTICS
- Labs: mild hemolytic anemia
- Thick and thin smear

TREATMENT
- Healthy patients:
  - Clindamycin and quinine po
  - **Quinine contraindicated in pregnant patients**
- Immunocompromised or elderly patients:
  - IV clindamycin and oral quinine
  - Or IV azithromycin and atovaquone
- Severe cases:
  - Consider exchange transfusion

Ehrlichiosis

ETIOLOGY
- Ehrlichial anaplasma—gram-negative organism that resemble *Rickettsia*

SIGNS AND SYMPTOMS
- Fever, headache, malaise, rigors, nausea, myalgias, nausea, vomiting
- Rash is rare
- Hepatosplenomegaly

DIAGNOSTICS
- Ehrlichia titer
- Coinfection with Rocky Mountain Spotted Fever and babesiosis possible
- Hyponatremia found in 40% of patients

TREATMENT
- Doxycycline × 10 to 14 days
- Rifampin if doxycycline contraindicated

Rocky Mountain Spotted Fever

ETIOLOGY
- *Rickettsia rickettsii*
- Second most common tick-borne disease, primarily in the North west United States

SIGNS AND SYMPTOMS
- Fever, maculopapular rash, eventually petechial
- Involves palms and soles, flexor surfaces of wrists and ankles
- Also nausea, vomiting, myalgia, HA, encephalitis
- Triad: fever, headache, and rash in 55% to 65% of patients

DIAGNOSTICS
- Titers often negative
- Skin biopsy: immunofluorescent antibody staining very sensitive but less specific

TREATMENT
- Doxycycline po for mild cases and IV for moderate-severe disease
- Chloramphenicol in children and pregnant patients

Tularemia

ETIOLOGY
- Infectious zoonosis caused by aerobic, gram-negative, bacillus *F. tularensis*
- Transmission: tick-borne, mosquitoes, flies
- Also from animal bites and exposure to contaminated water and mud

SYMPTOMS
- Sudden onset of flu-like symptoms: fever, chills, headache, myalgias, malaise, cough, pharyngitis, abdominal pain
- Fever lasts for several days, will cease briefly, then resume
- Macular → maculopapular rash → pustular rash
- **Pulse temperature dissociation:** relative bradycardia in the setting of fever (also seen in typhoid fever, dengue fever, avian flu, and Q fever)

DIAGNOSTICS
- Labs including tularemia antibody titer

TREATMENT
- Streptomycin is drug of choice
- Fluoroquinolones can also be used (limited data)

West Nile Virus

ETIOLOGY
- Flavivirus, mosquito-borne
- Less than 1% of people infected go on to develop severe illness

SIGNS AND SYMPTOMS
- Mild illness: fever, nausea, anorexia, malaise, myalgia, headache
- Severe illness: muscle weakness, photophobia, seizures, flaccid paralysis, mental status changes

DIAGNOSTICS
- Hyponatremia secondary to SIADH
- Serum or CSF West Nile IgM

TREATMENT
- Supportive

Eastern Equine Encephalitis

BASICS
- Also called "sleeping sickness"

ETIOLOGY
- Zoonotic alphavirus, mosquito-borne

SIGNS AND SYMPTOMS
- Headache, nausea, vomiting, confusion, nuchal rigidity, seizures, somnolence, cranial nerve palsies (most commonly VI, VII, and XII), fever, chills, myalgia

DIAGNOSTICS
- Hyponatremia due to SIADH, elevated WBC
- Serum EEE IgM
- Viral culture or PCR of CSF

TREATMENT
- Supportive

Brucellosis

ETIOLOGY
- Zoonotic infection caused by *Brucella*
- Most common zoonotic infection
- *Brucella melitensis* most common and virulent worldwide
- Transmission: from animals to humans through ingestion of infected food products or direct contact with affected animal
- Most commonly from sheep, goats, pigs, cattle, and dogs

SIGNS AND SYMPTOMS
- Fever, chills, arthralgia, sweats, anorexia
- Hepatosplenomegaly common on exam
- Neuro: meningoencephalitis with MS change, coma, neurologic defects, seizures, or coma
- GI: dyspepsia, abdominal pain, hepatic abscess

DIAGNOSTICS
- Tube agglutination test (other bacterial illnesses may trigger false positive), serum *Brucella* IgG or PCR
- Isolation of *Brucella* organism: blood or bone marrow culture
- CSF studies

TREATMENT
- Mild cases: doxycycline po
- Moderate to severe cases: multidrug IV regimens

NOTES

Toxicologic Disorders—4%

Heather R. Becker, Hannah S. Dodd, and Rachel Frances

● ACETAMINOPHEN TOXICITY, SALICYLATES, NONSTEROIDAL ANTI-INFLAMMATORY DRUGS

Acetaminophen

BASICS
- Common drugs: Tylenol
- **Acetaminophen poisoning has become the most common cause of acute liver failure in the United States**
- Pediatric toxicity >250 mg/kg/24 hours
- Adult toxicity >12 g ingestion

SIGNS AND SYMPTOMS
- Nausea, vomiting within 2 hours, elevated liver enzymes, rise in prothrombin time/international normalized ratio

DIAGNOSTICS
- Serum level
- If 4-hour Tylenol level >140 mg per dL then treat

TREATMENT
- N-acetylcysteine (NAC)
  - Works by restoring hepatic glutathione stores
  - Best if started within the first 8 hours

Salicylates

BASICS
- Common drugs
  - Aspirin

SIGNS AND SYMPTOMS
- Respiratory alkalosis, tinnitus, anion gap metabolic acidosis

DIAGNOSTICS
- Serum level

TREATMENT
- Bicarb
- Dialysis

Nonsteroidal Anti-Inflammatory Drugs

BASICS
- Common drugs
  - Ibuprofen, piroxicam

SIGNS AND SYMPTOMS
- Most common: gastrointestinal upset
- Less common: drowsiness, lethargy, ataxia, nystagmus, tinnitus
- Rare and only with massive amounts: seizure, coma, renal failure

DIAGNOSTICS
- Based on detailed history
- No specific levels available

TREATMENT
- Antacids for mild gastrointestinal upset
- Treats seizures, coma, hypotension if they occur
- No antidote

● ANTICHOLINERGICS

BASICS
- Common drugs
  - Antihistamines, tricyclic antidepressant, atropine, Donnatal, Lomotil, oxybutynin, scopolamine, jimson weed

SIGNS AND SYMPTOMS
- Dry as a bone, mad as a hatter, blind as a bat, hot as a hare

DIAGNOSIS
- Clinical exam findings
- Physostigmine trial

TREATMENT
- Physostigmine

● DRUGS OF ABUSE

See substance abuse and overdose in Chapter 12: Psychobehavioral Disorders—3%

Opioids

BASICS
- Common drugs
  - Oxycodone, morphine, heroin

SIGNS AND SYMPTOMS
- Central nervous system and respiratory depression, miosis

DIAGNOSTICS
- Serum level

TREATMENT/ANTIDOTE
- Narcan

Cocaine/Amphetamines

BASICS
- Common drugs
  - Cocaine, ritalin, speed

SIGNS AND SYMPTOMS
- Agitation, dilated pupils, diaphoresis, irritability, decreased appetite, cardiac arrhythmia

DIAGNOSTICS
- History
- Toxicology screen

TREATMENT
- Supportive
- If chest pain, give benzodiazepines
- Avoid β-blockers in cocaine and chest pain

● METALS

Lead

BASICS
- Common drugs
  - Found in household paints

SIGNS AND SYMPTOMS
- Abdominal pain, microcytic anemia with basophilic stippling, ataxia, purple lines on gums

DIAGNOSTICS
- Serum level

TREATMENT
- Ca EDTA

Mercury

BASICS
- Common drugs
  - Thimerosal
  - Thiazide

SIGNS AND SYMPTOMS
- Insomnia, delirium, pulmonary edema

DIAGNOSTICS
- Blood level

TREATMENT
- Bicarb
- Dialysis

Organophosphates

BASICS
- Common drugs
  - Insecticides
  - Herbicides for flowers and plants
  - Nerve gases

SIGNS AND SYMPTOMS
- Impaired memory, disorientation, confusion, headache, nausea, weakness, appetite loss

DIAGNOSTICS
- Serum test

TREATMENT
- Anticholinergic drugs

●TRICYCLICS, MAOI, ANTIPSYCHOTICS, LITHIUM, BENZODIAZEPINES

Tricyclics

BASICS
- Common drugs
  - Amitriptyline, doxepin, nortriptyline

SIGNS AND SYMPTOMS
- Anticholinergic symptoms, QRS >100 ms, **torsades des pointes**

DIAGNOSTICS
- Blood level

TREATMENT
- Bicarb drip

Monoamine Oxidase Inhibitors

BASICS
- Common drugs
  - Isocarboxazid, phenelzine, selegiline

SIGNS AND SYMPTOMS
  - Hypertension, delirium, hyperthermia, dysrhythmia, seizures

DIAGNOSTICS
  - Clinical exam findings

TREATMENT
- Supportive
- Treat hypertension with α-blockers or combined α- and β-blockers

Antipsychotics

BASICS
- Common drugs
  - Chlorpromazine, haloperidol, droperidol, olanzapine, promethazine, quetiapine, risperidone

SIGNS AND SYMPTOMS
- Mild: sedation, small pupils, orthostatic hypotension
- Severe: coma, seizures, respiratory arrest

DIAGNOSTICS
- History of ingestion combined with physical exam findings and prolonged QT on EKG

TREATMENT
- Supportive
- QT prolongation may respond to Mg

Lithium Carbonate

BASICS
- Common drugs
  - Lithium

SIGNS AND SYMPTOMS
- Lethargy, muscle weakness, slurred speech, ataxia, tremor

DIAGNOSTICS
- Serum level

TREATMENT
- Supportive
- Dialysis for severe cases

Benzodiazepines

BASICS
- Common drugs
  - Alprazolam, clonazepam, diazepam, lorazepam, midazolam

SIGNS AND SYMPTOMS
- Rapid onset of weakness, ataxia, drowsiness, respiratory arrest

DIAGNOSTICS
- Serum levels

TREATMENT
- Flumazenil

NOTES

Traumatic Disorders—12%

Nicole Kostarellas and Kristen Vella Gray

● FACIAL TRAUMA

Mandibular Fracture

BASICS
- Most commonly caused by assault or motor vehicle crash

SIGNS AND SYMPTOMS
- Malocclusion
- Floor of mouth ecchymosis
- Lower lip/chin paresthesias

DIAGNOSTICS
- X-ray two views or Panorex view
- Maxillofacial CT preferred

TREATMENT
- Referral to Oral and Maxillofacial Surgery
- Prophylactic antibiotics: needed only if oral involvement (penicillin or first-generation cephalosporin, clindamycin)

Maxillary Fracture (Midface Fracture)

BASICS
- Look for malocclusion
- Nasal intubations and nasogastric tubes are contraindicated
- Associated with significant traumatic mechanism

DIAGNOSTICS
- Maxillofacial CT
- **Le Fort fracture classification** (Figure 17.1)
  - Le Fort I: transverse, through the maxilla
  - Le Fort II: extends superiorly involving the nasal bridge, maxilla, lacrimal bones, orbital floor, and rim
  - Le Fort III: craniofacial dissociation; involves bridge of the nose and extends posteriorly along the medial wall and floor of the orbit, lateral orbital wall, zygomatic arch to the base of the sphenoid. May involve the cribriform plate; check for cerebrospinal fluid (CSF) leak

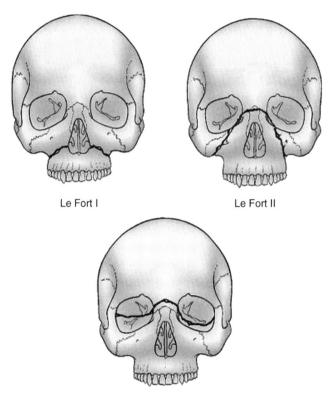

Le Fort I   Le Fort II

Le Fort III

FIGURE 17.1. Le Fort fractures of the midface. (From Auerbach PS, ed. *Wilderness Medicine*. 6th ed. Philadelphia, PA: Elsevier Mosby; 2011. Figure 31-18 MD Consult. Redrawn from the American Association of Oral and Maxillofacial Surgeons. *Oral and Maxillofacial Surgery Services in the Emergency Department*. Rosemont, IL: American Association of Oral and Maxillofacial Surgeons; 1992, With permission.)

TREATMENT
- ABCs (airway, breathing, circulation), supportive, antibiotics
- Plastic surgery, Oral and Maxillofacial Surgery consults
- **Neurosurgery consult for Le Fort III**
- Keep head of bed >30 degrees

Zygomatic Fracture

BASICS
- Tripod fractures (infraorbital rim, zygomaticofacial and zygomaticotemporal suture lines)

DIAGNOSTICS
- Maxillofacial CT

TREATMENT
- ENT, plastics consult
- Delayed open reduction internal fixation

Orbital Fracture

BASICS
- Most involve the orbital floor and medial wall

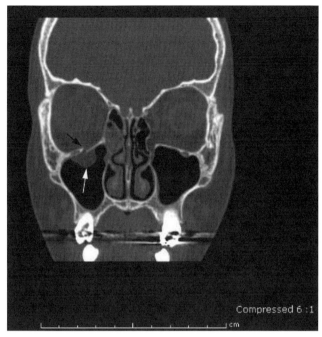

FIGURE 17.2. CT shows a right inferior orbital fracture (blowout fracture). (Neuman ML. Orbital fractures. In: Post TW, ed. *UpToDate*. Waltham, MA: UpToDate; 2014. Graphic 53238 Version 3.0. Courtesy of Mark Neuman, MD.)

SIGNS AND SYMPTOMS
- Periorbital swelling and tenderness
- Numbness over cheek
- Can cause muscle and nerve entrapment

DIAGNOSTICS
- CT with clinical findings

TREATMENT
- Surgery within 24 hours, unless there is too much edema, then within 5 to 7 days
- Discharge with sinus precautions and Augmentin for 7 days or azithromycin
- **Blowout fracture (Figure 17.2)**

Nasal Fracture

BASICS
- The most common fracture of the face

SIGNS AND SYMPTOMS
- Pain, history of trauma
- Nasal deformity
- **Assess for septal hematoma:** requires immediate evacuation to prevent necrosis

DIAGNOSTICS
- Mostly clinical, can get x-ray

TREATMENT
- Reduction in 5 to 7 days by plastics or ENT

● MUSCULOSKELETAL TRAUMA

BASICS
- Most fractures can be diagnosed with at least two-view x-rays; however, some need CT or MRI (especially elderly with continued pain)
- The neurovascular exam is essential on initial assessment and after splint placement; always document this
- Orthopedic consult should be considered for fractures that are open, intra-articular, unstable, require surgical repair, or with neurovascular compromise
- General treatment: pain control, elevation, immobilization, follow–up, and rehabilitation
- Always examine joint above and below injury
- **Bone anatomy (Figure 17.3)**
  - Epiphysis: ends of a bone
  - Physis: growth plate
  - Metaphysis: upper and lower third of a bone
  - Diaphysis: middle third of a bone

Shoulder Dislocation

BASICS
- Anterior: most common, arm is externally rotated and slightly abducted
- Posterior: 2% to 4%, arm held in adduction and internal rotation
- Inferior: 0.5%, arm held above the head, high risk for fracture and nerve damage
- Complications that need ortho referral
  - Humerus fracture
    - Hill–Sachs deformity: humeral head cortical depression
    - Bankart lesion: avulsion fracture
    - Greater tuberosity fracture
  - **Axillary nerve:** always test on exam for injury

DIAGNOSTICS
- X-ray pre- and postreduction
- In some cases, there is no need for x-ray if the patient meets all of these criteria: age <40, atraumatic, and history of multiple shoulder dislocations

TREATMENT
- Reduction (many techniques)
  - Scapular manipulation, external rotation, traction-countertraction
- Immobilization with sling and swath
- Occasional surgery

Radial Ulna Fractures/Dislocation

BASICS
- Colles fracture: radial styloid fracture and distal radius fracture with dorsal displacement of the distal fragment
- Smith fracture: distal radial fracture with palmar displacement
- Galeazzi: midshaft radius fracture with dislocation at the distal radioulnar joint
- Monteggia: fracture at the junction of the proximal and middle thirds of the ulna, with an anterior dislocation of the radial head

TREATMENT
- Reduce displaced fracture
- Splint, ortho follow-up

Location of the bone

Integrity of skin and soft-tissue envelope around fracture

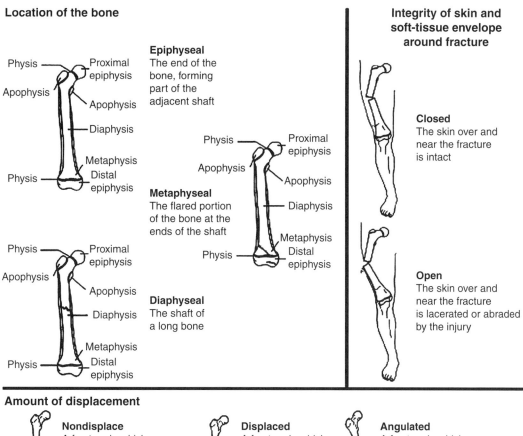

Epiphyseal
The end of the bone, forming part of the adjacent shaft

Metaphyseal
The flared portion of the bone at the ends of the shaft

Diaphyseal
The shaft of a long bone

Closed
The skin over and near the fracture is intact

Open
The skin over and near the fracture is lacerated or abraded by the injury

Amount of displacement

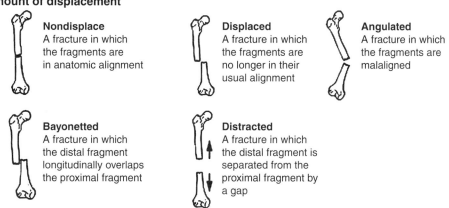

Nondisplace
A fracture in which the fragments are in anatomic alignment

Displaced
A fracture in which the fragments are no longer in their usual alignment

Angulated
A fracture in which the fragments are malaligned

Bayonetted
A fracture in which the distal fragment longitudinally overlaps the proximal fragment

Distracted
A fracture in which the distal fragment is separated from the proximal fragment by a gap

FIGURE 17.3. Bone anatomy and fracture classifications. (From Beutler A, Mark Stephens. General principles of fracture management: bone healing and fracture description. In: Post TW, ed. *UpToDate*. Waltham, MA: UpToDate; 2014. Graphic 56313 Version 2.0. Reproduced with permisiion from: Johnson TR, Steinback, LS. eds. *Essentials of Musculoskeletal Imaging*. Rosemonst, IL: Amercan Academy of Orthopedic Surgeons; 2004:40–41. Copyright 2004 American Academy of Orthopaedic Surgeons.)

Radial Head Fracture

DIAGNOSTICS

- X-ray:
  - Anterior fat pad: can be normal, but if sail shape, always indicative of fracture
  - Posterior fat pad: never normal, indicative of fracture

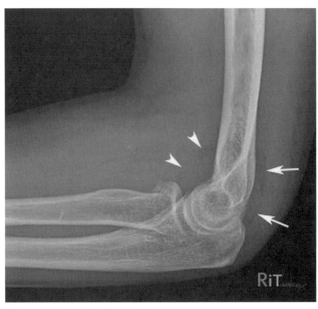

FIGURE 17.4. Radial head fracture.

■ In adults:
 • **Assume radial head fracture if anterior sail shape or posterior fat pad (Figure 17.4)**
■ In children:
 • Assume supracondylar fracture if anterior sail shape or posterior fat pad

TREATMENT
■ Sling and ortho follow-up

Boxer's Fracture

BASICS
■ Fifth metacarpal neck fracture, sometimes involves the fourth metacarpal
■ Mechanism is usually direct trauma to a clenched fist such as punching
■ Dorsal angulation of the fracture causes metacarpophalangeal joint depression (loss of the knuckle)

DIAGNOSTICS
■ X-ray

TREATMENT
■ May need reduction with a hematoma block
■ Ulnar gutter splint
■ Hand surgery follow-up
■ Complications
 • Open fracture
  ○ Antibiotics within 6 hours to prevent osteomyelitis (cefuroxime or fluoroquinolone, consider methicillin-resistant *Staphylococcus aureus* coverage)
 • **"Fight bite"**: skin tear near the metacarpal head from a tooth
  ○ Irrigation, must give antibiotic coverage
  ○ First line: Augmentin
  ○ Second line: doxycycline, Bactrim, fluoroquinolone, cefuroxime, or penicillin *plus* Flagyl or clindamycin

Scaphoid Fracture (Navicular)

BASICS
- Mechanism is usually a fall onto an outstretched hand
- Classified as distal, central, or proximal
- Tenderness at the radial, dorsal aspect of hand, anatomical snuff box

DIAGNOSTICS
- X-ray scaphoid views

TREATMENT
- Thumb spica splint
- **If suspected, but x-ray is negative, still splint it!**

Gamekeeper's/Skier's Thumb

BASICS
- Ulnar collateral ligament injury of the thumb
- Caused by hyperextension
- Common in skiers, volley ball players, goalies

TREATMENT
- Thumb spica splint

Rib Fracture

BASICS
- From trauma or exertion, such as, coughing
- Ribs 1 to 3 associated with mediastinal injury (i.e., aorta)
- Ribs 9 to 12 associated with intra-abdominal injury
- **Flail chest**
  - Three or more consecutive ribs fractured in two or more places
  - "Floating" segment, paradoxical movement on inspiration
- Complications
  - Pneumonia
  - Pneumothorax
  - Hemothorax
  - Respiratory failure
    - More rib fractures = longer ventilation duration and increased mortality

DIAGNOSTICS
- Chest x-ray, ultrasound, CT

TREATMENT
- Most heal in 6 weeks
- Less than three rib fractures: outpatient pain control, incentive spirometry
- Three or more rib fractures: inpatient, elderly with six or more admit to ICU, pain control, continuous pulse oximetry, multidisciplinary care

Pneumothorax

BASICS
- *Primary pneumothorax (PTX):* occurs without a causing event or an underlying lung disease
  - Risk factors: smoking, family history, Marfan syndrome
  - Usually in early 20s to 30s
- *Secondary PTX:* occurs with an underlying lung disease
  - Risk factors: chronic obstructive pulmonary disease, cystic fibrosis, cancer, necrotizing pneumonia

- *Traumatic PTX:* may occur with a hemothorax
- *Tension PTX:* hypotension, tracheal deviation, elevated jugular venous pressure, requiring emergent needle decompression, and/or chest tube

SIGNS AND SYMPTOMS
- Shortness of breath, tachypnea, tachycardia, hypoxia, decreased breath sounds, subcutaneous emphysema; tracheal deviation is a late finding
- Hemodynamic instability may indicate a tension PTX

DIAGNOSTICS
- Chest x-ray, ultrasound, CT

TREATMENT
- Small (<15% volume): observation, high-flow O_2 with non-rebreather face mask, repeated chest x-ray
- Large (2 cm on upright posterior to anterior chest x-ray equals a 50% PTX)
  - Needle decompression (14G IV catheter into the pleural space at the second intercostal space, midclavicular line)
  - Chest tube (see Chapter 18 for procedure details)
- VATS (video-assisted thoracoscopic surgery) pleurodesis
- ABCs, supportive, smoking cessation education

Hip and Pelvic Fracture

BASICS
- Benign to life-threatening
- Examine the genital and rectum for signs of open fracture
- Always perform rectal exam before Foley placement

SIGNS AND SYMPTOMS
- Affected side: **shortened, externally rotated, and abducted**
- Presentation is pathognomonic

DIAGNOSTICS
- X-ray, CT (gold standard)
- Complications: urethral, vaginal, or rectal injuries

TREATMENT
- ABCs, pain control, resuscitation
- Pelvic binder, external fixation
- Orthopedic consult for open reduction internal fixation

Hip Dislocation

BASICS
- Posterior: most common, leg flexed and adducted
- Anterior: leg abducted and externally rotated

DIAGNOSTICS
- X-ray

TREATMENT
- Reduction with postreduction films

Femur Fracture

BASICS
- High-energy trauma
- High risk for hemorrhage

DIAGNOSTICS
- X-ray

TREATMENT
- ABCs, pain control, resuscitation
- Immobilization and traction
- Ortho consult for surgery

Tibial Plateau Fracture

BASICS
- Most commonly from a direct blow to the lateral knee
- Seen often in pedestrian struck by vehicle

DIAGNOSIS
- X-ray

TREATMENT
- Brace in extension, non-weight-bearing with crutches
- Ortho follow-up

Ankle Fracture

BASICS
- Anterior talofibular ligament is most common ligament injured in sprained ankle, from inversion injury
- Always examine knee looking for Maisonneuve fracture
  - A spiral fracture of proximal fibula and medial malleolus associated with a tear of the distal tibiofibular syndesmosis
- **Ottawa ankle rules:** x-rays indicated if one of the following:
  - Tenderness over the medial or lateral malleolus
  - Tenderness over the midfoot
  - Tenderness over the base of the 5th metatarsal
  - Unable to weight bear immediately and take four steps in the emergency department

DIAGNOSTICS
- X-ray

TREATMENT
- Short-leg posterior splint or boot
- Ortho consult and surgery if unstable

Foot Fractures

BASICS
- *Jones:* transverse fracture of the diaphyseal region of the base of the 5th metatarsal
- *Lisfranc:* fracture/dislocation of the tarsometatarsal joint
- Caution: avulsion fracture of base of 5th metatarsal concerning for malunion given peroneus brevis ligament attachment site

TREATMENT
- Most nondisplaced shaft fractures of metatarsal 2 to 5 do not require reduction or casting

Achilles Tendon Rupture

BASICS
- Usually caused by force during physical activities that involve sudden pivoting on a foot or rapid acceleration

SIGNS AND SYMPTOMS

- Patient may describe feeling struck in the back of the ankle or hearing a "pop"
- Severe acute pain when pushing off with his or her foot, although the absence of pain does not rule out rupture

DIAGNOSTICS

- Do *not* assume rupture is absent because the patient can plantar flex or walk; 20% to 30% ruptures are missed because of this assumption
- **Thompson test:** the patient lies prone with his or her feet hanging off the end of the examination table, or kneels on a chair; clinician squeezes the gastrocnemius muscle belly while watching for plantar flexion; absence of plantar flexion when squeezing the gastrocnemius muscle marks a positive test = rupture
- Clinical exam diagnosis

TREATMENT

- Complete tendon rupture: ice, rest, pain control, plantar flexion splint, crutches, non-weight-bearing
- Ortho consultation
- Partial tendon rupture: RICE (rest, ice, compression, elevation), 3 to 6 months of conservative treatment, if failed then ortho consultation

Compartment Syndrome

BASICS

- Increased pressure between muscle and fascia layers caused by bleeding or edema usually from trauma or burns
- Results in venous congestion and arterial insufficiency
- Late findings are associated with irreversible nerve and muscle damage

SIGNS AND SYMPTOMS

- Swelling with tight compartments
- Pain out of proportion from exam (early)
- Early signs: numbness, tingling, and paresthesias
- Late signs: loss of function, and decreased pulses or pulselessness
- 7 Ps
  - Pain
  - Pallor
  - Paresthesia
  - Paralysis
  - Poikilothermia (inability to regulate temperature)
  - Pulselessness
  - Pressure

DIAGNOSTICS

- Handheld manometer (Stryker)
  - Normal pressure is 0 to 8 mm Hg

TREATMENT

- Remove all splints/casts
- Do not elevate or lower the limb; it should be level with the heart
- Pain control, IV fluids, treat hypotension to reduce hypoperfusion
- Emergent surgery consult for fasciotomy

● NEUROLOGIC TRAUMA

Head Trauma

(see also Chapter 10, Nervous System Disorders)

BASICS

■ Brain ischemia is caused by decrease in cerebral perfusion pressure

■ If intracranial pressure sharply increases, it can result in herniation

DIAGNOSTICS

■ Decision to obtain head CT scan should be based upon Canadian or National Emergency X-Ray Utilization Study (NEXUS) II Head CT rules
  • Canadian CT Head Rule (consider CT if yes to any of the following):
    ○ Glasgow Coma scale (GCS) <15 two hours after injury
    ○ Suspected open skull fracture
    ○ Sign of a basal skull fracture
    ○ Two or more episodes of vomiting
    ○ Age more than 65
    ○ Thirty minutes of preimpact amnesia
    ○ Dangerous mechanism
  • NEXUS II CT Head Rule (consider CT if yes to any of the following):
    ○ Evidence of skull fracture
    ○ Scalp hematoma
    ○ Neuro deficit
    ○ Altered level of consciousness
    ○ Abnormal behavior
    ○ Coagulopathy
    ○ Persistent vomiting
    ○ Age more than 65

■ GCS
  • GCS <8: severe head trauma
  • GCS 9 to 13: moderate head trauma
  • GCS 14 to 15: minor head trauma
    ○ Eye opening
      – 4 spontaneous
      – 3 to verbal commands
      – 2 to pain
      – 1 no response
    ○ Verbal response
      – 5 oriented
      – 4 confused
      – 3 inappropriate
      – 2 incomprehensible sounds
      – 1 no response
    ○ Motor response
      – 6 obeys commands
      – 5 localizes to pain
      – 4 flexion withdrawal
      – 3 decorticate posturing
      – 2 decerebrate posturing
      – 1 no response

TREATMENT
- ABCs
- Neurosurgery consult
- Keppra, Dilantin (seizure prevention)
- Correct coagulopathy as indicated (fresh frozen plasma, platelet, vitamin K, profile 9)
- Goal systolic blood pressure <140
- Mannitol is sometimes used to decrease cerebral edema
- **Uncal herniation**
  - Most common
  - Ipsilateral uncus herniation compresses cranial nerve (CN) III
  - Dilated ipsilateral pupil, ptosis, nonreactive pupil
- **Central transtentorial herniation**
  - Central biphasic herniation though tentorium caused by a lesion in the vertex or frontal lobe
  - Signs: altered mental status, bilateral motor weakness, pinpoint pupils that eventually become dilated and nonreactive
- **Cerebellotonsillar herniation**
  - Cerebellar tonsils herniate through the foramen magnum
  - Signs: quadriplegia caused by compression of the corticospinal tracts, cardiopulmonary collapse from brainstem compression
- **Subdural hematoma (SDH)**
  - Tearing of veins between the brain and dura occurring with acceleration-deceleration
  - Risk factors: people with brain atrophy (elderly, alcoholics)
  - CT: concave density adjacent to the skull, crosses suture lines
- **Epidural hematoma (EDH)**
  - Bleeding between the dura and skull, usually from the middle meningeal artery
  - Usually from direct trauma over the temporoparietal region
  - CT: biconvex density adjacent to skull, does not cross suture lines
- **Subarachnoid hemorrhage (SAH)**
  - **Most common abnormality seen on CT posttrauma**
  - CT: hyperdensity within subarachnoid space, prominent in the sulci or cerebral peduncles
  - See SAH under Headache for more information

Basilar Skull Fracture

BASICS
- Most commonly involves the temporal bone
- High risk for intracranial hemorrhage

SIGNS AND SYMPTOMS
- **Battle sign:** ecchymosis over the mastoid area
- Raccoon eyes: periorbital ecchymosis

DIAGNOSTICS
- Head CT

COMPLICATIONS
  - Temporal bone fracture
  - Check for CSF leak, "halo" or "ring" test, risk for meningitis
  - Dural tear (intracranial hemorrhage)
  - CN palsies

TREATMENT
- Head of bed 60 degrees if concerned for CSF leak
- Admission for observation and consider neurosurgery consult

● PEDIATRIC TRAUMA

BASICS
- When in doubt, splint and follow up with orthopedics
- May need sedation, consider ketamine
- Current state and federal laws support the treatment of minors with an emergent medical condition, regardless of consent issues

Salter–Harris Fracture Classification (Based on the Growth Plate)
- Type I: **S**eparation at the physis
- Type II: **A**bove, separation at the physis with partial metaphyseal fracture
- Type III: **L**ower, partial separation of the physis with intra-articular epiphyseal fracture
- Type IV: **T**hrough, intra-articular fracture extending across the physis into the metaphysis
- Type V: **E**verything **R**uined, crush of the growth plate (Figure 17.5)

Clavicle Fracture

BASICS
- Most common pediatric fracture
- **Middle-third clavicle fracture: most common** (80%), treat with a sling
- Distal-third clavicle fracture: sling, displaced fracture may require surgery
- Medial-third clavicle fracture: sling, displaced fracture needs ortho referral for reduction, consider intrathoracic injuries

DIAGNOSTICS
- X-ray

TREATMENT
- Usually comfort measures, sling
- Rarely surgery

Nursemaid's Elbow

BASICS
- Radial head subluxation
- Usually age 1 to 4
- Mechanism is usually someone pulling on the child's pronated forearm while the elbow is in extension, commonly while he or she is falling or pulling away

SIGNS AND SYMPTOMS
- Child not using his or her arm and holding it close to the body
- Pain with forearm supination

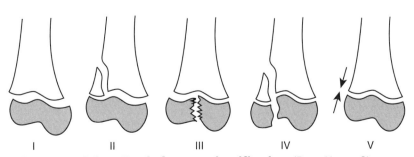

FIGURE 17.5. Salter–Harris fracture classification. (From Young SJ, Barnett PLJ, Oakley EA. Fractures and minor head injuries: minor injuries in children II. *Med J Aust.* 2005;182(12):644–648.)

DIAGNOSTICS
- Clinical exam findings
- X-ray: if suspected fracture or dislocation of the radius or ulna or after multiple failed reduction attempts

TREATMENT
- Reduction
  - **Supination/flexion method**
  - Hyperpronation method
  - When reduced, a click can be felt over the radial head or a pop may be heard

● TRAUMA IN PREGNANCY

BASICS
- Differences in the pregnant patient
  - Anatomy: greater than 20 weeks bowels are mostly in the upper abdomen
  - Blood volume and composition
    - Increase in plasma volume, clotting factors, and white blood cell
    - Decrease in hematocrit and serum albumin
  - Hemodynamics
    - Cardiac output (CO)
      - After 10 weeks, increases 1 to 1.5 L per min
      - Uterus receives 20% of CO in third trimester
      - **Supine position: inferior vena caval compression can decrease CO by 30%**
    - Heart rate: increases 10 to 15 bpm
    - EKG: left axis deviation, flat or inverted T waves in III and AVF, ectopic beats
    - Blood pressure, heart rate, complete blood count must be interpreted carefully in the pregnant trauma patient
  - Respiration
    - Increase in minute ventilation and tidal volume
    - Hypocapnia common
  - Gastrointestinal
    - Prolonged gastric emptying
    - Assume the patient's stomach is full, early gastric tube decompression prevents aspiration
  - GU
    - Glycosuria
    - Increase in glomerular filtration rate, renal blood flow
    - Decrease in blood urea nitrogen and Cr
    - Dilation of the right renal collection system
  - Endocrine
    - Increase in the pituitary gland size
    - Shock can cause gland necrosis and result pituitary insufficiency
  - Musculoskeletal
    - Widening of the symphysis pubis 4 to 8 mm and sacroiliac joints (consider when looking at pelvis x-ray)
  - Neuro:
    - Eclampsia can mimic head injury

TREATMENT

- Initial treatment: optimal resuscitation and stabilization of the mother and then early assessment of fetus
- Consult obstetric and surgery
  - Always turn mother onto her left side to displace the uterus and relieve pressure on the inferior vena caval
  - Crystalloid intravenous fluids: mother can lose a significant amount of blood before signs of hypoperfusion occur; therefore, the fetus may be in distress and the placenta deprived of perfusion while mother's condition and vital signs appear stable
  - Fetal monitoring
  - **Rhogam** for all Rh-negative pregnant woman, unless there is a remote injury away from the uterus (distal extremity)
  - Always consider tetanus

NOTES

Procedures and Skills—7%

Patricia Gatcomb, Michelle Higgins, and Kristen Vella Gray

● AIRWAY MANAGEMENT

Indications for Intubation

BASICS
- Failure to oxygenate or ventilate
- Failure to protect airway
- Anticipated clinical course

Rapid Sequence Intubation

BASICS
- Preoxygenate
- Pretreat
  - Lidocaine if reactive airway disease or increased intracranial pressure (ICP)
  - Fentanyl in increased ICP or cardiovascular disease
- Paralysis with induction agent
  - Etomidate 0.3 mg per kg
- Intubation paralytic agent
  - Succinylcholine 1.5 mg per kg
    - **Contraindications**
      - History of malignant hyperthermia
      - Burns
      - Crush injury
      - Stroke or spinal cord injury <6 months
      - Neuromuscular disease (multiple sclerosis, amyotrophic lateral sclerosis)
      - Intra-abdominal sepsis
  - Rocuronium 1 mg per kg

TREATMENT
- Intubate
  - Confirm with end tidal CO_2
- Sedation

Surgical Airway

BASICS
- Creation of opening in trachea to oxygenate and ventilate

INDICATIONS
- When a failed airway has occurred and the patient cannot oxygenate
- Severe facial or nasal trauma and unable to intubate through mouth or nose

CONTRAINDICATIONS
- Young age
- Laryngeal or tracheal tumor, abscess, other pathology

TECHNIQUE
- Identify the cricothyroid membrane
- Above the thyroid cartilage and below the cricoid cartilage
- Create a vertical incision
- Apply traction
- Intubate
- **Other techniques**
  - Seldinger technique
    - Used when provider is inexperienced or uncomfortable with surgical technique
  - Needle cricothyrotomy
    - Used in children

●CARDIAC PACING, DEFIBRILLATION, AND CARDIOVERSION
Cardiac Pacing
BASICS
- Goal is to reestablish cardiac hemodynamics until cardiac problem is resolved or permanent pacing is applied
- Regular pulses of electrical current are applied transcutaneously to stimulate heart muscle contractions

INDICATIONS
- Hemodynamically unstable bradyarrhythmias
  - Myocardial infarction
  - Complete heart block
  - Sinus node dysfunction
- Tachyarrhythmias refractory to drug therapy or electrical cardioversion
- Not recommended for asystole

CONTRAINDICATIONS
- Severe hypothermia
- Severely confused or agitated patients who may not be able to keep pads in place

METHOD
- May be uncomfortable for the patient, consider sedation with analgesic or anxiolytic
- Anterior-posterior or anterior-lateral pad placement
- Fixed rate pacing: electrical stimulus is delivered at preset intervals
- Synchronous pacing: pacer fires only when no impulse is sensed within a predetermined time

Defibrillation
BASICS
- Defibrillation is nonsynchronized delivery of energy applied usually transcutaneously to cardiac muscle during any phase of cardiac cycle

INDICATIONS
- Pulseless ventricular tachycardia
- Ventricular fibrillation
- Cardiac arrest due to or resulting in ventricular fibrillation

CONTRAINDICATIONS
- Multifocal atrial tachycardia
- Digitalis toxicity or catecholamine-induced arrhythmias

METHOD
- Anterior-posterior or anterior-lateral pad placement
- Manual defibrillator for infants <1 year of age
- Pediatric attenuator pads for children aged 1 to 8
- Due to variability among manufacturers for biphasic waveform shock configurations, use the manufacturer's recommended energy dose for its waveform

Cardioversion

BASICS
- Cardioversion is delivery of energy synchronized to the large R waves or QRS complex

INDICATIONS
- Supraventricular tachycardia
- Atrial fibrillation
- Atrial flutter
- Ventricular tachycardia
- Any unstable patient with reentrant tachycardia with narrow or wide QRS complex

CONTRAINDICATIONS
- Multifocal atrial tachycardia
- Digitalis toxicity or catecholamine-induced arrhythmias
- Ventricular fibrillation

METHOD
- Almost always performed under induction or sedation
- Atrial flutter: initial dose of 50 to 100 J of monophasic or biphasic energy
- Atrial fibrillation: initial dose of 200 J of monophasic or 120 to 200 J biphasic energy
- Monomorphic ventricular tachycardia: initial dose of 100 J of monophasic or biphasic energy, increased in a stepwise fashion

● CHEST TUBE PLACEMENT

BASICS
- Used to remove air or fluid from pleural space

INDICATIONS
- Pneumothorax, hemothorax, pleural effusion, pleurodesis

CONTRAINDICATIONS
- Anticoagulation or coagulopathy if nonemergent; sometimes pleural effusions from liver failure adhesions; need for thoracotomy

PROCEDURE
- Elevate head of bed 30 degrees to minimize possibility of injuring intra-abdominal organs
- Prep, sterilize, and anesthetize the skin with lidocaine

- Incision at the 4th or 5th intercostal space at the anterior axillary or midaxillary line
- Blunt dissection into the pleural space
- Direct 8 to 14 Fr tube posteriorly and superiorly
  - 36 to 40 Fr for tension pneumothorax
  - Direct inferiorly for hemothorax
- Set to suction or water device (usually—20 cm of water)
- Confirm with chest x-ray

● INTRAOSSEOUS ACCESS

BASICS
- Analgesia: can use lidocaine 2% over 1 minute in awake patients
- Administer IV drugs or resuscitation fluid, followed by flushing
- Prolonged intraosseous infusions after 24 hours are associated with increased risk of osteomyelitis
- Can be used for diagnostic studies
- Sites:
  - Proximal tibia (recommended first attempt)
    - Children: 2 cm below tibial tuberosity and up to 1 cm medially on the tibial plateau
    - Adults: 2 cm medial and 1 cm above the tibial tuberosity
  - Distal femur
    - Used as an alternative site in infants and small children
    - Midline, 1 to 2 cm above the superior border of the patella with leg extension
  - Distal tibia or fibula
    - 1 to 2 cm superior to the malleoli in the midline, medial malleoli preferred
  - Proximal humerus
    - Greater tubercle, 2 cm below the acromion process, adduct and internally rotate the upper arm to palpate the tubercle
  - Manubrium
    - Adults, superior one-third of the sternum
- Complications
  - Less than 1% rate of serious complications
  - Tibia fracture
  - Compartment syndrome
  - Skin necrosis
  - Osteomyelitis
  - Subcutaneous abscess
  - Theoretical long-term: bone marrow damage, disturbance of bone growth, fat embolism

INDICATIONS
- Infants, children, or adults in full cardiopulmonary arrest or severe shock without IV access
- It is recommended in all children after two failed attempts of IV access
- Emergent or urgent situations where reliable venous access cannot be achieved quickly

CONTRAINDICATIONS
- Bone fracture or previously penetrated bone (if unsuccessful at first attempt, go to another area or extremity for a second attempt)
- Extremity with vascular interruption from trauma or venous cut down
- If possible, avoid intraosseous in the following patients:
  - At the site of a cellulitis, burn, or osteomyelitis
  - Osteogenesis perfecta or osteopetrosis
  - Right-to-left intracardiac shunts, may increase risk for bone marrow or fat emboli

● LUMBAR PUNCTURE

BASICS
- Sterile procedure to remove cerebrospinal fluid
- Most common complication is a post–lumbar puncture (LP) headache (HA) (10% to 30%)
  - Using a smaller needle is the only proven intervention that decreases the risk of post-LP HA
- Head CT *first* if:
  - Suspect a brain mass
  - One or more of these risk factors
    - Seizure in the last week
    - Altered mental status
    - Papilledema
    - Focal neurologic signs
    - Immunosuppressed
- Position
  - Lateral recumbent (preferred)
  - Upright (this position cannot accurately measure opening pressure)
- Iliac crests align with L4
- 20 to 22 G needle insertion into the subarachnoid space of the interspace of L3 to L4 or L4 to L5
  - Avoid higher vertebral levels to ensure that you stay away from the spinal cord
- 8 to 15 mL cerebrospinal fluid collected, more if sending for cytology or unusual cultures
  - Tube 1 and 4: cell count/diff
  - Tube 2: glucose, protein
  - Tube 3: Gram stain, culture, hold the rest
- See HA/meningitis for LP interpretation

INDICATIONS
- Central nervous system infections
- Subarachnoid hematoma

CONTRAINDICATIONS
- Zero absolute
- Coagulopathy
- Raised ICP
- Spinal epidural abscess

● NASOGASTRIC TUBES

INDICATIONS
- Evacuation and decompression of stomach contents
- Diagnostic aspiration of contents
- Monitoring blood loss in gastrointestinal bleed (GIB)
- Decreasing pulmonary aspiration, treating gastric distention, and delivering meds in intubated patient

CONTRAINDICATIONS
- Facial fracture
- Severe coagulopathy
- Ingestions likely to cause upper GI perforation such as alkaline substances
- Esophageal strictures
- Recent bariatric surgery

TECHNIQUE
■ **Placement:**
- Estimate tube length by measuring from xiphoid process to earlobe to tip of nose and add 15 cm
- Check nare patency
- Anesthetize
  - Lidocaine spray to oropharynx
  - Viscous lidocaine to nares, consider nasal vasoconstrictor to decrease traumatic bleeding
- Lubricate tube, insert into nare along floor close to 90-degree angle to the face, directed parallel to floor of nose
- Advance with gentle pressure and once in the posterior pharynx, ask patient to swallow sips of water to aid tube into esophagus
- Stop and secure at premeasured length

■ **Verifying tube placement:**
- Plain films most sensitive but not standard of care
- Three bedside measures to verify placement:
  - Insufflation of air, causing gurgling sounds over epigastrium
  - Aspiration of gastric fluid pH < 4
  - Normal clear speech without coughing in a conscious patient
- Kidney, ureter, and bladder if any question on placement and always before formula or meds given

■ **Complications:**
- Epistaxis
- Tracheal or bronchial placement
- Pneumothorax
- Intracranial placement
- Esophageal perforation
- Gastric or duodenal rupture
- Esophageal obstruction or rupture
- Pulmonary aspiration

● WOUND MANAGEMENT
Soft Tissue Wounds and Repair

LOCATION TIPS
■ Face: can repair up to 24 hours without serious infection risk (except animal bites), select cases 48 to 72 hours
- 8 to 12 hours for the rest of the body
■ Lip: first suture the vermillion border
■ Muscle/mucous membranes: 4-0 or 5-0 absorbable sutures
■ Facial skin: 6-0 nonabsorbable
■ Primary closure
- Consider if deep and dirty
- If >6 hours and patient is at high risk for infection

SUTURE TYPE
■ Absorbable
- Vicryl or Chromic Gut: single or layered closure of tongue, oral mucosa, or nail bed
- Vicryl or Monocryl: deep facial laceration
■ Nonabsorbable
- Silk: rarely used
- Nylon (Dermalon, Ethilon)

- Polypropylene (Surgilene, Prolene): accommodates swelling
- Polybutester (Novafil): expands with wound edema

SUTURE REMOVAL
- Eye lids: 3 days
- Face: 4 to 6 days
- Scalp: 7 days
- Chest, hand, fingers: 8 to 10 days
- Back, forearm: 10 to 14 days
- Legs: 8 to 12 days
- Foot: 10 to 12 days

ANIMAL/HUMAN BITES
- Irrigation with warm normal saline is the most effective way to decrease bacterial load and remove foreign body material
- Broad-spectrum antibiotics (i.e., Augmentin covers polymicrobial, consider methicillin-resistant *Staphylococcus aureus* coverage)
- If debrided then can close, most cannot be closed primarily

ANESTHESIA
- Two classes of local anesthetics include esters and amines
- Esters:
  - Benzocaine
  - Procaine
  - Tetracaine
  - Cocaine
- Amides:
  - Lidocaine
  - Bupivacaine: longest acting
  - Prilocaine
- When used with epinephrine do not use in fingers, toes, nose, genitals
- Consider buffering with bicarb

NOTES

Other Components—3%

19

Tara Itrich and Audrey Ranieri

● POSTEXPOSURE PROPHYLAXIS

BASICS
- Infectious bodily fluids
  - Blood
  - Cerebrospinal fluid
  - Semen
  - Vaginal fluid
  - Amniotic fluid
  - Pericardial, peritoneal, pleural, synovial fluids
- Noninfectious bodily fluids (unless contaminated with blood)
  - Tears, saliva, sweat, feces, vomitus, urine

MODE OF TRANSMISSION
- Percutaneous
- Cutaneous
- Mucous membrane

MANAGEMENT
- Immediate decontamination with soap and water or irrigation
- Source person: voluntary testing for HIV Ab, hepatitis C virus (HCV) Ab, HBsAg
  - If HIV positive, obtain disease stage
- Exposed person: baseline labs including HIV Ab, HCV Ab, hepatitis B virus (HBV) surface Ag, HBV surface Ab
  - If postexposure prophylaxis (PEP), consider
    - Pregnancy test for childbearing age females
    - Complete blood count, blood urea nitrogen, Cr, alanine amino transferase
- **If indicated, PEP starts ASAP (≤72 hours after exposure)**

TREATMENT
- Preferred HIV three-drug PEP regimen × 28 days:
  - Raltegravir (Isentress) 400 mg po twice daily plus
  - Truvada (tenofovir disoproxil fumarate 300 mg per emtricitabine 200 mg) 1 po once daily
- HBV: begin hepatitis B immune globulin series if not previously vaccinated
- HCV: no PEP recommended, follow ALT

VACCINATIONS (TABLES 19.1 AND 19.2)

TABLE 19.1. **Vaccination Guidelines: Adult**						
	19–21	22–26	27–49	50–59	60–64	65+
Influenza	Annually					
Td/Tdap	Every 10 y with one time substitution Tdap					
Varicella	2 doses					
HPV female	3 doses					
HPV male	3 doses					
Zoster					1 dose	
MMR	1 or 2 doses					
PPSV23	1 or 2 doses[a]					1 dose
PCV13	1 dose[b]					
Meningococcal	1 or more doses[c]					
Hepatitis A	2 doses (in at-risk patients)					
Hepatitis B	3 doses (HCWs and at-risk patients)					

[a]Under 65 with chronic illness, reside in nursing home, smokers.
[b]Over age 19 with immunocompromise.
[c]Asplenia, complement deficiency, military recruits, college students living in dormitories.
HPV, human papillomavirus; MMR, measles, mumps, and rubella; PPSV, pneumococcal polysaccharide vaccine; PCV, pneumococcal conjugate vaccine; HCW, health care workers.

TABLE 19.2. **Vaccination Guidelines: Children**	
Vaccination	**Age Recommended**
Hepatitis B	3 doses (birth, 1–2 mo, 6–18 mo)
Rotavirus	2–3 doses between 2 and 6 mo
DTaP (<7 y)	3 doses 2–6 mo, 4th dose 15–18 mo, 5th dose 4–6 y
Tdap (>7 y)	1 dose 11–12 y
Haemophilus influenza type b (Hib)	2 doses 2–4 mo, 3rd dose 12–15 mo
PCV 13	3 doses 2–6 mo, 4th dose 12–15 mo
PCV 23	For high-risk kids over age 2 y
Inactivated poliovirus	2 doses 2–4 mo, 3rd dose 6–18 mo, 4th dose 4–6 y
Influenza	Annual starting at 6 mo
MMR	1st dose 12–15 mo, 2nd dose 4–6 y
Varicella	1st dose 12–15 mo, 2nd dose 4–6 y
Hepatitis A	2 doses between 1 and 2 y
HPV	3 doses between 11 and 12 y
Meningococcal	1st dose 11–12 y., booster age 16

HPV, human papillomavirus; MMR, measles, mumps, and rubella; PCV, pneumococcal conjugate vaccine.

NOTES

NOTES

Questions and Answers

20

1. A 72-year-old female presents to the emergency department (ED) with 4 hours of substernal crushing chest pain, that radiates to the back. She reports associated shortness of breath, diaphoresis, and nausea. After getting a thorough history, you realize that her medical history includes hypertension, hyperlipidemia, coronary artery disease with percutaneous coronary intervention, and tobacco use. In the ED an EKG is performed, showing significant ST elevation in EKG leads II, III, and aVF. You act quickly and page the on-call cardiologist and activate the cath lab. While waiting for the cardiology team, you realize that the most likely location of her MI is:

    A. Anterior wall
    B. Lateral wall
    C. Inferior wall
    D. Posterior wall

Correct Answer C: *Inferior wall*. Acute inferior wall MI will likely show ST elevation in leads II, III, and aVF. This tells us that the blood vessels geographically located on the inferior part of the myocardium likely are affected. An acute anterior wall MI will show ST elevation in the precordial leads (V1 to V6), whereas a lateral wall MI will have ST elevation in leads I and aVL. A posterior wall MI will be represented by ST depression in the precordial leads (mainly V1 to V4) and may coincide with an inferior wall MI due to the closely shared blood supply in these locations.

2. A 52-year-old male with a medical history significant for coronary artery disease, hypertension, hyperlipidemia, and diabetes mellitus type II presents to the emergency department with left arm paresthesias, mild back pain, and some dull left-sided chest pain. His 12-lead EKG shows ST elevation in his precordial leads. You quickly realize that reperfusion is crucial for this patient. What are the recommended guidelines for door-to-balloon time from the time the patient enters the emergency room (ER) and receives first medical contact to when he should undergo catheterization?

    A. <30 minutes
    B. <60 minutes
    C. <90 minutes
    D. <120 minutes

Correct Answer C: *<90 minutes*. ACCF/AHA guidelines recommend that patients with acute ST elevation myocardial infarction door-to-balloon time be no >90 minutes from the first contact upon arrival to the ER. Patients who are unable to receive percutaneous coronary intervention can receive fibrinolytic therapy if no contraindication. Guidelines recommend that if fibrinolytic therapy is the choice for reperfusion it should be done in no >30 minutes.

3. A 38-year-old African American female, with no reported significant medical history, presents to the emergency department (ED) with shortness of breath (SOB), which has been worsening over the past 2 days. She has associated pleurisy, cough, and very poor po intake. This morning she believes she saw blood-tinged sputum in a napkin she coughed into. After obtaining a thorough history, you realize that she has recently returned from a business trip to Japan 3 days prior. The only medications she uses are birth control and Advil prn. Her vitals are significant for temp, 98.6°F; HR, 108; BP, 132/80; RR, 24; and O_2 sat, 91% on RA. Laboratory studies are significant for white blood cell of 11.2, Cr of 2.3, blood urea nitrogen of 64, and D-dimer of 660. Based on this information, which is the most appropriate diagnostic test that could help to figure out what is going on?

A. V/Q perfusion scan
B. Chest CT angiography
C. Chest x-ray
D. EKG

Correct Answer A: *V/Q perfusion scan.* Based on the provided information, this patient likely has a pulmonary embolism. She is tachycardic and tachypneic, with reported SOB and hemoptysis. She also recently has had prolonged stasis on a trip and is on birth control pills. Her D-dimer is high on initial labs. The best and most sensitive test would be a CTA of the chest to diagnose pulmonary embolism (PE), but with her renal insufficiency, it is contraindicated. A chest x-ray may be helpful to show sequelae of PE, but is nondiagnostic. An x-ray may show atelectasis, cardiomegaly, Hampton's hump, Westermark's sign, or possibly effusion. An EKG also would not be diagnostic for PE, and some of the findings that could be present on an EKG with pulmonary emboli can also be present in patients who do not have a PE. If a massive PE is present, it is possible patients may have S1Q3T3 pattern and possibly right ventricular strain or new incomplete right bundle branch block. The most appropriate choice for the diagnosis of PE in this particular patient is a V/Q perfusion scan to check for ventilation mismatch. If the V/Q scan is negative, there is a low probability that this is an acute PE.

4. A 45-year-old obese male presents to the emergency department (ED) with generalized chest pain, fatigue, and shortness of breath. He has been unable to sleep over the past 2 days since the pain started. He reports the only thing that mildly helps to alleviate the pain is sitting up and leaning forward. When he lies down flat or takes a deep breath, he reports that the pain is intensified. After obtaining a thorough history, you realize that he recently had a Non-ST elevation myocardial infarction 2 weeks prior and had a drug-eluting stent placed to his left anterior descending artery. On exam you note him to have a pericardial friction rub and lungs clear throughout. He is tachycardic on admission, but afebrile. Laboratory studies are significant for white blood cell count of, 13.1; erythrocyte sedimentation rate, 52; troponin; and B-type natriuretic peptide (BNP) normal. Chest x-ray is unremarkable. EKG demonstrates diffuse ST elevation throughout all leads. Based on your findings, the most likely diagnosis is:

A. ST elevation myocardial infarction
B. Acute congestive heart failure (CHF)
C. Myocarditis
D. Dressler's syndrome

Correct Answer D: *Dressler's syndrome.* This patient recently had a myocardial infarction with stent placement a few weeks prior to these symptoms. He presents back to the ED with chest discomfort, which is improved with sitting forward. This finding is common in patients with pericarditis, or Dressler's syndrome (pericarditis following a myocardial infarction [MI]). Other key findings include pericardial friction rub and diffuse ST elevation on EKG. These patients may have nonspecific findings as well, including low-grade fever, leukocytosis, and elevated inflammatory markers. Even though there is ST elevation on the EKG, when the elevations are seen throughout.

Diffuse ST elevations on EKG are consistent with pericarditis. No clinical findings support CHF (lungs clear, x-ray normal, BNP normal). This is unlikely myocarditis even though it can present with similar chest pain symptoms such as pericarditis. Myocarditis is also generally associated with troponin elevation. EKG findings may show nonspecific ST-T wave changes, but with myocarditis, there usually is no diffuse ST elevation.

5. A 74-year-old female is seen in the emergency department for weakness, which has been ongoing for about a week. She denies chest pain, palpitations, or shortness of breath. Medical history includes hypertension, diabetes mellitus type II, and history of rheumatic heart disease. She also reports that her primary care physician told her she has an "abnormal heart exam." Upon auscultation of her heart, you hear a high-pitched systolic murmur that is best heard at the apex of the heart. Based on these findings, which is the most likely type of murmur present?

   A. Mitral stenosis
   B. Mitral regurgitation
   C. Aortic stenosis
   D. Aortic insufficiency

Correct Answer B: _Mitral regurgitation._ Rheumatic heart disease can affect all valves of the heart, but most commonly affects the mitral valve. Mitral regurgitation is a high-pitched, blowing, holo-systolic murmur heard best at the apex. Mitral stenosis is a low-pitched, mid-diastolic rumble murmur heard best at the apex. Aortic stenosis is a midsystolic, crescendo-decrescendo murmur heard best at right upper sternal border. Aortic stenosis also usually is harsh, high-pitched, and radiates to the carotids. Aortic insufficiency is an early diastolic decrescendo murmur heard best at left upper sternal border.

6. A 74-year-old male with a medical history of colon cancer, status post bowel resection, hypertension, hyperlipidemia, and Parkinson's disease presents to the emergency department with 2 days of right lower extremity swelling, erythema, and tenderness. On admission his vital signs are stable. A lower extremity ultrasound of the right leg is performed and shows a new deep venous thrombosis. Which of the following is not part of Virchow's triad?

   A. Venous stasis
   B. Vessel wall injury
   C. Malignancy
   D. Hypercoagulable state

Correct Answer C: _Malignancy._ Virchow's triad describes the three broad categories of factors thought to contribute to thrombosis. These factors are hypercoagulability, hemodynamic changes (stasis), and endothelial injury/dysfunction. Although malignancy is a risk factor for thrombosis, it is not part of this triad.

7. A 67-year-old female is brought to the emergency department after a car accident. She was the unrestrained driver, and emergency medical services report that she hit a telephone pole and her airbag did not deploy. On admission she reports chest pain and shortness of breath, and she appears to be in significant distress. Vital signs: temp, 98.9°F; HR, 106; BP, 86/54; RR, 26; and O_2 sat 92% on RA. You do note that with inspiration there is a 14-mm Hg drop in systolic pressure. Exam is notable for distant heart sounds and faint crackles at the lung bases. Based on this information, what is the gold standard for treatment?

   A. Admit to hospital with urgent cardiology evaluation
   B. Nonsteroidal anti-inflammatory drugs, colchicine, and supportive care with pain medication
   C. Cardiac catheterization
   D. Pericardiocentesis

Correct Answer D: *Pericardiocentesis.* This is the mainstay of treatment for cardiac tamponade. This patient will likely need hospital admission and cardiology evaluation, but this is not the mainstay of treatment. Supportive care should be used during the hospital stay for pain control. Cardiac catheterization will have no benefit since there is no vessel occlusion with tamponade, although this is often carried out in the cardiac catheterization laboratory.

8. A 58-year-old male reports to the emergency department with chest pain and shortness of breath. While obtaining a history, he reports to you that in the past he had open heart surgery complicated by cardiac tamponade. Which is not part of Beck's triad?

   A. Pulsus paradoxus
   B. Muffled heart sounds
   C. Distended neck veins
   D. Hypotension

Correct Answer A: *Pulsus paradoxus.* Beck's triad is associated with cardiac tamponade, an emergent condition in which fluid accumulates around the heart. It is classified by hypotension, distended neck veins, and muffled heart sounds. Pulsus paradoxus is an abnormally large decrease in systolic blood pressure and pulse wave amplitude during inspiration. Even though this can be found with cardiac tamponade, it is not part of Beck's triad. Pulsus paradoxus can also be found with pericarditis and obstructive lung disease.

9. A 58-year-old male with a medical history significant for hypertension and hyperlipidemia presents to the emergency department with acute onset of severe chest and back pain. He reports that the pain is sharp and "takes his breath away." He reports feeling like he is being ripped open and is unable to tolerate the pain. On exam he appears ill and in severe distress. Vital signs are significant for BP of 84/62 and HR of 112. Based on your initial findings and workup, what would be the most appropriate imaging study to diagnose this potentially life-threatening disorder?

   A. Chest CT with contrast
   B. Transesophageal echocardiogram (TEE)
   C. Coronary angiography
   D. Thoracic MRI

Correct Answer B: *Transesophageal echocardiogram (TEE).* Based on initial workup, he likely has an unstable aortic dissection. All of these studies are very sensitive for detection of aortic dissection, but the TEE is the test of choice for any unstable patient and it can be done at bedside.

10. A 64-year-old male, with a known history of hypertension and medical noncompliance, presents to the emergency department with gradual onset of visual changes associated with dizziness and headache. He has not taken any of his home antihypertensives for over a month due to reported financial issues. On admission BP is 188/96 and HR is 85. On fundoscopic exam, which is *not* a finding associated with hypertensive retinopathy?

   A. Copper/silver wiring
   B. Cotton wool spots
   C. Cherry-red spot in macula
   D. Papilledema

Correct Answer C: *Cherry-red spot in macula.* A cherry-red spot found in the macula is not associated with hypertensive retinopathy but rather with central retinal vein occlusion. Copper/silver wiring is found in grade I hypertensive retinopathy, cotton wool spots in grade III, and papilledema in grade IV. Urgent evaluation by an ophthalmologist should occur.

11. A 70-year-old female presents to the emergency department (ED) with back pain for 2 days. She has a medical history significant for hypertension (HTN) and tobacco use. In the ED she is tachycardic, but BP is stable. She appears in acute distress, and on exam, you note a palpable mass in the abdomen. A bedside ultrasound is being ordered, and you are concerned for an aneurysm. Which of the following is not a risk factor for abdominal aortic aneurysm (AAA)?

   A. Diabetes
   B. HTN
   C. Tobacco use
   D. Hyperlipidemia

Correct Answer A: *Diabetes*. The risk factors for AAA include smoking (past or current), advancing age, male gender, HTN, hyperlipidemia, atherosclerosis, Caucasian race, family history AAA, or other large artery aneurysm. A decreased risk of AAA is associated with the female gender, diabetes mellitus type II, and non-Caucasian race.

12. A 32-year-old male with a medical history significant for intravenous drug use (IVDU) presents to the emergency department with continued fevers and chills at home for the past 3 days. His last IVDU was 5 days prior, and he uses IV heroin about one to two times per week. Vitals show the following: temp, 101.4°F; HR, 92; and BP, 138/90. On exam you note a murmur heard along the left sternal border. Patient reports he has never been told he has a murmur before. You also note petechiae in his lower extremities as well as raised, red, and tender nodules on his hands. He reports these are also new. Based on your clinical judgment, you are highly concerned for infective endocarditis. He does not have any prosthetic valves, and you order a stat echocardiogram to evaluate for vegetation. You start him on empiric antibiotic therapy with IV vancomycin and gentamicin. What is the most likely organism?

   A. *Streptococcus viridans*
   B. *Enterococcus*
   C. *Staphylococcus aureus*
   D. *Staphylococcus epidermidis*

Correct Answer C: *Staphylococcus aureus*. All of the options listed above are potential organisms found in infective endocarditis. The most common organism associated with IVDU native valve endocarditis is *Staphylococcus aureus* (about 68%). In IV drug users, the tricuspid valve is most commonly affected. If this were a non-IV drug user, the most common organism would be *Streptococcus viridans* (about 35%). In non-IV drug user, native valve endocarditis, the most commonly affected valve, is the aortic valve.

13. A 74-year-old female with a history significant for cerebrovascular accident (CVA), hypertension (HTN), and diabetes mellitus (DM) type II presents to the emergency department with acute onset of palpitations. She has experienced similar symptoms a few times over the past few years, but never to this extent. On admission she is tachycardic, with heart rate in the 120s. EKG demonstrates atrial fibrillation with rapid ventricular response. Patient reports that this is a new diagnosis for her. She is curious about the options for treatment. You order a dose of IV diltiazem for rate control, and you discuss anticoagulation with her. Based on the information, what is her CHADS2 score?

   A. 3
   B. 4
   C. 5
   D. 6

Correct Answer B: 4. Based on the provided information, the CHADS2 score is 4. Based on the criteria, 1 point is given for HTN, 1 point for DM, 1 point for age ≥75, 1 point for congestive heart failure, and 2 points for history of transient ischemic attack/CVA/thromboembolism. Guidelines recommend anticoagulation if CHADS2 score is 2 or more unless anticoagulation contraindicated.

14. A 60-year-old male with a history of amyloidosis presents to the emergency department with lower extremity swelling and shortness of breath. His primary care physician told him that he has a "cardiomyopathy," but he is unclear exactly what this is. On exam you note he has bilateral lower extremity swelling, crackles in his lung bases, and Kussmaul sign noted on exam. What is the most likely type of cardiomyopathy?
    A. Nonischemic hypertrophic cardiomyopathy
    B. Ischemic hypertrophic cardiomyopathy
    C. Dilated cardiomyopathy
    D. Restrictive cardiomyopathy

Correct Answer D: *Restrictive cardiomyopathy.* Rigid heart walls that restrict the heart from stretching and filling with blood properly classify this form of cardiomyopathy. Amyloidosis is one of the most common causes of this type of cardiomyopathy. This can easily be confused with constrictive pericarditis, in which Kussmaul sign is also noted (paradoxical rise in jugular venous pressure on inspiration). In amyloidosis clumps of protein build up in body tissues, and over time these proteins replace normal tissue, leading to organ failure. In the heart, this can cause electrical and conduction issues, as well as restrictive cardiomyopathy.

15. A 58-year-old male with a medical history significant for congestive heart failure (CHF), hypertension, and hyperlipidemia presents to the emergency department with shortness of breath (SOB). He reports he cannot lie flat due to difficulty breathing. He also reports waking up frequently at night with SOB and he needs to sleep upright in a recliner. On admission he appears in mild respiratory distress. Chest x-ray shows bilateral pleural effusions with Kerley B lines. Cardiac exam reveals a harsh systolic murmur in the right upper sternal border and he does have lower leg edema. Which of the following medications does not reduce the mortality for CHF?
    A. Lisinopril
    B. Metoprolol
    C. Spironolactone
    D. Lasix

Correct Answer D: *Lasix.* Lasix is a loop diuretic which most, if not all, patients with CHF take in acute CHF exacerbations as well as chronically. It is used for symptomatic management but has not proven to decrease mortality. Ace inhibitors, β-blockers, and aldosterone antagonists have shown to decrease overall mortality. Lisinopril will decrease afterload overall, reducing the amount of work the heart has to do. Metoprolol will improve left ventricular function and in the long run also decrease the amount of work the heart has to perform.

16. A 48-year-old female, with no significant medical history, presents to the emergency department complaining of a week of dizziness and fatigue. On admission heart rate is low at 50. Chest x-ray is unremarkable; EKG shows a progressive prolongation of the PR interval on consecutive beats followed by a dropped QRS. After the dropped QRS, the PR interval resets and the cycle repeats. Based on the EKG, which type of heart block is this?
    A. First-degree atrioventricular (AV) block
    B. Second-degree AV block type I
    C. Second-degree AV block type II
    D. Third-degree AV block

Correct Answer B: *Second-degree AV block type I (Mobitz 1, aka Wenckebach).* With a first-degree AV block, the PR interval is constantly prolonged (>0.20 seconds) but every QRS is conducted. In second-degree AV block type II (Mobitz 2, aka Hay), the PR interval remains unchanged prior to the P, which suddenly fails to conduct to the ventricles. Third-degree AV block is complete dissociation between P waves and QRS complexes. Both third-degree block and second-degree block type II will likely need pacemaker placement.

17. A 35-year-old male with a past medical history significant for Marfan syndrome presents to the emergency department after a car accident with acute onset of severe chest and back pain. On admission his BP is 156/94 and HR is 76. Chest CTA demonstrates an acute aortic dissection. Which medication should be given first for blood pressure control?

    A. IV labetalol
    B. IV sodium nitroprusside
    C. IV hydralazine
    D. IV nicardipine

Correct Answer A: *IV labetalol.* With acute aortic dissection without shock, a β-blocker is used initially to decrease cardiac contractility and to prevent reflex tachycardia. By reducing shear force, it will help to prevent further damage. Reflex tachycardia will increase pressure and worsen the dissection if not prevented/controlled. The goal is to reduce the heart rate to about 60 beats per minute (or lowest tolerated by patient), and the BP should be reduced to mean arterial pressure of 60 or systolic BP of 100 to 120 (or the lowest tolerated by the patient). Sodium nitroprusside is an effective vasodilator with a short half-life and should be used after initial meds to decrease heart rate. Ca channel blockers can be used to decrease systolic BP and contractility in patients that β-blockade is contraindicated (not first-line therapy). Hydralazine is used for BP reduction, but is not a medication used commonly with aortic dissection.

18. A 68-year-old male who presents with chest pain is found to have a ST elevation myocardial infarction (STEMI) in the precordial leads. Unfortunately your hospital does not have reperfusion available. You discuss the different treatment options with the patient and his family and they agree to fibrinolysis. The patient is also in the appropriate time frame to receive the medication. Which of the following is not an absolute contraindication to receiving fibrinolysis?

    A. Intracranial hemorrhage 9 months prior
    B. Ischemic stroke 5 months prior
    C. Active gastrointestinal bleed
    D. Suspected aortic dissection

Correct Answer B: *Ischemic stroke 5 months prior.* The absolute contraindications to receiving fibrinolysis therapy for STEMI include any prior intracranial hemorrhage, intracranial neoplasm/arteriovenous malformation/aneurysm, nonhemorrhagic stroke or closed head trauma within 3 months, active internal bleeding or known bleeding diathesis, or suspected aortic dissection. The relative contraindications include history of severe hypertension, ischemic stroke over 3 months, prolonged cardiopulmonary resuscitation, trauma/major surgery within 3 weeks, recent internal bleed/active peptic ulcer disease, noncompressible vascular punctures, pregnancy, or current use of anticoagulants.

19. A 36-year-old male presents with "flu-like symptoms" and is found to be febrile on admission with a temperature of 101.1. EKG shows sinus tachycardia with nonspecific changes; biomarkers are elevated. After further workup, the patient is diagnosed with myocarditis and

admitted to the hospital for treatment with supportive care. What is the most common cause of myocarditis?

- **A.** Idiopathic
- **B.** Chemotherapy
- **C.** Connective tissue disease
- **D.** Infectious

Correct Answer D: *Infectious.* Myocarditis is an inflammation of the myocardium and commonly is associated with pericarditis. Even though all the choices are causes for myocarditis, the most common cause is viral infection (particularly coxsackie B virus). The treatment for myocarditis typically is supportive care.

20. A 62-year-old female presents to the emergency department for worsening leg swelling. On exam you note she has pitting edema in her lower legs. She also has mild right upper quadrant pain and jugular venous distention (JVD). EKG is unremarkable; chest x-ray shows cardiomegaly; B-type natriuretic peptide is elevated. What is the most common cause of right-sided heart failure?

- **A.** Left-sided heart failure
- **B.** Left-to-right shunt
- **C.** Pulmonary embolism
- **D.** Coronary artery disease

Correct Answer A: *Left-sided heart failure.* When the left ventricle fails, increased fluid pressure is transferred back through the lungs, ultimately damaging the heart's right side. With a left-to-right shunt, the right ventricle (RV) eventually becomes volume overloaded. With pulmonary emboli and chronic lung disease, high blood pressure in the pulmonary arteries will cause RV failure, and with coronary artery disease, if there is a right-sided infarct, the right ventricle will fail and cause blood to back up into the systemic system.

21. A 58-year-old male with a history of coronary artery disease, hypertension, hyperlipidemia, diabetes mellitus type II, and tobacco use presents to the emergency department with left arm paresthesias, numbness, and dull left-sided chest pain. He also reports dyspnea on exertion, nausea, and diaphoresis. On admission his vitals are stable. EKG shows new ST elevation in V1 to V6. Based on the type of myocardial infarction (MI), which coronary artery likely is blocked?

- **A.** Right coronary artery
- **B.** Left anterior descending artery
- **C.** Right circumflex artery
- **D.** Left circumflex artery

Correct Answer B: *Left anterior descending artery.* With ST elevation in V1 to V6, this would represent an anterior wall MI. Based on the anatomical location of the heart, this would correlate with the left anterior descending artery (LAD). The LAD is a branch off the left main coronary artery. The LAD supplies the anterior and inferior portions of the heart and thus would be the affected vessel in an anterior wall MI. The left circumflex artery (LCX) is also a branch of the left main coronary artery. The LCX supplies blood to the left atrium and lateral/posterior portions of the left ventricle. It will be affected most commonly in a lateral wall MI. The right coronary artery (RCA) supplies blood to the right atrium, right ventricle, and the bottom portion of both ventricles and the back of the septum. The RCA most commonly is affected in inferior wall MI or right ventricular MI.

22. A 46-year-old male presents to the emergency department (ED) with palpitations and fatigue. In the ED his HR is elevated to the 160s. 12-lead EKG demonstrates narrow-complex supraventricular tachycardia. Since vital signs are stable, you attempt vagal maneuvers that are unsuccessful. Which is the first medication that should be administered?

    A. Adenosine 12 mg
    B. Adenosine 6 mg
    C. Atropine 0.5 mg
    D. Epinephrine 1 mg

Correct Answer B: *Adenosine 6 mg.* This patient has a stable tachyarrhythmia on admission. He is found to have a narrow-complex tachyarrhythmia, and since vagal maneuvers are unsuccessful, medical therapy should be used to break the arrhythmia. If this patient were unstable then cardioversion should be performed immediately. The first dose of adenosine is 6 mg, and if this is unsuccessful, the second dose is 12 mg. Atropine is used for bradyarrhythmias, and epinephrine is used in cardiac arrest.

23. A 58-year-old female is brought to the emergency department by her husband complaining of palpitations. On admission to the ED her HR is 146 and BP is 80/54. She starts to report chest discomfort on admission, and she appears fatigued and clammy. You immediately hook her up to a cardiac monitor, administer O$_2$, and obtain IV access. 12-lead EKG shows atrial fibrillation with rapid ventricular response. What is the initial treatment of choice?

    A. Synchronized cardioversion
    B. IV diltiazem
    C. IV labetalol
    D. Vagal maneuvers

Correct Answer A: *Synchronized cardioversion.* This is indicated for treatment of unstable supraventricular tachycardia, unstable atrial fibrillation, and unstable atrial flutter. Since this patient is hypotensive with chest discomfort, she is considered unstable and needs cardioversion. Both IV diltiazem and labetalol can be used for rate control in atrial fibrillation once stable. Vagal maneuvers should be attempted in stable wide QRS tachyarrhythmias only.

24. A 28-year-old male presents to the emergency department with dyspnea. He reports he recently had an echocardiogram as an outpatient and was diagnosed with hypertrophic cardiomyopathy. What type of murmur would you expect to hear on exam?

    A. Diastolic murmur that increases in intensity with Valsalva and standing
    B. Systolic murmur that increases in intensity with Valsalva and standing
    C. Diastolic murmur that decreases in intensity with Valsalva and standing
    D. Systolic murmur that decreases in intensity with Valsalva and standing

Correct Answer B: *Systolic murmur that increases in intensity with Valsalva and standing.* Hypertrophic cardiomyopathy (HOCM) is a disease resulting in abnormal myocardium thickening commonly in the interventricular septum. This is a concerning cardiomyopathy since it can result in sudden cardiac death. HOCM is also an autosomal dominant genetic disorder. On exam the murmur is a high-pitched, crescendo-decrescendo, systolic murmur heard best at left lower sternal border. This murmur does not radiate to the carotids (unlikely aortic stenosis). The murmur with HOCM becomes more intense with Valsalva and standing. These maneuvers decrease left ventricular filling, resulting in worsened left ventricular outflow tract obstruction since the septum is thickened making the murmur louder. With aortic stenosis, the murmur becomes softer with these positions since less blood is being ejected through the aortic valve.

25. A 57-year-old male presents to the emergency department after being sent from his primary care physician for uncontrolled hypertension (HTN). He reports a history of HTN but he has been noncompliant with his home antihypertensive medications. His BP is elevated on initial vitals. Which of the following represents hypertensive urgency?

    A. BP of 210/112 with papilledema
    B. BP of 168/122 with headache
    C. BP of 190/86 with acute renal failure
    D. Pregnant female with BP of 150/86

Correct Answer B: *BP of 168/122 with headache.* Hypertensive crises can present as hypertensive urgency or emergency. Hypertensive urgency is a condition defined by elevated BP (≥180 systolic and/or ≥110 diastolic), without evidence of end-organ damage. The patient may experience minor symptoms, including headache, shortness of breath, or anxiety. Hypertensive emergency is a condition marked by elevated BP with evidence of end-organ damage. This includes stroke, change in mental status, myocardial infarction, acute renal failure, aortic dissection, angina, pulmonary edema, or eclampsia. For hypertensive urgency, treatment should be to decrease BP over hours with oral meds if possible (target to normalize BP in 1 to 2 days). When there is concern for hypertensive emergency, treatment should aim to decrease mean arterial pressure by about 25% in minutes to 2 hours with IV antihypertensives.

26. A 10-year-old male presents to the emergency department with his mother with lethargy, fever, nausea, and proptosis. His mother reports that for the past 5 days he has been complaining of nasal drainage and congestion, but no reports of cough for sore throat. On exam the patient is lethargic and febrile to 101°F. Head, eyes, ears, nose, and throat exam is significant for no sinus tenderness, nonerythematous tonsils without exudate. What is the likely cause?

    A. Acute sinusitis
    B. Cavernous sinus thrombosis (CVT)
    C. Meningitis
    D. Urinary tract infection (UTI)

Correct Answer B: *Cavernous sinus thrombosis (CVT).* CVT usually accompanies an untreated odontogenic or sinus infection sources. Acute sinusitis may have been the predisposing infection; however, it does not cause cranial nerve deficits. With fever and neurologic deficits on exam, meningitis is a likely answer; however, with the known history, it is lower on the differential. UTI, though part of the workup in a febrile pediatric patient, does not present with the following symptoms, history, or exam findings.

27. A 25-year-old female presents to the ED complaining of a sore throat, difficulty swallowing, and fever. She was recently seen in an urgent care 2 days ago and diagnosed with *Streptococcus pharyngitis* and started on a course of penicillin, but reports no improvement in her symptoms. She reports taking ibuprofen 600 mg 1 hour prior to presentation. On exam her Vital signs: temp, 99.0°F; HR, 90; BP; 110/50; RR, 20; and O$_2$ sat 99% on RA. She looks ill, but not toxic appearing. Throat exam reveals normal-appearing tonsils without erythema or exudate. What is the next likely course of action to be taken?

    A. Continue course of antibiotics and follow-up with her primary care physician in 3 days
    B. Send a throat culture
    C. Order a CT scan of the neck
    D. Admit the patient for IV antibiotics

Correct Answer C: *Order a CT scan of the neck.* This is done to assess for a retropharyngeal abscess. The index of suspicion should be high as a patient with a retropharyngeal abscess may have a normal physical exam. The patient usually has improvement 24 hours after the start of antibiotic therapy. Even so, with worsening symptoms, the differential should be broadened for other causes. A throat culture may have been appropriate during the initial urgent care visit, but would not be the next step on this ED visit, as management would not be altered. Admission with IV antibiotics and ENT consult for I+D in the operating room is the ultimate disposition of the patient, and is not the next likely step in this patient's workup.

28. What is the antibiotic of choice for the treatment of *Streptococcus pharyngitis* in an adult patient who is allergic to penicillin and macrolide antibiotics?
    A. Clindamycin
    B. Ciprofloxacin
    C. Cefadroxil
    D. Erythromycin

Correct Answer C: *Cefadroxil.* For a patient who is penicillin allergic, the current recommendations would be to start a macrolide antibiotic, such as erythromycin or azithromycin. In a patient who is both penicillin and macrolide allergic, the next antibiotic of choice is a first-generation cephalosporin.

29. A 65-year-old male presents to the emergency department complaining of sudden onset of right eye pain. He reports decreased vision, photophobia, and pain. The patient has had bilateral cataract surgeries and has since had fixed pupils on exam. When concerned for an acute ophthalmologic emergency, what is the next exam test that should be performed?
    A. Visual acuity
    B. Slit lamp exam
    C. Measurement of intraocular pressure
    D. Fluorescence staining

Correct Answer C: *Measurement of intraocular pressure.* The most concerning diagnosis for this patient's symptoms would be acute narrow-angle glaucoma, and as such, measurement of intraocular pressure would be the next test that should be performed. A slit lamp exam should be done to assess for cells in the anterior chamber in uveitis, which may lead to glaucoma, but in acute narrow-angle glaucoma, delay of treatment may result in complete vision loss. The patient did not have any history of trauma to suspect a corneal abrasion. A visual acuity should be done on all patients presenting with an eye complaint.

30. A 28-year-old female presents after being struck in the left eye with a baseball. Exam is notable for normal visual acuity, periorbital ecchymosis, and blood in the anterior chamber. You diagnose her with a hyphema. What is the most appropriate treatment?
    A. Warm compresses to the affected eye
    B. Nonsteroidal anti-inflammatory drugs (NSAIDs) to reduce inflammation and to treat pain
    C. Rest with the head of the bed elevated
    D. No further treatment recommended

Correct Answer C: *Rest with head of bed elevated.* Most cases of hyphemas resolve on their own, but current recommendations are to rest with the head of the bed elevated. Warm compresses are not contraindicated, but are not the most appropriate treatment. NSAIDs should be avoided to prevent prolonged bleeding.

31. An 18-year-old male presents to the emergency department complaining of pain and redness in the left eye, which started when he woke up. He has no history of any sexually transmitted diseases. The patient admits to regularly wearing his soft contact lens while sleeping. Slit lamp examination reveals significant conjunctival injection and discharge. Fluorescein

staining shows a large oval defect in the central cornea with an underlying white haze. What is the most likely diagnosis?

A. Herpes simplex keratitis
B. Corneal abrasion
C. Corneal ulcer
D. Conjunctivitis

Correct Answer C: *Corneal ulcer.* The findings on the slit lamp exam, combined with his history of contact lens use, prove this diagnosis, which is an ophthalmic emergency. Herpes simplex keratitis will show dendritic lesions on slit lamp. Corneal abrasion is a very superficial injury seen on slip lamp. Conjunctivitis can have a red, irritated eye, but it is usually associated with drainage and without defects seen on slit lamp exam.

32. A patient presents complaining of progressive left ear hearing loss. On exam there is impacted cerumen in the affected ear. What other physical exam findings would you have in determining conductive hearing loss?

    A. On the Weber test, sound lateralizes to the unaffected ear and sound is heard longer through the bone than through air.
    B. On the Rinne test, sound is heard longer on the bone than through air to the affected ear and sound does not lateralize.
    C. On the Rinne test, sound is heard longer through the bone than through air to the affected ear and sound lateralizes to the affected ear.
    D. On the Weber test, sound lateralizes to the affected ear and sound is heard longer through air than through bone.

Correct Answer D: *On the Weber test, sound lateralizes to the affected ear and sound is heard longer through air than through bone.* In conductive hearing loss, the sound lateralizes to the affected ear on the Weber test and sound is heard longer through the bone than through air on the Rinne test. In sensorineural hearing loss, the sound lateralizes to the unaffected ear on the Weber test and sound is heard longer through air than through bone.

33. A 68-year-old male presents complaining of right eyelid swelling and redness. He denies any fevers, changes in vision, and only minimal irritation. On exam there is erythema and swelling to his upper right eyelid with normal conjunctivae. What is the most appropriate next step?

    A. Discharge the patient home advising warm compresses and frequent washing
    B. Start the patient on oral antibiotics
    C. Order a CT scan
    D. Consult an ophthalmologist

Correct Answer A: *Discharge the patient home advising warm compresses and frequent washing.* The patient likely has blepharitis, which can be managed with proper eyelid hygiene. Oral antibiotics can be used, but generally blepharitis resolves without antibiotic use. If an antibiotic were to be used, a topical antibiotic would be the initial choice. Oral antibiotics are indicated with early periorbital cellulitis; however, there were no physical exam findings consistent with that diagnosis. CT imaging would be necessary if concerned for orbital cellulitis as well as consulting ophthalmology, but in a patient presenting with isolated eyelid erythema and edema, without concerning exam findings, blepharitis is the likely diagnosis.

34. In a person diagnosed with whooping cough, at what stage are they infectious?

    A. Incubation stage
    B. Catarrhal stage
    C. Paroxysmal stage
    D. Convalescent stage

Correct Answer A: *Incubation stage.* A person can spread pertussis within the first 3 weeks of the start of cough, which begins in the catarrhal stage. During the incubation stage, patients are typically asymptomatic. Patients are no longer considered infectious after 5 days of antibiotics, or after the 3rd week from symptom onset.

35. A 50-year-old female with a history of atrial fibrillation, who is not on anticoagulation, presents with a complaint of sudden painless left eye vision loss. What physical exam finding are you most expecting to see on the fundoscopic exam?
    A. Cotton wool spots
    B. Irregular contours of the retina
    C. Cherry-red spot
    D. Cloudy lens

Correct Answer C. *Cherry-red spots.* A person with atrial fibrillation who is not on anticoagulation is at risk for a thrombotic event. A blanched retina and cherry-red spot are the classic physical exam findings. Cotton wool spots may be present, but are not associated with sudden onset of vision loss and are indicative of other disease states, such as hypertension or diabetes. Retinal detachments can also cause sudden painless vision loss; however, as discussed above, this person is at risk for a thrombotic event. A cloudy lens is seen in cataracts and is the most common cause for progressive painless vision loss.

36. A 55-year-old male presents for a vesicular lesion on the tip of his nose. This lesion was preceded by generalized fatigue and subjective fevers. What is an important test to do in the evaluation of this patient?
    A. Skin biopsy
    B. Otoscopic exam
    C. Slit lamp exam
    D. Tonometry

Correct Answer C: *Slit lamp exam.* In a patient with a vesicular lesion on the tip of his nose, the differential diagnosis includes herpes zoster. The tip of the nose is located in the V1 branch of cranial nerve V (trigeminal nerve), and an evaluation for herpes zoster ophthalmicus must be done. Timely diagnosis and referral to an ophthalmologist for persistent symptoms are necessary to limit visual morbidities. A skin biopsy can be done to help aid in diagnosis; however, most cases are clinically diagnosed based on history and physical exam. Additionally, if a patient is in need of a skin biopsy, proper dermatology referral should be performed. A slit lamp exam without staining will not reveal the dendritic lesions seen in herpes zoster ophthalmicus.

37. What criteria give you a negative value when evaluating for *Streptococcus pharyngitis* using the Centor score?
    A. Absence of cough
    B. Age 14 to 44
    C. Age >45
    D. Age <2

Correct Answer C: *Age >45.* Age >45 gives you a –1 value. Absence of cough gives you +1, age >15 but <44 gives you 0, and the rule cannot be applied to patients <2 years of age.

38. A 25-year-old female presents complaining of pain, swelling, and drainage from her right ear for the past 5 days. She reports decreased hearing, but denies fevers. On exam she has tenderness with palpation of the tragus, drainage from the ear, an erythematous and edematous

canal, clear tympanic membranes, no mastoid tenderness, and no trismus. What is the next likely course of treatment?

A. CT scan
B. ENT consultation
C. Oral antibiotics
D. Topical antibiotics

Correct Answer D: *Topical antibiotics.* The patient has otitis externa and should be started on topical otic antibiotics. TMs are clear and, therefore, do not suggest otitis media. A CT scan should be done if suspecting mastoiditis, but in a well-appearing patient without mastoid tenderness, it is less likely. An ENT consultation should be done for patients who have refractory otitis externa despite a complete course of topical antibiotics.

39. A 2-year-old girl presents with her father with 1 week of purulent drainage/discharge from the right nostril. No reports of fevers or coughs. The father reports a foul odor from the nose. What is the likely diagnosis?

A. Acute sinusitis
B. Upper respiratory infection
C. Nasal polyp
D. Retained foreign body

Correct Answer D: *Retained foreign body.* Without infectious symptoms or associated symptoms consistent with upper respiratory infection, the likely cause is a retained foreign body.

40. The steeple sign is associated with what disease state?

A. Croup
B. Epiglottis
C. Retropharyngeal abscess
D. Pertussis

Correct Answer A: *Croup.* The thumb print sign is associated with epiglottitis. A patient with a retropharyngeal abscess narrowing of the retropharyngeal space may be seen on plain films of the neck, but better seen on a CT scan. Pertussis does not have an associated radiographic sign.

41. A 37-year-old male presents to the emergency department after having been bitten by a bat that was in his basement. He appears well; vital signs include a temp, 98.4°F, HR, 85; and BP, 136/84. He has no medical history and no history of rabies exposure or rabies vaccination. His wound is without significant erythema or tenderness. What would be the most important intervention before discharging him from the emergency department?

A. IV antibiotics to cover for animal bites
B. One dose of intramuscular human rabies immune globulin (HRIG) and initiation of rabies vaccine with follow-up instruction to complete the series
C. Initiation of rabies vaccine with follow-up instruction to complete the series
D. Irrigation of the wound and debridement if necessary

Correct Answer B: *One dose of intramuscular human rabies immune globulin (HRIG) and initiation of rabies vaccine with follow-up instruction to complete the series.* Bats are high-risk animals carrying rabies; patients who are exposed need to receive the vaccine series. The patient should have HRIG and the vaccine on day one. The wound is not being described as infected; therefore, the patient does not need IV antibiotics or debridement.

42. A 19-year-old female arrives to the emergency department brought in by her boyfriend, complaining of diffuse lower abdominal pain and purulent/bloody vaginal discharge. Vital signs: temp, 102.7°F; HR, 107; and BP, 105/75. She has a history of multiple sexual partners without the use of barrier protection/birth control. Initial testing shows a negative urinalysis and the patient is not pregnant. She is diagnosed presumptively with pelvic inflammatory disease (PID), and cultures are sent for analysis. What would be the most appropriate treatment?

    A. Ceftriaxone 250 mg intramuscular (IM) × 1 dose plus doxycycline 100 mg po bid × 14 days
    B. Azithromycin 1 g po × 1 dose plus ceftriaxone IM × 1 dose
    C. Metronidazole 500 mg po tid × 10 days
    D. Do not treat, wait for culture results

Correct Answer A: *Ceftriaxone 250 mg IM × 1 dose plus doxycycline 100 mg po bid × 14 days.* This is the standard treatment for PID. Azithromycin plus ceftriaxone is the treatment when you suspect chlamydia or gonorrhea cervicitis. Metronidazole 500 is the treatment for vaginal trichomoniasis. It is not recommended to wait for cultures in any suspected sexually transmitted disease case.

43. What is the most common sexually transmitted disease in the United States?

    A. HPV (human papillomavirus)
    B. Gonorrhea
    C. Chlamydia
    D. Syphilis

Correct Answer A: *HPV (human papillomavirus).* Previously chlamydia had been the most common STD in the United States; however, the incidence for HPV has increased, making it the most common existing STD in the United States. Gonorrhea and Syphilis are less common.

44. A 45-year-old presents to the ED with complaints of fevers for 2 days and development of a rash over the last 24 hours. The rash is vesicular with a "dew drop on a rose petal" appearance noted on the bilateral upper and lower extremities as well as the trunk. The rash is pruritic and spares the palms and soles. What is your treatment plan?

    A. Admit for broad-spectrum IV antibiotics
    B. Doxycycline 100 mg po bid × 3 weeks
    C. Admit for supportive treatment, including Tylenol and IV Fluids
    D. Acyclovir 800 mg po qid × 5 days

Correct Answer D: *Acyclovir 800 mg po qid × 5 days.* This patient has a rash consistent with chickenpox. Acyclovir is the treatment in adult patients. In children, supportive treatment is the mainstay of therapy; however, it is recommended to treat adults with an antiviral medication. Antibiotics are not warranted, as this is not a bacterial rash. Doxycycline is incorrect because this is not a tick-borne illness.

45. A 19-year-old male presents to the emergency department with complaints of sore throat and generalized malaise. On exam the patient has exudates on tonsils and posterior cervical lymphadenopathy. What laboratory finding will help confirm the diagnosis?

    A. Elevated liver function tests (LFTs)
    B. Positive cold agglutinin test
    C. Positive heterophile antibody
    D. Elevated C-reactive protein

Correct Answer C: *Positive heterophile antibody.* This patient most likely has infectious mononucleosis. A positive heterophile antibody is the most specific test confirming the diagnosis. Although a patient may have elevated LFTs and an elevated C-reactive protein, these tests are not specific to mono. A positive cold agglutinin test does not assist in the diagnosis of infectious mononucleosis.

46. A 24-year-old male presents to the emergency room with diarrhea for the past 2 weeks. His primary care physician evaluated him 2 days previously and no antibiotics were started. Vital signs: temp, 100.5°F; HR 105; BP, 98/65; and patient appears profoundly dehydrated. He describes profuse watery diarrhea with generalized malaise and intermittent fevers. He has no medical history, but admits to recently returning from Africa, where he was doing missionary work. Laboratory studies are notable for the following: white blood cell, 22; Na, 132; K, 2.9; and creatinine, 1.80. Stool cultures sent by his PCP earlier this week have returned confirming *Giardia*. What is the next most appropriate treatment plan?

    A. Admit for symptomatic treatment intravenous fluids (IVF) and antidiarrhea medication
    B. Discharge home with continued supportive therapy
    C. Admit for IVF and metronidazole IV or po 500 mg bid
    D. Discharge home with a script for metronidazole 500 mg po bid × 5 days

Correct Answer C: *Admit for IVF and metronidazole IV or po 500 mg bid.* The patient requires antibiotic therapy for symptomatic diarrhea and admission for IVF for associated acute renal failure.

47. What opportunistic infection is an HIV patient most at risk to develop when CD4 counts drop to 190 μL?

    A. *Pneumocystis jiroveci* (carinii) pneumonia
    B. Toxoplasmosis
    C. Histoplasmosis
    D. Mycobacterium avium complex (MAC)

Correct Answer A: *Pneumocystis jirovecii (carinii) pneumonia.* Patients with CD4 counts <200 μL are at risk for *P. jiroveci* (carinii) pneumonia. Patients with CD4 counts <100 μL become higher risk for developing toxoplasmosis and histoplasmosis. When CD4 counts drop below 50 μL, the patient is at risk for MAC.

48. A 23-year-old active male presents to the ED with complaints of a rash. He began feeling joint pain and having fevers 2 days ago. His rash is diffuse, maculopapular, and is noted on his palms and soles. Upon further questioning, he reveals that he is an avid hiker and spent time camping in the mountains last weekend. What is the treatment of choice?

    A. Supportive care and NSAIDs
    B. Doxycycline 100 mg po bid
    C. Acyclovir 800 mg po qid
    D. Topical steroids

Correct Answer B: *Doxycycline 100 mg po bid.* This is classic Rocky Mountain spotted fever. Treatment is doxycycline. Steroids and Acyclovir are not indicated in this diagnosis.

49. Which of the following does *not* put a patient at risk for transmission of hepatitis B?

    A. Contact with blood or open sores of an infected person
    B. Sex with an infected partner
    C. Breast-feeding from an infected person
    D. Birth to an infected mother

Correct Answer C: *Breast-feeding from an infected person.* The Centers for Disease Control and Prevention guidelines state that hepatitis B can be transmitted through blood, bodily fluids, and mucous membranes, though not through breast milk.

50. A 21-year-old male college student presents to the emergency department with headache, photophobia, and generalized malaise. His intake vital signs include the following: temp, 102°F; HR, 110; BP, 100/62; and RR, 18. He appears toxic and uncomfortable. Upon examination he has nuchal rigidity. You suspect meningitis and perform a lumbar puncture. Cerebrospinal fluid cell count reveals white blood cell 1,300, protein 21, and glucose 30. What is the most likely bacterial source?

    A. Group B Streptococcus
    B. *Escherichia coli*
    C. *Listeria monocytogenes*
    D. *Streptococcus pneumoniae*

Correct Answer D: *Streptococcus pneumoniae.* This patient has meningitis. *S. pneumoniae* and *Neisseria meningitidis* are the most common types of bacteria seen in young adults as well as older adults. Group B Streptococcus, *E. coli*, and *L. Monocytogenes* are more common in newborns.

51. Which of the following will help support the diagnosis of viral meningitis when interpreting cerebrospinal fluid results?

    A. Predominance of lymphocytes
    B. Markedly decreased glucose
    C. Elevated opening pressure
    D. Elevated white blood cell

Correct Answer A: *Predominance of lymphocytes.* On a cell count/differential, there is typically a predominance of lymphocytes on patients with viral meningitis. With viral meningitis, you will typically see a normal glucose level with normal opening pressure.

52. A 67-year-old, with a medical history of benign prostatic hyperplasia and hypertension, presents to the emergency room with complaints of shortness of breath. His initial vital signs include the following: temp, 100.5°F; HR, 105; BP, 92/45; and RR, 25. Basic labs show white blood cell 12, creatinine 0.9, blood urea nitrogen 8, and C-reactive protein 12. His chest x-ray reveals left lower lobe pneumonia. The patient appears more comfortable after an albuterol nebulizer treatment and 1 L of intravenous fluids. What is the most appropriate intervention for this patient?

    A. Discharge the patient home with an antibiotic to treat of community-acquired pneumonia
    B. Discharge the patient home with a nebulizer machine, albuterol, and an antibiotic to treat of community-acquired pneumonia
    C. Admit the patient to the general medical floors, and initiate treatment for community-acquired pneumonia
    D. Admit the patient to the intensive care unit, and initiate broad-spectrum antibiotics to treat for hospital-acquired pneumonia

Correct Answer C : *Admit the patient to the general medical floors, and initiate treatment for community-acquired pneumonia.* The CURB-65 is often used to determine the risk of mortality in patients with pneumonia for clinical practice. This particular patient scores a 3 (1 point for increased respiratory rate, 1 point for low blood pressure, and 1 point for age >65). It is recommended to admit the patient with a score of 2 or more. However, given the patient's medical history, he does not appear to be at risk for hospital-acquired pneumonia.

53. A 32-year-old female with a medical history of asthma presents to the emergency department with fevers up to 102, chills, and a productive cough. Her chest x-ray confirms pneumonia. What is the most likely pathogen?

    A. *Streptococcus pneumoniae*
    B. *Haemophilus influenzae*
    C. *Chlamydophila pneumoniae*
    D. *Staphylococcus aureus*

Correct Answer A: *Streptococcus pneumoniae*. This is the most common cause of community-acquired pneumonia. *H. influenzae*, *C. pneumoniae*, and *Staphylococcus aureus* are also common causes of pneumonia; however, they are not the most common types seen in the community.

54. Which of the following is true regarding influenza treatment?

    A. Children under the age of 2 years, but older than 14 days are considered high risk and should receive Tamiflu (oseltamivir)
    B. Initiating Tamiflu (oseltamivir) has no benefit for a patient 48 hours after the onset of symptoms
    C. Tamiflu (oseltamivir) should not be initiated in pregnancy
    D. Tamiflu (oseltamivir) should not be initiated in immunosuppressed patients

Correct Answer A: *Children under the age of 2 years, but older than 14 days are considered high risk and should receive Tamiflu (oseltamivir)*. Children under 2 years old are considered high risk for developing complications of pneumonia. The Food and Drug Administration approved the drug for children older than 14 days in 2012. Tamiflu is safe in pregnancy and should be initiated in high-risk populations, including immunosuppressed patients. Although initiating the drug <48 hours of symptom onset shows the greatest benefit, however, there is still a benefit to initiating treatment after 48 hours of symptom onset.

55. A 24-year-old female with no medical history presents to the emergency department with an acute onset of right-sided facial weakness. She is unable to completely close her right eye and is worried that she may have suffered a stroke. She also admits to having a circular rash of the back of her neck, which has now resolved. She has an otherwise normal neurologic examination with 5/5 strength of all the extremities. Upon further questioning, she tells you that she has recently done landscaping work in her yard. What is the next most appropriate intervention?

    A. Admit to the hospital for stroke workup, including an MRI/MRA of her head and neck
    B. Obtain blood cultures, and admit to the hospital for treatment with IV antibiotics for septic arthritis
    C. Obtain Lyme serology, and initiate doxycycline to treat Lyme disease
    D. Obtain basic labs, and initiate acyclovir to treat Bell palsy

Correct Answer C: *Obtain Lyme serology, and initiate doxycycline to treat Lyme disease*. Based on this patient's history and physical exam, she most likely has Lyme disease. Although facial palsies may resolve without treatment, oral antibiotic therapy may prevent further sequelae. This patient's signs and symptoms are not consistent with Lyme meningitis or encephalitis, which would require 28 days of IV antibiotics (generally a cephalosporin). Although a workup for this patient may include imaging or blood cultures, it is not the most important next step for this patient's work up. The most likely source for the patient's Bell's palsy is Lyme and not a viral source; so acyclovir is not indicated.

56. A 22-year-old female, without any medical history, presents to the emergency department complaining of right-sided facial weakness that was first noticed about 8 hours ago. Her only complaint is that she is having difficulty closing her right eye, but otherwise feels well. She has

no other complaints. The exam is only significant for obvious facial weakness, and patient is unable to wrinkle her forehead. What is your next step?

A. MRI/MRA head and neck
B. Start prednisone and discharge home
C. Stat tPA
D. Carotid ultrasound

Correct Answer B: *Start prednisone and discharge home.* This patient has a history and exam consistent with Bell's palsy. Bell's palsy is a clinical diagnosis MRI/MRA and carotid ultrasound are not as helpful; however, in older patients with more risk factors for a stroke, imaging could be considered to rule out cerebrovascular accident (CVA). This is not an acute stroke given her lack of other findings, hence tPA, which would be used for acute stroke, is not indicated.

57. What physical exam finding would you expect to find in a patient with Bell's palsy?

A. Positive *pronator* drift
B. Inability to elevate right side of forehead
C. Carotid bruit
D. Anisocoria

Correct Answer B: *Inability to elevate right side of forehead.* Bell's palsy is a motor seventh cranial nerve palsy; so patients are unable to elevate or raise their forehead. You would otherwise have a normal neurologic exam. Carotid bruit is not something you would typically find in Bell's palsy.

58. A 74-year-old male with a history of hypertension, atrial fibrillation, and hyperlipidemia is complaining of acute onset of severe headache. Patient states that this headache is much worse than his typical headaches. Patient is awake, alert, but appears to be uncomfortable and in mild distress. Vital signs: temp, 97.8°F; HR, 96; BP, 192/104; RR, 22; and O_2 sat 96% on RA. A head CT confirms a subarachnoid hemorrhage (SAH). Neurosurgery has been consulted. Which of the following is the most important next step?

A. Start nicardipine drip
B. Start Keppra
C. Intubate
D. Obtain an MRI/MRA

Correct Answer A: *Start nicardipine drip.* Blood pressure control is the most important next step in a patient with a SAH. MRI/MRA, although may be warranted, will most likely take several hours and is not the most important next step. Patient is awake, alert, and maintaining his airway; so there is no indication to intubate at this time. Starting Keppra to prevent seizures is indicated, but not as important as blood pressure control.

59. An 89-year-old male, with a history of prostate cancer, is transferred to the ED from his nursing home with mental status change. The patient has become more confused, aggressive, and combative ever since being discharged from the hospital where he was admitted for 2 days for urinary retention. While in the hospital, he had a Foley placed and was started on Flomax. Today in the ED, vital signs are significant for temp, 102.1°F; HR, 116; BP, 95/54; RR, 24; and O_2 sat 97% on RA. What is the most likely cause for this patient's mental status change?

A. Medication effect
B. Urinary tract infection (UTI)
C. Dehydration
D. Metastatic disease to the brain

Correct Answer B: *Urinary tract infection (UTI).* The presence of fever, tachycardia, and hypotension likely indicates infection, and the recent Foley placement makes him high risk for UTI. The other options are possible causes of mental status change; however, his history and vital signs make UTI much more likely.

60. A 16-year-old female is brought in by emergency medical services after having her first seizure. She was witnessed to have a 2-minute tonic-clonic seizure with urinary incontinence. There was no head trauma. In the ED patient is postictal, but no focal neurologic findings. Vital signs: temp, 99°F; HR, 67; BP, 110/54; RR, 16; O_2 sat 99% on RA. All of the following are indicated in the ED except:

    A. EEG
    B. Chest x-ray
    C. Head CT scan
    D. Complete blood count, Chem 7, toxicology screen, urinalysis, hCG

Correct Answer A: *EEG.* Chest x-ray, lab work, and head CT are all indicated in the ED to rule out infection, toxic metabolic disorder, intracranial bleed, edema, or mass etiologies for first-time seizures. EEGs are not routinely done in the ED and obtained by the outpatient neurologist during follow-up.

61. All are findings you could find in a patient with a cerebellar infarct except:

    A. Gait disturbance
    B. Dysmetria
    C. Nystagmus
    D. Visual field defect
    E. Vomiting

Correct Answer D: *Visual field defect.* Visual field defects are noted in middle cerebral artery strokes. All other options are all typical findings in a patient with a cerebellar infarct.

62. A 24-year-old female comes to the emergency department (ED) complaining of severe left-sided headache, left eye pain, and left facial numbness. The headache is throbbing and associated with nausea and vomiting. She also complains of "seeing spots." She has had similar headaches in the past, but she has never seen a specialist or been given a diagnosis for these symptoms. Her only medication is levothyroxine. Her vital signs are as follows: temp, 99.2°F; HR, 100; BP, 120/88; RR, 24; and O_2 sat 100% on RA. Her neuro exam is nonfocal. What is her most likely diagnosis?

    A. Bell's palsy
    B. Transient ischemic attack (TIA)
    C. Venous sinus thrombosis (VST)
    D. Complex migraine

Correct Answer D: *Complex migraine.* The presence of aura, facial numbness, nausea, and vomiting are typical in a complex migraine. TIA and VST are incorrect in that she is a young woman with no risk factors and she has a normal neuro exam. Bell's Palsy is a cranial nerve VII palsy, and you would not see the above symptoms with this.

63. A 42-year-old male comes to the emergency department complaining of bilateral lower extremity weakness that began in his feet but has quickly spread proximally up the legs. He is now having difficulty walking. Besides a recent flu-like illness, he is otherwise healthy. All are physical exam findings you could find except:

    A. Hyperreflexia
    B. Lumbar tenderness

C. Respiratory distress

D. Facial weakness

Correct Answer A: *Hyperreflexia.* Guillain–Barré syndrome usually presents with lower extremity and back pain with rapidly progressing lower extremity weakness. Reflexes are usually decreased or absent. Facial weakness and respiratory distress can occur as the weakness progresses.

64. What diagnostic measure could you do in the emergency department (ED) for the diagnosis of Guillain–Barré syndrome?

A. MRI of the spine

B. Lumbar puncture

C. Vascular ultrasound

D. Head CT

Correct Answer B: *Lumbar puncture.* Cerebrospinal fluid analysis showing elevated protein with normal white blood cell count is indicative of Guillain–Barré and can easily be done in the ED. MRI, vascular ultrasound, and head CT would not confirm the diagnosis and would likely be normal.

65. A 38-year-old female comes to the emergency department complaining of sudden onset of dizziness, described as the room spinning, with nausea and vomiting. Symptoms are worse sitting up and standing. All are signs of a peripheral etiology except:

A. Resolution of symptoms with Epley maneuver

B. Horizontal nystagmus

C. Normal gait

D. Increased symptoms with Epley maneuver

Correct Answer D: *Increased symptoms with Epley maneuver.* The Epley maneuver is done to remove otoconia (otolith) crystals from the semicircular canals that have become dislodged, causing benign paroxysmal positional vertigo. If done correctly, the Epley maneuver would cause resolution of symptoms, not worsening. Horizontal nystagmus and normal gait are both common in peripheral etiologies.

66. A 74-year-old male is brought in by an ambulance after found down by his family. Patient is awake, answering questions, but disoriented to time and place. Medical history: hypertension, coronary artery disease, atrial fib, high cholesterol. Patient is on aspirin, lisinopril, Zocor, Coumadin, hydrochlorothiazide, amlodipine. Vital signs: temp, 97°F; HR, 88; BP, 130/60; RR, 22; and O$_2$, sat 96% on RA. Head CT done in the emergency department confirms a subdural hemorrhage (SDH). What is your next step for management?

A. Intubation

B. Arterial line and nicardipine

C. Vitamin K, fresh frozen plasma, platelets

D. Keppra

Correct Answer C: *Vitamin K, fresh frozen plasma, platelets.* In a patient with a SDH, it is most important to correct anticoagulation. Given that patient is awake, answering questions, and has a normal O$_2$ sat, intubation is not indicated. With a normal BP, nicardipine and arterial line are not indicated. Reversing anticoagulation is more important than starting Keppra to prevent seizures.

67. A 37-year-old male with a history of hepatitis C, intravenous drug use (IVDU), comes to the emergency department complaining of back pain and leg weakness. He states that he cannot walk because of the pain in his back and legs, to the point where he is unable to go to the bathroom. In ED, vital signs are as follows: Temp, 101.4°F; HR, 128; BP, 160/67; RR, 22; and

O_2 sat 100% on RA. Exam is significant for focal lumbar spine tenderness at L3 and 3/5 strength testing in his lower extremities bilaterally. His most likely diagnosis is:

A. Epidural abscess
B. Cauda equina syndrome
C. Guillain–Barré
D. Muscle strain

Correct Answer A: *Epidural abscess.* Tachycardia, fever, and focal lumbar tenderness, with risk factor of IVDU, suggest an infectious etiology. Cauda equina, though it can cause symptoms of back pain and leg weakness, also causes bowel or bladder dysfunction, and you typically would not see a fever. Guillain–Barré presents with ascending leg weakness. Muscle strain would not typically cause weakness or midline tenderness.

68. A 42-year-old female with history of seizures is brought in by emergency medical services having a seizure. Her family states that she ran out of her Keppra 3 days ago and has now been seizing for about 45 minutes. Patient received 2 mg IV Ativan en route. On exam, vital signs are as follows: Temp, 99.2°F; HR, 110; BP, 140/72; RR, 20; and O_2 sat 91% on RA. She is having a tonic-clonic seizure. What is your next step for management?

A. Ativan drip
B. Keppra loading dose
C. Head CT
D. Intubation

Correct Answer D: *Intubation.* This patient is in status epilepticus. Securing the airway is the first step. Ativan drip, Keppra load, and head CT can be done after securing the airway.

69. A 36-year-old female with metastatic breast cancer to lung and bone presents complaining of leg weakness and difficulty ambulating for 1 day. Her exam is notable for 1/5 strength testing in her bilateral lower extremities. What other findings could you expect to find to support your diagnosis?

A. Hyperreflexia
B. Normal rectal tone
C. Bladder scan with 1,500 cc urine
D. Perineal hyperesthesia

Correct Answer C: *Bladder scan with 1,500 cc urine.* The patient described most likely as Cauda equina syndrome from a metastatic lesion. Urinary retention is common in Cauda equina syndrome. You would also expect to find decreased or absent reflexes, decreased rectal tone, and perineal hypoesthesia.

70. A 79-year-old male is brought to the emergency department by family, who state they are having difficulty taking care of him over the last 8 months. He is having memory loss, difficulty with ADLs, and has been wandering out of the house. The family is concerned something is wrong with him. The patient has no complaints and would not have come if it were not for his family. On exam, vital signs are as follows: Temp, 98.5; HR, 86; BP, 123/72; RR, 16; and O_2 sat 99% on RA. His physical exam is unremarkable. You do a broad workup, including complete blood count, comprehensive metabolic panel, toxicology screen, urinalysis, chest x-ray, head CT. All of the following support the diagnosis of dementia over delirium except:

A. Chronic and progressive onset
B. White blood cell (WBC) 9
C. Na 119
D. CT showing white matter changes

Correct Answer C: *Na 119*. Metabolic disorders including hyponatremia are a common cause of acute delirium. Dementia is chronic in nature, while delirium is acute and rapid onset. A WBC of 9 is within the normal range, making infection-causing delirium less likely. Chronic white matter changes are typical in an elderly person, and do not represent anything acute.

71. A 28-year-old female, who is G2P1, presents with 2 days of vaginal bleeding with a confirmed urine pregnancy test in the clinic at approximately 8 weeks pregnant from last menstrual period. She reports the bleeding to be light with some spotting and no pain. Vital signs: temp, 98.2°F; HR, 86; BP, 108/58; RR, 16; and O_2 sat 100% on RA. On exam: she has a soft, non-tender abdomen, and pelvic exam shows trace blood in the vaginal vault, cervical os is closed, no discharge, no adnexal tenderness or cervical motion tenderness. Pelvic ultrasound report: single, intrauterine pregnancy, fetal heart rate present, crown-rump length measuring 1.67 cm. What is the most likely diagnosis?

    A. Complete miscarriage
    B. Threatened miscarriage
    C. Missed miscarriage
    D. Inevitable miscarriage

Correct Answer B: *Threatened miscarriage*. Threatened miscarriage is early pregnancy <20 weeks with bleeding and a closed cervical os. There may also be mild pain and cramping. Complete miscarriage occurs when products of conception have passed and is associated with heavy bleeding and cramping, Ultrasound may only see debris (blood) with open os. Missed miscarriage is often detected at the first ultrasound when there is no heartbeat present. No preceding bleeding or pain have occurred. Inevitable Miscarriage is when the cervical os is open (dilated) and bleeding is often heavier, and associated pain and cramping. There is a transition from inevitable miscarriage to complete miscarriage.

72. A 24-year-old female presents to the emergency department with 5 days of left-sided pelvic pain, vaginal discharge, and fevers to 101. She denies urinary symptoms or other infectious symptoms. She was seen in the clinic 5 days ago and treated for pelvic inflammatory disease (PID). Her last menstrual period was 10 days ago. Medications include oral contraceptive and Tylenol. Vital signs: temp, 101.2°F; HR, 114; BP, 105/58; RR, 18; and O_2 sat, 97% on RA. Labs demonstrate white blood cell, 14K; red blood cell, 5.15; hematocrit, 38; HG, 12. Urinalysis negative for infection and urine hCG negative. What is the most likely diagnosis?

    A. Ectopic pregnancy
    B. Ovarian cyst
    C. Diverticulitis
    D. Tubo-ovarian abscess

Correct Answer D: *Tubo-ovarian abscess*. Complication of PID, usually in reproductive-age females with a history of upper genital infections, can be potentially life-threatening infection with management requiring parenteral antibiotics and often drainage. Ectopic pregnancy risk is increased with history of PID/sexually transmitted infection, but pregnancy test is negative, making ectopic unlikely. Ovarian cysts are fluid-filled sacs that form within the ovaries. They are also non-infectious but can be painful. Diverticulitis can cause similar symptoms with fever and pain, but given her young age, it makes this less likely.

73. What is the recommended first-line treatment for gonorrhea infection?

    A. Ciprofloxacin 500 mg twice a day for 7 days
    B. No treatment recommended
    C. Ceftriaxone 2 mg IV × 1
    D. Ceftriaxone 250 mg intramuscular (IM) × 1

Correct Answer D: *Ceftriaxone 250 mg IM ×1.* Centers for Disease Control and Prevention recommends ceftriaxone 250 mg IM ×1 as the initial first-line treatment for gonorrhea for both men and women. Fluoroquinolones are no longer recommended due to high resistance rates. Treatment of gonorrhea is strongly recommended as untreated infection can lead to pelvic inflammatory disease, scarring of the reproductive organs, ascending to the upper pelvic organs and rarely into the bloodstream. Ceftriaxone IV is not recommended for outpatient treatment.

74. A 32-year-old female presents to the emergency department with right-sided pelvic pain that has been worsening over the past 3 days. She describes the pain as waxing and waning with episodes of severe pain that caused her to double over. She denies fevers or urinary symptoms, but has nausea with severe pain episodes. Her last menstrual period was 9 days ago, and she is not currently sexually active. She was unable to get relief with over-the-counter medications and presents to the emergency department for evaluation. Her medical history includes depression, anxiety, endometriosis, and history of ovarian cysts. Surgical history includes exploratory laparotomy for endometriosis, cystectomy. Vital signs: temp, 98.7°F; HR, 122; BP, 135/78; RR, 18; and O$_2$ sat 99% on RA. What is the initial emergency treatment for the suspected diagnosis.
    A. Consult gynecologist (GYN), stat pelvic ultrasound
    B. FAST ultrasound exam for free fluid
    C. Laboratory tests
    D. General surgical consultation for bowel obstruction

Correct Answer A: *Consult gynecologist (GYN), stat pelvic ultrasound.* This patient is most likely having ovarian torsion, which is a surgical emergency. She has a history of ovarian cyst as well as past cystectomy. Consulting GYN and obtaining stat ultrasound should not be delayed. Viability of the ovary is time sensitive and any delay for further testing could compromise its viability. Obtaining a fast exam for free fluid is reasonable if concern for ectopic rupture though the patient states she is not sexually active, with a recent menstrual period and vital signs notable only for tachycardia. Do not delay GYN consultation for lab testing with a high clinical suspicion for ovarian torsion. Appropriate workup for bowel obstruction can be obtained only after evaluation for ovarian torsion is negative.

75. A 32-year-old female, G3 P2, approximately 18 weeks pregnant, presents with vaginal bleeding that started today. She had some mild cramping and then the bleeding that has slowed down upon her arrival in the emergency department. She is feeling otherwise well. She reports that she has had prenatal care at another hospital and reports her blood type is O negative. Vital signs: temp, 97.6°F; HR, 86; BP, 108/58; RR, 16; and O$_2$ sat 100% on RA. Exam: Abdomen soft nontender, pelvic exam: small amount of blood in the vaginal vault, os closed, and no active bleeding. There is no cervical motion tenderness or adnexal tenderness. Pelvic ultrasound shows a small sub-chorionic hematoma, fetal heart rate 158, no free fluid. Urinalysis is negative, and urine culture is pending. Complete blood count: white blood cell, 10; red blood cell, 5.1; hematocrit, 34; Hgb, 11. What does the patient need before being discharged?
    A. Counseling on subchorionic hematoma
    B. Treatment for asymptomatic cystitis in a pregnant person
    C. Rhogam
    D. Blood transfusion

Correct Answer C: *Rhogam.* Rhogam injection is given to prevent hemolytic disease of the newborn in this pregnancy and any subsequent pregnancy given her Rh screen is negative. Counseling on subchorionic hematoma is also recommended as increased risk of pregnancy loss with increased size of hematoma, increased maternal age, as well as increased gestational age. Urinalysis is negative; so she does not need empiric antibiotics. She has mild anemia in pregnancy, but does not require a transfusion as the hematocrit is stable and she has no further bleeding

76. A 23-year-old female presents with 6 days of vaginal itching and thick, white discharge. She denies fevers. She is not sexually active. She denies urinary symptoms. Vital signs are normal. On exam, there is thick white discharge in the vaginal vault, no cervical motion tenderness, and no adnexal tenderness. pH is 4.0. Wet prep with + hyphae after KOH. What does the patient have?

   A. Bacterial vaginosis
   B. *Chlamydia*
   C. Candida vulvovaginitis
   D. *N. Gonorrhea*

Correct Answer C: *Candida vulvovaginitis.* The patient has classic symptoms for yeast infection, which include itching, pain, thick white discharge, and wet prep with positive hyphae. pH is usually low/normal for yeast. She has no pain and is not sexually active, but it is recommended to send gonorrhea/*Chlamydia* test on all patients with vaginal discharge and pain. Bacterial vaginosis can cause itch and discharge, but there is presence of clue cells on wet prep.

77. A 37-year-old healthy female, approximately 35 weeks gestation, is a restrained driver in an automobile accident. She is brought to the ED with symptoms of neck and back pain. Her initial set of vital signs was reported to be normal. While in the ED, she reports sudden onset of abdominal pain and cramping with vaginal bleeding. Vital signs are notable for tachycardia and hypotension. What is the likely diagnosis?

   A. Muscle strain
   B. Abdominal wall contusion
   C. Placental abruption
   D. Threatened miscarriage

Correct Answer C: *Placental abruption.* Placental abruption is a condition where the placental lining has separated from the uterus. This separation can be partial or complete. Patients are often tachycardic and hypotensive given blood loss. Muscle strain and abdominal wall contusion may also be present, but given pregnancy and vaginal bleeding, less likely the cause of the abdominal pain. Threatened miscarriage occurs during the early stages of pregnancy, not in third trimester.

78. In the above scenario, what is the next step in the emergency department management of the patient?

   A. Admit to the antepartum floor
   B. Discharge home
   C. Consult obstetric (OB) for stat evaluation and potential emergent C-section
   D. Comprehensive OB ultrasound

Correct Answer C: *Consult OB for stat evaluation and potential emergent C-section.* This patient is hemodynamically unstable and may need stat delivery. She will need two large-bore IVs with aggressive fluid resuscitation to maintain perfusion, supplemental O_2, possible blood transfusion. If hemodynamic instability is prolonged, then risk of hypoperfusion to the fetus increases. It is recommended for emergent delivery of fetus if mother or fetus becomes unstable. If the patient were stable, consider admission to the antepartum floor. OB ultrasound is a consideration may be delayed or prolong definitive intervention. Recommend bedside focused assessment with sonography for trauma exam to evaluate for bleeding.

79. A 35-year-old female, G1 P0, who is 37 weeks 3 days gestation, presents to the emergency department with headache and abdominal pain. She was not able to get in touch with her obstetrician, and her husband is concerned about her. Her evaluation is notable for BP, 157/78; HR, 103; urine notable for 3+ protein; and her liver function tests are normal. What is the diagnosis?

  A. Urinary tract infection
  B. Preeclampsia
  C. Hypertension in pregnancy
  D. **H**emolysis, **E**levated **L**iver enzymes, **L**ow **P**latelet count (HEELP) syndrome

Correct Answer B: *Preeclampsia.* Preeclampsia is defined as elevated blood pressure and proteinuria in pregnancy >20 weeks gestation. UTI is a complication in pregnancy and can contribute to preterm labor though no reported bacteria or urinary symptoms to consider this. Pregnancy-induced hypertension is elevated blood pressure in pregnancy >20 weeks gestation without proteinuria. HELLP is a complication of preeclampsia and is a severe life-threatening condition with constellation of lab abnormalities, including HEELP. Delivery of the fetus is the only known way to treat HELLP.

80. A 63-year-old homeless male with history of daily ETOH ingestion and 20 pack-year smoking history presents with 9 days of productive cough of gelatinous sputum, sweats, and shortness of breath. Vital signs: temp, 101.3°F; HR, 110; BP, 99/60; RR, 28; and O_2 sat 90% on RA. Exam reveals crackles in all lung fields, with decreased breath sounds and dullness to percussion in the right upper lobe. Which of the following is most true about his diagnosis?

  A. This patient can be managed outpatient with oral Azithromycin.
  B. Patient likely has community-acquired pneumonia due to *Pseudomonas aeruginosa.*
  C. Patient's chest x-ray will show a lobar infiltrate with accompanying pleural effusion, which is the pathognomonic radiographic presentation for pneumonia.
  D. Patient likely has community-acquired pneumonia due to *Klebsiella pneumoniae.*

Correct Answer D: *Patient likely has community-acquired pneumonia due to K. pneumoniae.* *K. pneumoniae* is the pathogen most likely to cause infection in those with chronic illnesses, including alcohol abuse, and in those with underlying lung disease. *P. aeruginosa*, on the other hand, is a common pathogen found in hospital-acquired pneumonia. The patient should not be managed as an outpatient since he exhibits hemodynamic instability. There is no pathognomonic radiographic presentation for pneumonia.

81. A 32-year-old, nonverbal female, with history of cerebral palsy and dysphagia with G-tube, presents with her caretaker after 1 month of cough. Patient completed 5 days of Z-pack after diagnosis of pneumonia 2 weeks ago, but continues with cough. According to the caretaker, patient spiked a temp two nights ago. Exam reveals poor oral dentition with gingivitis, cervical lymphadenopathy, and decreased sounds with crackles in lower lobes. Vital signs: temp, 102.0°F; HR, 102; BP, 108/70; RR, 20; and O_2 sat 91% on RA. What is the most likely diagnosis?

  A. Lung abscess
  B. Acute bronchitis
  C. Pneumonia that failed outpatient treatment
  D. Pulmonary embolism

Correct Answer A: *Lung abscess.* Lung abscesses are caused by pulmonary necrosis and are most likely to occur in the setting of aspiration pneumonia due to the anaerobes present in the gingiva. While bronchitis is characterized by persistent cough, it does not usually have accompanying fever or other constitutional symptoms. Pneumonia that failed outpatient treatment is a possible consideration, but the key features to this case are the history of dysphagia with poor dental hygiene, which predisposes this patient to lung abscess. Pulmonary embolism would be a consideration given that the patient does present with tachycardia and hypoxia. However, it does not fit in this clinical picture. Those with pulmonary emboli will exhibit pleuritic chest pain, dyspnea, hemoptysis, and accentuated pulmonic component to the second heart sound.

82. A 19-year-old female presents with 1-day history of intermittent cough, expiratory wheeze, and tachypnea. The patient is able to answer questions, but can only say three- to four-word sentences. Vital signs: temp, 98.6°F; HR, 100; BP, 155/105; RR, 28; and O_2 sat 95% on RA. What is the emergent treatment for this patient?

    A. Metoprolol
    B. Nebulized albuterol sulfate
    C. Get a STAT chest x-ray
    D. IV diphenhydramine

Correct Answer B: *Nebulized albuterol sulfate.* β-Adrenergic agonists such as albuterol sulfate are the first-line agents to treat acute bronchospasms from asthma. β-Blockers such as metoprolol, on the other hand, can exacerbate asthma. Chest x-rays are only helpful in the asthmatic setting if there is any concern for infectious causes such as pneumonia. But, in either case, it is not the next step in managing this patient emergently. Antihistamines such as diphenhydramine can reduce the patient's ability to clear secretions.

83. A very concerned mother brings her 2-month-old son after 2-day history of coughing, fever, rhinorrhea, and "breathing funny." On exam, you see the child has nasal flaring, accessory muscle use with retractions, and diffuse wheezing on auscultation. Vital signs: 99.9°F, HR, 160; BP, 80/50; RR, 40; and O_2 sat 94% on RA. Which of the following is *not* true?

    A. Respiratory syncytial virus is the most common cause of bronchiolitis.
    B. Heliox should *not* be considered to manage respiratory distress in infants.
    C. Nebulized epinephrine (1:1,000) should be considered if albuterol fails.
    D. Corticosteroid will be helpful in infants with previous history of reactive airway disease.

Correct Answer B: *Heliox should not be considered to manage respiratory distress in infants.* Heliox (helium-oxygen) has been found to be helpful in children with bronchiolitis, or those with postextubation stridor, respiratory distress syndromes, or bronchopulmonary dysplasia.

84. A 63-year-old male presents to the emergency department for the eighth time over 6 months. Patient is complaining of persistent dry cough with each visit. However, with today's visit, patient complains of worsening shortness of breath over the past week. Patient states he is now having difficulty ambulating to the bathroom without taking a break to catch his breath. On exam, he appears to have slight cyanosis around the mouth, inspiratory crackles, and clubbing. Chest x-ray reveals atelectasis and diffuse fibrosis of the lung. Chest CT reveals diffuse pleural honeycombing. What is the most likely diagnosis?

    A. Congestive heart failure (CHF)
    B. Pulmonary embolism
    C. Idiopathic fibrosing interstitial pneumonia
    D. Pulmonary hypertension

Correct Answer C: *Idiopathic fibrosing interstitial pneumonia.* Idiopathic fibrosing interstitial pneumonia given the progressive nature of the symptoms, worsening dyspnea on exertion, and pleural honeycombing on CT is a characteristic of interstitial lung disease. Congestive heart failure will also present with dyspnea on exertion. However, the radiographic findings are not consistent with CHF. Chest x-ray of a CHF patient will likely show cardiomegaly, pleural effusions, or Kerley B lines from interstitial edema. Pulmonary hypertension also presents with progressive exertional dyspnea; however, those with pulmonary hypertension may also complain of exertional angina and often with exertional syncope.

85. A 67-year-old male with longstanding chronic obstructive pulmonary disease (COPD) presents in the ED by emergency medical services with worsening dyspnea over the past 3 hours. Patient was provided with continuous bronchodilator nebulizers en route. Vital signs on arrival to the ED: temp, 97.6°F; HR, 100; BP, 167/98; RR, 26; and O_2 sat 90% on 2 L. Patient has diffuse wheezes on exam. You obtain an arterial blood gas, which shows pH 7.25, PCO_2 50. Patient is answering questions appropriately but lethargic and only able to answer two to three-word questions at a time. What is the first step in this patient's management?

    A. Increase the patient's supplemental oxygen
    B. Provide noninvasive positive pressure ventilation
    C. Chest x-ray
    D. Emergently intubate patient

Correct Answer B: *Provide noninvasive positive pressure ventilation.* Providing noninvasive positive pressure ventilation is beneficial for patients with acute exacerbations of COPD with hypercapnic acidosis. Positive results should be seen within 1 to 2 hours. Providing supplemental oxygen to a chronic COPD patient can be harmful. Providing too much oxygen can exacerbate the patient's hypercapnia. Goal should be to maintain an oxygen level between 88% to 92%. While obtaining a chest x-ray will be important in his emergent care, it is important to stabilize the patient first. Intubation and mechanical ventilation should be the last resort. It should be a consideration if the noninvasive positive pressure ventilation fails or is not tolerated by the patient, or if the patient has respiratory failure.

86. A 21-year-old college student presents with 2 months of progressive cough, shortness of breath, and intermittent chest pain. She reports a 5 to 10 pound weight loss over 2 months with increasing fatigue. Vital signs: temp, 98.6°F; HR, 80; BP, 110/70; RR, 16; and O_2 sat 95% on RA. On exam, patient has pupils equal, round, reactive to light, slight swelling to parotid gland, dry oral mucosa, no cervical lymphadenopathy, heart regular rate and rhythm (RRR), lungs exhibit slight expiratory wheeze, soft nontender abdominal, no significant muscle trophy, cranial nerve II-XII grossly intact. Chest x-ray shows bilateral hilar adenopathy and reticular opacities. Which of the following should be excluded from your differential?

    A. Sarcoidosis
    B. Tuberculosis
    C. Pulmonary histoplasmosis
    D. Horner syndrome

Correct Answer D: *Horner syndrome.* Horner syndrome does not fit the clinical picture. It is a neurologic syndrome that can occur from a wide variety of reasons, including stroke, injury to brachial plexus, cranial fossa neoplasm, as well as a Pancoast tumor (lung apex). Symptoms include ptosis, anhidrosis, miosis. Sarcoidosis typically presents between ages 20 and 60. Bilateral lymphadenopathy is common with sarcoidosis, while parenchymal findings can vary, but include reticular opacities. Sarcoidosis also causes other constitutional symptoms, including visual changes, dry mouth, parotid swelling, and muscle weakness. Tuberculosis can present with cough, occasional hemoptysis, fever, substernal or interscapular pain, night sweats, anorexia, and weight loss. Exam findings may include posttussive rales. Radiographic findings for tuberculosis include hilar lymphadenopathy, pleural effusions or infiltrates. Pulmonary histoplasmosis should be considered whenever sarcoidosis or tuberculosis are on the differential. Young healthy patients typically have mild symptoms, including chest pain, cough, arthralgias, fever, and rash, including erythema nodosum. Immunocompromised, or elderly patients can also exhibit pericarditis or lung infections. Radiographic findings include pneumonia with mediastinal or perihilar lymphadenopathy, cardiomegaly suggesting pericarditis, pulmonary nodules, or cavitary lung lesions.

87. A 74-year-old male, with a history of diabetes and hypertension, presents with worsening shortness of breath and cough. Patient states that for the past 4 days he has worsening dyspnea on exertion. On exam, decreased breath sounds in the right middle and right lower lobes, and rales on the left lower lobe. Abdomen is soft, nontender. Lower extremities show 1+ pitting edema bilaterally. Vital signs: temp, 98.2°F; HR, 82; BP, 164/78; RR, 22; and O_2 sat 94% on 2 L. Chest x-ray shows no cardiomegaly, large, bilateral pleural effusions (R>L). Labs show the following: white blood cell, 10.9; Hgb, 14.2; hematocrit, 41.4; Platelet, 226; Na, 139; K, 4.0; blood urea nitrogen, 14; Cr, 0.6; B-type natriuretic peptide (BNP) is within normal limits. What is the treatment?

    A. Provide more supplemental oxygen
    B. Provide nebulized albuterol
    C. Perform a thoracentesis
    D. Perform pulmonary function testing

Correct Answer C: *Perform a thoracentesis*. Thoracentesis is indicated in patients with presence of large pleural effusion without known cause, dyspnea, normal BNP, or clinically obvious heart failure. It will allow for relief of symptoms, as well as fluid examination and improved radiographic visualization of lung parenchyma. Giving additional supplemental oxygen, nebulized bronchodilators, and pulmonary functioning testing is not necessary.

88. A 35-year-old schoolteacher presents with persistent dry cough for the past 4 weeks. Patient states that the illness started with general malaise, increased lacrimation, rhinorrhea, and injected conjunctiva. While these symptoms resolved after a few days, her cough persists. She states the cough is paroxysmal in nature and can occur during the day or night. During your exam, lungs are clear with inspiration, but during expiration, the patient has multiple episodes of vigorous coughing, resulting in vomiting. Vital signs are within normal limits. What is the likely diagnosis?

    A. Viral upper respiratory infection
    B. Acute bronchitis
    C. Community-acquired pneumonia (CAP)
    D. Pertussis

Correct Answer D: *Pertussis*. Pertussis is a contagious respiratory illness that causes persistent cough with one or more of the classical symptoms: inspiratory whoop, paroxysmal cough, and posttussive emesis and best describes how the patient presented. Upper respiratory infections are viral infections that affect the nasal passages, pharynx, larynx, or sinuses. Symptoms include nasal congestion, cough with or without sputum production, low-grade temp, and postnasal drip. Illness is self-limited and usually resolves after 2 weeks. Acute bronchitis is a viral infection resulting in inflammation of the trachea, bronchi, and bronchioles. Symptoms include cough with or without sputum production, dyspnea, general malaise, sore throat, and expiratory rhonchi or wheeze. For healthy patients, symptoms resolve after 2 weeks. Pneumonia results from the inflammation and infection of the alveoli and interstitium of the lung. Symptoms include productive cough, dyspnea, fever, sweats, and rigors. Symptoms for bacterial CAP will continue to worsen until managed with antibiotics.

89. A healthy 28-year-old female who takes only oral contraceptive pills presents with 5 days of nonproductive cough, sore throat, headache, and arthralgias. On exam, head, eyes, ears, nose, and throat are unremarkable, no cervical lymphadenopathy, heart is regular rate and rhythm (RRR), lungs exhibit slight wheeze. Vital signs: temp, 99.1°F; HR, 82; BP, 120/70; RR, 16; and O_2 sat 98% on RA. How should you manage this patient?

    A. Ceftin
    B. Supportive treatment, including hydration, cough suppressants, and β-2 agonists
    C. Azithromycin
    D. Bactrim

Correct Answer B: *Supportive treatments, including hydration, cough suppressants, and β-2 agonists.* Acute bronchitis is a viral illness of the trachea, bronchi, and bronchioles. In healthy individuals, supportive measures are the proper treatment. Antibiotics are used in those with acute exacerbations of chronic bronchitis, the elderly, those with cardiopulmonary diseases or who are immunocompromised, or those with cough for more than 7 to 10 days.

90. A 27-year-old male, with a known history of a shellfish allergy, presents to your emergency room by ambulance after accidently eating a shrimp-based sauce. The emergency medical technician reports he was found to have lip swelling, wheezing, and complaints of feeling his throat closing. They quickly administered epinephrine and were able to bring him to your emergency department within 10 minutes. He is still symptomatic; however, he is able to speak to you and his vital signs (VS) are normal. What is the next appropriate treatment for this patient?

    A. 0.3 mg epinephrine 1/1,000 intramuscular (IM) q10 to 15 minutes, if still symptomatic, consider epinephrine drip
    B. 0.3 mg epinephrine 1/100 IM × 1, then start an epinephrine drip
    C. 0.3 mg epinephrine 1/1,000 subcutaneous (SC) q10 to 15 minutes, if still symptomatic, consider epinephrine drip
    D. 0.3 mg epinephrine 1/100 SC q10 to 15 minutes, if still symptomatic, consider epinephrine drip

Correct Answer A: *0.3 mg epinephrine 1/1,000 intramuscular (IM) q10 to 15 minutes, if still symptomatic, consider epinephrine drip.* Studies have shown that in a state of anaphylaxis, intramuscular injection of epinephrine is more rapidly absorbed than other routes. This patient does not necessarily need to be started on a drip; this decision is also based on his clinical appearance and VS. Therefore, you should consider only after re-evaluating the patient after IM injections.

91. A 66-year-old male, noninsulin-dependent diabetic, presents to his primary care doctor complaining of a pruritic insect bite to his right leg that has now become red and warm. He also admits to feeling subjective fevers and fatigue. His vital signs are normal, and on exam he has a warm, erythematous 5 × 6 cm area to his lower leg that is painful. What is recommended for the initial treatment of this patient?

    A. Start hydrocortisone ointment and take nonsteroidal anti-inflammatory drugs as needed for pain
    B. Start cephalexin 500 mg qid, advised elevate and f/u in 48 for reevaluation
    C. Admit for IV Ancef, dermatology consult, and leg immobilization
    D. Admit for IV vancomycin, leg elevation, and monitoring

Correct Answer B: *Start cephalexin and reevaluate in 2 days.* This patient has cellulitis, and although describing, some systemic symptoms have normal vital signs. It is recommended to treat for staph/strep and should follow up to reevaluate if symptoms have improved. If they have not, it may be warranted to admit for more broad-spectrum and parental antibiotics.

92. A 15-year-old male presents to your emergency department with his mother complaining of an itchy rash on his back. Otherwise she has admitted that he is in a normal state of health and recently started playing soccer. On exam you see a circular erythematous raised border with central clearing. Skin looks dry. What is the next appropriate treatment?

    A. Start Keflex 500 mg po qid × 7 days
    B. Start doxycycline 100 mg po bid × 21 days
    C. Start clotrimazole 1% topically × 14 days
    D. Start fluconazole 100 mg po qd × 14 days

Correct Answer C: *Start clotrimazole 1% topically × 14 days.* This topical antifungal is used in cases of suspected tinea corporis or ringworm. This is an immunocompetent patient with a probably fungal infection especially after starting soccer. There is no indication to start oral antifungals. Also there are no signs or symptoms of a bacterial infection or cutaneous manifestations of Lyme.

93. A 46-year-old female nurse comes to your emergency department after a possible blood-borne exposure while at work today. She was wearing gloves while placing an IV; she accidently stuck herself with the 22-gauge needle. She immediately took off her gloves and saw a tiny puncture wound with minimal bleeding. She washed her wound copiously and states she is up-to-date with all her vaccines, but the source is high risk. What is the most appropriate treatment?

    A. Raltegravir
    B. Truvada
    C. Tenofovir-emtricitabine and Raltegravir
    D. Does not meet criteria for postexposure prophylaxis treatment at this time

Correct Answer C: *Tenofovir-emtricitabine and Raltegravir.* Truvada is the coformulated name for Tenofovir-emtricitabine, which is non-nucleoside reverse transcriptase inhibitors. These work best with either an integrase inhibitor.

94. A patient presents to your emergency department within 72 hours of being possibly exposed to HIV. Postexposure prophylactic treatment (PEP) for HIV is recommended in which case(s).

    A. Repetitive vaginal intercourse with a high-risk person
    B. Reparative anal intercourse with a high-risk male
    C. Repetitive oral sex with a high-risk female
    D. All of the above

Correct Answer D: *All of the above.* It may be appropriate to recommend PEP for anyone exposed sexually to a high-risk person within 72 hours. Based on the ability to test, the source and the duration of treatment may vary.

95. A 39-year-old laboratory technician reports to the emergency department after spilling a urine sample over her hands. She states the patient has HIV, hepatitis C, and high-risk behaviors. On exam, there are no lacerations or skin disruption visible. What is the next most appropriate treatment?

    A. Wash area with soap and water, start postexposure treatment for HIV/hepatitis C, administer Tdap, follow-up with occupational health
    B. Start postexposure treatment for HIV/hepatitis C, obtain rapid serum HIV test
    C. Wash area with soap and water, start oral antibiotics, and follow-up with occupational health
    D. Wash the affected areas with soap and water

Correct Answer D: *Wash the affected areas with soap and water.* The Centers for Disease Control and Prevention does not recommend postexposure prophylaxis (PEP) in the following conditions: after 72 hours of exposure or when there is no visible blood to fluids (urine, nasal secretions, saliva, sweat, or tears). It does recommend PEP for exposures to someone's genitals, eyes, mouth, or mucous membranes, nonintact skin, or percutaneous exposures. There is no indication for antibiotics at this time.

96. A 65-year-old male with history asthma presents with a rash for 1 year. Patient has several areas of dry, red, and itchy skin mostly located on his face, neck, and also to the insides of his elbows and knees. What is the most likely diagnosis?

    A. Psoriasis
    B. Eczema
    C. Rosacea
    D. Contact dermatitis

Correct Answer B: *Eczema.* Psoriasis presents more as erythematous plagues with silvery, white scales, and does not necessarily need to be on the insides of joints. Rosacea is usually on the face. Contact dermatitis affects only the area of the body that was in contact with a particular allergen; it is usually associated with pustules, sometimes linear.

97. A 23-year-old female presents to the emergency department complaining of joint pain, swelling over the last 2 months. She also feels fatigue, poor appetite, and has recently developed an erythematous rash on the cheeks of her face. She just spent a week vacationing at the beach and feels her rash is now worse. What is the most likely diagnosis?

    A. Rosacea
    B. Systemic lupus erythematosus
    C. Eczema
    D. Melasma

Correct Answer B: *Systemic lupus erythematosus.* Although rosacea, melasma, and eczema may present with similar rashes, we would not expect to have any joint pain, swelling, fatigue with this etiologies. The above are some of the more common presentations of Lupus; however, they are not limited.

98. An 80-year-old female with history of hypertension and osteoarthritis presents to the emergency department with a painful rash × 2 days. Patient admits that she had just recovered from pneumonia and finished taking Levaquin. Her rash is on the left side of her back; she describes that her rash is extremely painful and sensitive to touch. On exam she has multiple erythematous lesions, some with vesicles, some with scabbing, and very tender to touch. Which is the most appropriate treatment for her diagnosis?

    A. Valacyclovir 1,000 mg po q8h × 7 days
    B. Acyclovir 800 mg po q8h × 7 days
    C. Acyclovir 500 mg po 5×/day × 7 days
    D. Valacyclovir 1,000 mg q12h × 7 days

Correct Answer A: *Valacyclovir 1,000 mg po q8h × 7 days.* Acyclovir would be an appropriate treatment for herpes zoster; however, it is dosed at 800 mg po 5×/day × 7 days. Antiviral treatment has been shown to have benefit when administered within 72 hours of symptom onset. Prednisone is not always recommended.

99. An 18-year-old female in otherwise good health reports to the emergency department after a syncopal episode following a long run. She complains of feeling lightheaded and itchiness all over. She has obvious swelling to her hands and feet. Her blood pressure is 80/40, and pulse is 148. Lung exam reveals diffuse wheezing. Her blood sugar is 102 mg per dL. The most important initial IV therapy would be:

    A. Epinephrine
    B. Diphenhydramine HCL

C. Methylprednisolone succinate

D. Normal saline

Correct Answer A: *Epinephrine*. The patient presents with exercise-induced anaphylaxis. With hypotension and tachycardia, the patient's most important initial therapy is epinephrine. Epinephrine has an α-1 adrenergic response that has vasoconstrictor effects, which decreases mucosal edema, elevates blood pressure, and prevents and relieves shock.

100. A young man presents to the emergency room after eating sushi 30 minutes prior with facial flushing, headache, abdominal pain, nausea, vomiting, diarrhea, and palpitations. What is the most likely diagnosis, and what is the treatment?

   A. Campylobacter—IV fluids and azithromycin

   B. *Clostridium difficile*—IV fluids, metronidazole, and antiemetics

   C. Scombroid—IV fluids, diphenhydramine

   D. Staph—IV fluids, loperamide

Correct Answer C: *Scombroid—IV fluids, diphenhydramine*. Scombroid usually results from ingesting Tuna and Mackerel. It causes histamine intoxication. It is best treated with IV fluids and Benadryl. Campylobacter usually presents 3 to 5 days after ingestion from undercooked meat or contaminated water. *C. difficile* usually results from recent antibiotic use. *Staphylococcus* usually presents 1 to 6 hours after ingestion.

101. An 80-year-old male on Coumadin for a pulmonary embolism presents to emergency department status post a mechanical fall 4 hours ago. He fell hitting his face. He has multiple abrasions to the side of the face. There was no reported loss of consciousness. His head CT was negative. His international normalized ratio (INR) is elevated to 6.0. What is the proper management that should be initiated in the emergency room?

   A. Omit warfarin altogether

   B. Administer 1 mg vitamin K orally and check INR in 24 hours

   C. Omit one to two doses of warfarin and administer fresh frozen plasma (FFP); recheck INR in 24 hours

   D. Omit one to two doses of warfarin, administer 1 mg vitamin K orally, and recheck INR in 24 hours

Correct Answer D: *Omit one to two doses of warfarin, administer 1 mg vitamin K orally, and recheck INR in 24 hours*. An INR >5 and <9 without signs of bleeding include omitting one or two doses of warfarin and more frequent INR checks. Oral vitamin K is indicated. FFP is not indicated without any life-threatening bleeding.

102. A 14-year-old girl suffers from severe menorrhagia since menarche at the age of 12. Her Hgb is 6.9 (normal 12 to 16 g per dL). Her labs indicate a hypochromic microcytic anemia. Her pregnancy test is negative. The most common coagulopathy associated in adolescents with menorrhagia is:

   A. Hemophilia A

   B. Hemophilia B

   C. Von Willebrand

   D. Factor V Leiden

Correct Answer C: *Von Willebrand*. Von Willebrand is the most common hereditary disorder. It represents 1%. It is the leading coagulopathy in adolescent menorrhagia. The treatment includes intranasal or IV desmopressin acetate if mild or von Willebrand factor concentrate if severe. Oral contraceptive pill may provide control. Hemophilia is rare in girls. Factor V Leiden is a disorder that increases the risk of clots.

103. A 63-year-old female presents with a fever, anemia, renal failure, and mental status changes. On exam you note fever to 101, petechiae on legs. Labs reveal a differential that notes schistocytes. What is your likely diagnosis?

   A. Idiopathic thrombocytopenic purpura (ITP)
   B. Thrombotic thrombocytopenic purpura (TTP)
   C. Meningitis
   D. Endocarditis

Correct Answer B: ***Thrombotic thrombocytopenic purpura (TTP).*** For TTP just remember FATRN. The pneumonic represents fever, hemolytic anemia, thrombocytopenia, renal failure, and neurologic dysfunction. It is a condition where blood clots form in the small blood vessels throughout. The red blood cells break apart faster than the body can produce them. Treatment involves fresh frozen plasma and plasma exchange. ITP does not present with anemia. The morphology of red blood cells and leukocytes are normal. Meningitis and endocarditis are less likely to cause all of the symptoms in her presentation.

104. A 58-year-old male with history of hypertension on lisinopril for 5 years presents with sudden onset of swelling of the tongue and uvula. On exam, vital signs remain stable. His O_2 level is 98% on room air. His respiratory rate is 18. He appears in no distress. He is not drooling. The most appropriate management for this patient is:

   A. Immediate intubation
   B. IV methylprednisolone, IV fluids, O_2, and observation for 1 hour
   C. Epinephrine subcutaneous, IV Benadryl, IV fluids, and O_2, and observation for 12 to 24 hours
   D. Discharge with antihistamines and steroid taper

Correct Answer C: ***Epinephrine subcutaneous, IV Benadryl, IV fluids, O_2, and observation for 12 to 24 hours.*** The patient needs observation of his airway for at least 12 hours with ace inhibitor angioedema. He is stable with no distress; therefore, intubation is not warranted. He should not be discharged with airway swelling.

105. A 46-year-old female undergoing outpatient oral chemotherapy for metastatic ovarian cancer presents with 24 hours of fever, diarrhea, and fatigue. She has no indwelling catheters. Her fever is 101.3; BP is 128/58; heart rate is 92; O_2 sat is 98% on room air. Labs reveal an absolute neutrophil count of <500 cells per μL. Hepatic and renal functions are normal. Chest x-ray is normal. Urinalysis is normal. The best management of this patient initially is:

   A. IV moxifloxacin × 1 dose, and discharge on Augmentin and ciprofloxacin orally with close follow-up
   B. IV cefepime 2 g IV q8h and oncology admission
   C. IV vancomycin (15 mg per kg) IV q12h and oncology admission
   D. IV Unasyn 3 g IV and discharge on Augmentin and ciprofloxacin

Correct Answer B: ***IV cefepime 2 g IV q8h and oncology admission.*** Initiation of monotherapy with an antipseudomonal β-lactam agent has been shown to be effective. Other agents such as vancomycin can be added with complicated presentations such as hypotension, pneumonia, indwelling catheters, or significant history of Methicillin-resistant *Staphylococcus aureus*. Fluoroquinolones is not the first line. Unasyn is not recommended, as it is not a broad-spectrum antibiotic.

106. A 57-year-old male presents to the emergency department status post discharge from the hospital yesterday following an admission for a lower gastrointestinal (GI) bleed. During his stay over the past 5 days, he had a hematocrit as low as 19. He was transfused two units of packed red blood cells upon admission and went to the GI service for a colonoscopy, where

the bleeding was stopped. He presents to the emergency room today with possible transfusion reaction. The most common symptom present is:

A. Fever and chills
B. Urticaria
C. Thrombocytopenia
D. Wheezing

Correct Answer A: *Fever and chills.* The most common symptom of transfusion reaction is fever and chills. This can occur even when the blood is correctly matched. Urticaria and wheezing can occur, but less commonly than fever and chills. Hemolytic reactions are rare.

107. An 8-week pregnant, G1P0AB1, female presents with heavy vaginal bleeding, which began today. She has had no prenatal care thus so far. Upon exam, her vital signs are normal. There are clots in the vaginal vault, and her cervical os is open. Pelvic ultrasound reveals no intrauterine pregnancy. Her blood type reveals that she is Rh incompatible. It means that her blood type is:

A. Rh positive
B. Rh negative

Correct Answer B: *Rh negative.* Rh incompatibility is a condition that develops when a pregnant woman has Rh-negative blood and the baby in her womb has Rh-positive blood. Rhogam should be given to an Rh-negative woman during every pregnancy, during miscarriage or abortion, after prenatal tests such as amniocentesis and chorionic villus biopsy, after injury to the abdomen during pregnancy.

108. A 19-year-old male with hemophilia A presents to the emergency room with severe pain and swelling to his left knee after a mechanical fall while walking down the stairs. On exam, his vital signs are normal. He is in moderate pain. His left knee has an obvious effusion. The best management is:

A. Factor VII replacement, arthrocentesis, and pain control
B. Factor VII replacement and pain control
C. Factor VIII replacement, arthrocentesis, and pain control
D. Factor VIII replacement and pain control

Correct Answer D: *Factor VIII replacement and pain control.* Factor VIII is the correct concentrate. Hemarthrosis is considered a major hemorrhage in a hemophiliac. Arthrocentesis should be avoided unless pain is severe and synovial tension is present.

109. A 55-year-old male with history of hypertension, bipolar disorder on metoprolol, simvastatin, and lithium presents to the emergency room complaining of 3 months of progressive polydipsia and polyuria. Basic metabolic panel demonstrates a Na of 148, a creatinine of 2.2, and a serum glucose of 108. Urinalysis is negative for leukocyte esterase, nitrites, or blood, with a specific gravity of 1.005. The most likely diagnosis is:

A. Acute lower urinary tract infection
B. Obstructive uropathy
C. Diabetic nephropathy
D. Lithium-induced diabetes insipidus

Correct Answer D: *Lithium-induced diabetes insipidus.* Chronic lithium ingestion interferes with the normal response to antidiuretic hormone, leading to a decrease in the ability of the kidney to concentrate the urine by removing free water. This causes excessive thirst and excretion of large volumes of dilute urine. Diabetic nephropathy is unlikely given a normal serum glucose. A negative urinalysis eliminates acute urinary tract infection. Obstructive uropathy is unlikely in the absence of pain and microscopic hematuria.

110. Salicylate toxicity is characterized by the following acid-base abnormalities?

    A. Primary respiratory alkalosis plus a primary metabolic acidosis
    B. Respiratory alkalosis
    C. Metabolic acidosis
    D. Metabolic alkalosis

Correct Answer A: *Primary respiratory alkalosis plus a primary metabolic acidosis*. Salicylate toxicity is marked by an initial primary respiratory alkalosis (due to direct stimulation of respiratory centers), followed by a metabolic acidosis (mainly attributable to production of lactic acid), resulting in a mixed acid-base disorder.

111. A 26-year-old male presents to the emergency department with altered mental status after running a marathon. Exam is notable for temp 98.8°F, HR 110, BP 118/62, RR 26, O_2 sat 98% on RA without focal neurologic deficits. Basic metabolic panel demonstrates Na of 117. Which is the next step in management?

    A. Immerse the patient in cold water
    B. IV normal saline (NS) infusion
    C. IV 3% saline infusion
    D. IV D5 NS infusion

Correct Answer C: *IV 3% saline infusion*. In severely symptomatic patients with hyponatremia, hypertonic (3% saline) is first-line treatment. Normal saline can exacerbate hyponatremia in patients with syndrome of inappropriate antidiuretic hormone secretion. Dextrose solutions are not useful in treating hyponatremia. Cooling techniques are used in acute heat stroke, but are not helpful for hyponatremia.

112. A 76-year-old female recently treated with high-dose prednisone for polymyalgia rheumatica presents to the emergency department complaining of nausea, vomiting, and confusion, with 4/4 systemic inflammatory response syndrome criteria and systolic blood pressures in the mid-80s refractory to fluid resuscitation. Aside from appropriate antibiotics for presumed sepsis, the most important treatment is which of the following?

    A. Additional IV normal saline bolus
    B. IV norepinephrine infusion via central access
    C. 100 mg IV hydrocortisone
    D. 50 mEq IV sodium bicarbonate

Correct Answer C: *100 mg IV hydrocortisone*. This patient's refractory hypotension is likely due to adrenal crisis. The most important treatment in this case is stress dose hydrocortisone. Additional IV fluids and pressors, while important, will not work in the absence of glucocorticoids. While sodium bicarbonate may have a role in treating concomitant hyperkalemia, it is not the best answer here.

113. The most common metabolic abnormalities associated with Addison disease include which of the following?

    A. Hypernatremia/hypokalemia
    B. Hyponatremia/hyperkalemia
    C. Hyponatremia/hyperglycemia
    D. Hypernatremia/hypocalcemia

Correct Answer B: *Hyponatremia/hyperkalemia*. Addison disease is a chronic endocrine disorder in which the adrenal glands do not produce adequate glucocorticoids (and at times, mineralocorticoids). These patients develop hyponatremia due to the kidneys' inability to excrete free water in the absence of cortisol. Hyperkalemia is also common due to insufficient aldosterone production.

114. What is the most common cause of hypoparathyroidism?

    A. Hemochromatosis
    B. Hypothyroidism
    C. Autoimmune disease
    D. Surgical procedures of the neck/throat

Correct Answer D: *Surgical procedures of the neck/throat.* Surgical procedures of the neck remain the most common cause of acquired hypoparathyroidism. Although with improvements in surgical techniques, autoimmune processes may overtake iatrogenic causes in the near future. There is no causal relationship between hypothyroidism and disorders of the parathyroid. Hemochromatosis can lead to parathyroid dysfunction, but is not the most common cause.

115. A 47-year-old female, post-op day two from thyroidectomy, presents to the emergency department complaining of fatigue, muscle cramps, as well as paresthesias of her fingertips and perioral area. Which will be most helpful in establishing a diagnosis?

    A. Comprehensive metabolic panel
    B. Noncontrast head CT
    C. Electrocardiogram
    D. Chest x-ray

Correct Answer A: *Comprehensive metabolic panel.* This patient's symptoms appear to be consistent with hypocalcemia, which is most easily diagnosed with laboratory studies. In addition to serum Ca, measurement of serum albumin is paramount to distinguish true hypocalcemia from factious hypocalcemia. Computed tomography scans, ECG, and chest x-ray may otherwise be indicated in this patient's workup, but will not be the most helpful of the diagnostic tools listed.

116. Which of the following is a life-threatening complication of treating hyponatremia?

    A. Acute coronary syndrome
    B. Central pontine myelinolysis
    C. Subarachnoid hemorrhage
    D. Diabetes insipidus

Correct Answer B: *Central pontine myelinolysis.* Correcting serum Na too rapidly can precipitate central pontine myelinosis, a neurologic complication that can produce spastic quadriparesis, swallowing dysfunction, and mutism. The rate of correction should not exceed 8 to 12 mEq/L/day. Subarachnoid hemorrhage (SAH) is associated with cerebral salt wasting, which is a potential cause of hyponatremia. However, SAH is not a complication associated with hyponatremia treatments. Acute coronary syndrome and diabetes insipidus are not known complications of hyponatremia treatments.

117. Which of the following agents most rapidly counteracts the cardiac effects of hyperkalemia?

    A. Albuterol
    B. Calcium gluconate
    C. Kayexalate
    D. Insulin-dextrose

Correct Answer B: *Calcium gluconate.* Calcium gluconate counteracts the cardiac effects of hyperkalemia by stabilizing the cardiac cell membrane against undesirable depolarization. Insulin administered with dextrose acts to facilitate the uptake of glucose into cells, bringing K with it. Albuterol also facilitates the shift of K intracellularly. Kayexalate binds K in the gut, with an onset of action of 2 to 24 hours.

118. Pseudohyponatremia is caused by which of the following?

    A. Diarrhea
    B. Marked hyperlipidemia/hypertriglyceridemia
    C. Hypocalcemia
    D. Use of loop diuretics

Correct Answer B: *Marked hyperlipidemia/hypertriglyceridemia.* Extraordinarily high blood levels of lipid can interfere with certain laboratory tests of serum Na concentration, resulting in an erroneously low Na measurement. Loop diuretics are sometimes used with intravenous normal saline to treat hyponatremia. Large-volume diarrhea may cause hypovolemic hyponatremia. Hypocalcemia is not associated with pseudohyponatremia.

119. A 60-year-old male, with a history of prostate cancer, presents to the emergency department with atraumatic low back pain for 2 weeks with new left lower extremity weakness and urinary incontinence. What is the first thing you would do for this patient?

    A. Order IV steroids
    B. Perform a postvoid residual urine volume
    C. Order lumbar spine x-rays
    D. Order an emergent cord compression protocol MRI

Correct Answer D: *Order an emergent cord compression protocol MRI.* The patient's symptoms are concerning for cord compression which he is at risk for with his prostate cancer; so emergency MRI is necessary. A postvoid residual volume would be helpful in this patient to determine whether he is retaining urine, but is not the first thing that should be done in his management. Lumbar x-rays would not be helpful in this diagnosis as they will not be able to assess the spinal cord. While IV steroids may be part of the treatment plan, confirming the diagnosis of cord compression as soon as possible is most important.

120. A 65-year-old male, with history of hypertension (HTN) and gout, presents with atraumatic left great toe pain, erythema, and warmth for 3 days, similar to his gout flares in the past. He takes lisinopril, metoprolol, hydrochlorothiazide, and hydralazine for his HTN. What mediation would you recommend so that he stops taking to prevent future flares?

    A. Hydrochlorothiazide (HCTZ)
    B. Lisinopril
    C. Metoprolol
    D. Hydralazine

Correct Answer A: *Hydrochlorothiazide (HCTZ).* HCTZ can precipitate acute gout flares or hyperuricemia in patients with a history of gout, a familial predisposition to gout, or chronic renal failure. The other antihypertensive medications do not have this adverse reaction.

121. What test would you perform to further confirm that a patient has carpel tunnel syndrome?

    A. Adson test
    B. Thompson test
    C. Phalen test
    D. Empty can test

Correct Answer C: *Phalen test.* Phalen test as well as Tinel test can help confirm the diagnosis of carpel tunnel. Phalen test is performed by having the patient fully flex the palms at the wrist with the elbow in full extension to provide extra pressure on the median nerve. Alternatively, the backs of the hands are placed against each other to provide hyperflexion of the wrist and the elbows remain flexed. A positive Phalen sign is defined as pain and/or paresthesias in the median-innervated fingers, with 1 minute of wrist flexion. Adson test is performed to assist in the diagnosis of thoracic outlet syndrome, while the Thompson test helps facilitate the diagnosis over Achilles rupture. Empty can test evaluates the strength and integrity of the supraspinatus muscle and tendon for rotator cuff injury.

122. A 35-year-old female presents with atraumatic left foot pain for 3 weeks. The pain is primarily over the bottom of her foot and is worse when she has to get up to go to the bathroom in the middle of the night and the morning. What is your working diagnosis?

   A. Heel spur
   B. Plantar fasciitis
   C. Peripheral neuropathy
   D. Osteoarthritis

Correct Answer B: *Plantar fasciitis.* Many patients with plantar fasciitis have the "first step in the morning" symptom, in which the pain occurs for the first few minutes after getting out of bed and then resolves, but as the disease progresses, the pain can continue throughout the day. While a heel spur can cause heel pain, there is no direct relationship to heel spurs and plantar fasciitis. It would be unusual for a 35-year-old to have osteoarthritis as well as neuropathy without diabetes, and this is an atypical presentation of both.

123. A 25-year-old male with a history of intravenous drug use presents to the emergency department with atraumatic low back pain, and there is concern for osteomyelitis. What lab studies would be helpful in the diagnosis?

   A. Wound culture
   B. Erythrocyte sedimentation rate (ESR)
   C. Lactate dehydrogenase (LDH)
   D. Rheumatoid factor

Correct Answer B: *Erythrocyte sedimentation rate (ESR).* ESR is nonspecific; however, it is elevated in 90% of cases. Superficial wound or sinus tract cultures often do not correlate with the bacteria that are causing osteomyelitis and have limited use. LDH is useful in the diagnosis of red blood cell hemolysis, is elevated in nonspecific tissue damage and liver damage, and is also one of the factors correlating with reduced survival in patients with non-Hodgkin lymphoma. Rheumatoid factor is used as a marker for patient with suspected rheumatoid arthritis or other immunologic conditions.

124. What would you expect to see on joint aspiration in a patient with pseudogout?

   A. Uric acid crystals
   B. Calcium pyrophosphate crystals
   C. Calcium oxalate
   D. Calcium phosphate

Correct Answer B: *Calcium pyrophosphate crystals.* Calcium pyrophosphate is found in synovial fluid in pseudogout. Uric acid crystals are found in gout. About 70% of kidney stones are made of calcium oxalate, and about 10% are made of calcium phosphate.

125. A 35-year-old female who works as a house cleaner presents to the emergency department with atraumatic right knee pain for 2 weeks with swelling, but she continues to have full range of motion. What is your working diagnosis?

   A. Osteoarthritis
   B. Prepatellar bursitis
   C. Iliotibial band syndrome
   D. Septic arthritis

Correct Answer B: *Prepatellar bursitis.* Prepatellar bursitis, also known as "housemaid's knee," "coal miner's knee," "carpet layer's knee," is inflammation of the prepatellar bursa and can be caused by an acute traumatic event or repeated trauma, such as one kneeling daily. Iliotibial band syndrome causes lateral knee pain typically in runners or cyclers. Osteoarthritis would be less likely in a 35-year-old, and septic arthritis would be less likely with full range of motion.

126. A 10-year-old boy presents to the emergency department with atraumatic right knee pain for 1 week with a lump. What is your working diagnosis?
    A. Osgood Schlatter disease
    B. Avascular necrosis
    C. Legg-Calvé–Perthes disease
    D. Hemarthrosis

Correct Answer A: *Osgood Schlatter disease.* Osgood Schlatter disease is an inflammation of the patellar ligament at the tibial tuberosity, which presents as painful lumps below the knee and most common in young adolescents during skeletal development, typically aggravated by running and jumping. Avascular necrosis usually involves the epiphysis of long bones, such as the femoral and humeral heads, and most commonly affects the hip and the fourth and fifth decade of life. Legg–Calvé–Perthes disease is avascular necrosis of the proximal femoral head resulting from compromise of the blood supply to this area, usually occurring in children aged 4 to 10 years. It has an insidious onset and may occur after an injury to the hip. Hemarthrosis typically occurs in a patient who has a blood disorder such as hemophilia or someone who is anticoagulated.

127. What medication is not indicated for the acute treatment of gout?
    A. Indomethacin
    B. Colchicine
    C. Allopurinol
    D. Prednisone

Correct Answer C: *Allopurinol.* All of these medications are indicated in the acute treatment of gouty arthritis except for allopurinol as it can cause an acute attack or worsen the existing attack.

128. What blood test is not helpful in the diagnosis of rheumatoid arthritis?
    A. RF (rheumatoid factor)
    B. ANA (antinuclear antibody)
    C. Erythrocyte sedimentation rate
    D. Lactate dehydrogenase (LDH)

Correct Answer D: *Lactate dehydrogenase (LDH).* All of these tests are helpful except LDH. LDH is useful in the diagnosis of red blood cell hemolysis, is elevated in nonspecific tissue damage and liver damage, and is also one of the factors correlating with reduced survival in patients with non-Hodgkin lymphoma.

129. A 15-year-old boy is brought to the emergency department by his mother with atraumatic worsening right hip pain over the past 2 weeks. He denies fever/chills. Labs show white blood cell (WBC) 5k; x-ray shows distal femoral lytic lesion with "onion-skin" appearance. Which of the following is the most likely diagnosis?
    A. Slipped capital femoral epiphysis
    B. Legg–Calvé–Perthes disease
    C. Ewing sarcoma
    D. Septic arthritis
    E. Osteomyelitis

Correct Answer C: *Ewing sarcoma.* Ewing sarcoma is correct given the "onion-skin" appearance of periosteal reaction. Ewing sarcoma is a rare malignant bone tumor seen in teenagers and young adults, typically found in the femur or pelvis. Osteomyelitis and septic arthritis can present similarly, but less likely given absence of fever or elevated WBC. Slipped capital femoral epiphysis would show displacement of the femoral head on x-ray, and Legg–Calvé–Perthes disease would show sclerosis of the femoral head, indicating avascular necrosis.

130. A 45-year-old male with a history of noninsulin-dependent diabetes mellitus and peptic ulcer disease presents with an atraumatic right knee pain and swelling for 18 hours associated with erythema, warmth, and painful ROM. Denies fever or chills. You perform arthrocentesis, and synovial fluid is cloudy, yellow, white blood cell (WBC) 35K, with needle-shaped crystals. What is the best initial treatment option?
    A. IV antibiotics
    B. Colchicine
    C. Oral corticosteroids
    D. Indomethacin
    E. Opiates

Correct Answer B: *Colchicine.* The patient has gout given the needle-shaped crystals and findings consistent with inflammatory synovial fluid. Antibiotics would be indicated in septic arthritis, which is diagnosed when fluid has WBC >50k without crystals. Typically, first-line therapy would be NSAIDs such as indomethacin, but in this case, it is contraindicated given history of peptic ulcer disease causing concern for bleeding risk. Opiates are added only for breakthrough pain, not initial therapy. Oral corticosteroids may be used to treat gout, but should be reserved for inability to take or failure of nonsteroidal anti-inflammatory drugs and colchicine. Colchicine is most effective when administered within the first 24 hours of symptom onset.

131. A 22-year-old female, who delivered a healthy baby by C-section 1 day ago, presents to the emergency department with lower abdominal pain. Her vitals are as follows: temp, 102°F; HR, 110; BP, 130/70; RR, 20; and O_2 Sat 100% on RA. On exam, she has lower abdominal tenderness, cervical motion tenderness, and foul-smelling vaginal discharge. What is the appropriate medication to start?
    A. Magnesium sulfate 4 to 6 g in 100 mL of fluid over 20 minutes, followed by 1 to 2 g per hour
    B. Ampicillin 1 g IV every 6 hours and gentamicin 15 mg per kg IV every 8 hours
    C. Ceftriaxone 250 mg IM and doxycycline 100 mg bid × 14 days
    D. Metronidazole 500 mg bid × 7 days

Correct Answer B: *Ampicillin 1 g IV every 6 hours and gentamicin 15 mg per kg IV every 8 hours.* The patient has postpartum endometritis and should be admitted for broad-spectrum antibiotics. Risk factors include cesarean delivery, prolonged ruptured membranes, and younger maternal age. Magnesium sulfate would be used for treatment in severe preeclampsia or eclampsia. Rocephin and doxycycline would be appropriate outpatient treatments for pelvic inflammatory disease. Metronidazole would be an appropriate treatment for bacterial vaginosis.

132. A 32-year-old female, G4 P3003, who is 32 weeks gestation, presents with vaginal bleeding. Her vitals are as follows: temp, 98.6°F; HR, 82; BP, 120/60; RR, 18; and O_2 sat 100% on RA. On exam, her abdomen is soft and nontender. What is the most appropriate next step?
    A. Discharge home and schedule a follow-up appointment with obstetrician/gynecologist in the morning
    B. Perform a sterile digital and speculum exam
    C. Order a transabdominal ultrasound
    D. Administer magnesium sulfate

Correct Answer C: *Order a transabdominal ultrasound.* An ultrasound is the safest test in suspected placenta previa, which usually presents with painless bright red vaginal bleeding. Risk factors include multiparity and prior cesarean section. The placenta previa is present on ultrasound. The patient is in active labor, and arrangements should be made for immediate delivery. A speculum and digital examination should be avoided because they can lead to disruption of the placenta and can lead to bleeding. Magnesium sulfate would be used in treatment of preeclampsia.

133. A 39-year-old female, 33 weeks gestation, presents with vaginal bleeding and abdominal pain. Her medical history is significant for smoking 1 ppd. Her vitals are as follows: temp, 98.6°F; HR, 110; BP, 90/60; RR, 20; and O_2 sat 100% on RA. Which of the following is *false*?

    A. Lab tests should include a complete blood count, type/cross match, and coagulation studies.
    B. Crystalloids should be administered.
    C. Emergency obstetrical consultation is necessary.
    D. Administer Magnesium 2 gm IV.

Correct Answer D: *Administer Magnesium 2 gm IV.* The patient has abruptio placentae (or placental abruption), which is a separation of the placenta from the uterine wall. It accounts for 30% of bleeding in the second half of pregnancy. Magnesium is used in the treatment of seizures. Lab tests should be performed, crystalloids should be started, and emergent obstetric/gynecologic consultation should be obtained, because complications could include fetal death, maternal death from hemorrhage, or disseminated intravascular coagulation.

134. A 25-year-old female, 35 weeks gestation, arrives with epigastric pain and a headache. Vitals include the following: temp, 98.7°F; HR, 82; BP, 158/98; RR, 16; and O_2 sat 100% on RA. She is Rh positive. Her labs were significant for proteinuria. Which of the following statements is *not true*?

    A. Administer Rhogam
    B. May administer magnesium sulfate IV followed by an infusion
    C. Hydralazine or labetalol may be administered.
    D. Betamethasone may be administered.

Correct Answer A: *Administer Rhogam.* This patient has preeclampsia. Rhogam is administered to Rh-negative mothers. Magnesium sulfate may be used in severe preeclampsia to prevent seizures. Hydralazine or labetalol may be used for blood pressure control. Betamethasone may be given under 34 weeks of gestation to enhance fetal lung maturity.

135. A 32-year-old female presents with vaginal spotting for 3 days and left pelvic pain for 2 hours. Her last menstrual period was about 7 weeks ago. Her vitals are stable. She has left adnexal tenderness on examination. Her serum β-hCG is 2,000 mU per mL. Pelvic ultrasound shows no intrauterine pregnancy, but a left adnexal mass is present. What is the next step in management of this patient?

    A. Laparoscopy
    B. Discharge home and reexamine in the morning
    C. Methotrexate
    D. Ceftriaxone 250 mg intramuscular (IM)

Correct Answer C: *Methotrexate.* This patient has an ectopic pregnancy with a triad of abdominal pain, amenorrhea, and vaginal bleeding. Methotrexate intramuscularly may be given with a treatment plan developed by the emergency department and obstetric/gynecologic department. A patient with an ectopic pregnancy should not be discharged home without treatment because of the risks of a ruptured ectopic pregnancy, hemorrhage, or death. Laparoscopy is useful in patients with suspected ectopic pregnancy and a nondiagnostic ultrasound. While laparoscopy is an option, this patient is stable and can be medically managed with methotrexate. Ceftriaxone IM is used in the treatment of *Neisseria gonorrhoeae.*

136. A 22-year-old female presents with vaginal itching and discharge for 2 days. Her vitals are stable, and she has no abdominal tenderness on examination. Pelvic examination reveals vaginal erythema and a frothy, malodorous discharge. What is the treatment for the patient?

    A. Fluconazole 150 mg orally as single dose
    B. Acyclovir 400 mg orally tid for 7 to 10 days
    C. Benzathine penicillin (PCN) G 2.4 million units intramuscular
    D. Metronidazole 2 g orally as a single dose

Correct Answer D: *Metronidazole 2 g orally as a single dose.* This patient has Trichomonas vaginitis. It may cause vaginal irritation, pelvic pain, or a yellow-green frothy discharge. A "strawberry cervix," punctate hemorrhages visible on the cervix, may be visible on examination. It may be diagnosed microscopically by the presence of motile flagellates. Fluconazole would treat candida vaginitis, which would reveal a "cottage cheese" discharge. Acyclovir would treat genital herpes, which would cause painful, fluid-filled vesicles which progress to shallow-based ulcers. Benzathine PCN G would treat syphilis, characterized by a painless ulcer with a clean base.

137. A 21-year-old female presents with pelvic pain and vaginal discharge for 2 days. She is sexually active with multiple partners and does not use any contraceptives. Her vitals are as follows: temp, 101.7°F; HR, 100; BP, 110/70; RR, 18; and O_2 sat 100% on RA. She has adnexal tenderness, cervical motion tenderness, and mucopurulent discharge on pelvic examination. Her β-hCG is negative. What is the best treatment?

    A. Ceftriaxone 250 mg intramuscular (IM) and doxycycline 100 mg bid for 14 days
    B. Ofloxacin 400 mg bid for 14 days
    C. Metronidazole 500 mg bid for 14 days
    D. Discharge the patient home without treatment and wait for culture results

Correct Answer A: *Ceftriaxone 250 mg IM and doxycycline 100 mg bid for 14 days.* This patient has pelvic inflammatory disease (PID). *Neisseria gonorrhoeae* and/or *Chlamydia trachomatis* are isolated in most cases. Ceftriaxone and doxycycline are appropriate oral/outpatient treatment regimens. Ofloxacin or metronidazole alone would not provide adequate coverage against anaerobes, gram-negative organisms, streptococci, as well as *N. gonorrhoeae* and *C. trachomatis*. PID should not be left untreated. PID is associated with serious sequelae: tubo-ovarian abscess, infertility, chronic pelvic pain, and ectopic pregnancy.

138. A 24-year-old female presents with vaginal pruritus and vaginal discharge for 3 days. Her vitals are stable. Examination reveals gray-white vaginal discharge. Clue cells are seen on a saline wet prep. Which of the following is *not* true about her diagnosis?

    A. It has been associated with preterm labor and premature rupture of membranes (PROM).
    B. Treatment is metronidazole 500 mg bid po for 7 days.
    C. Treatment should be delayed for pregnant patients.
    D. Fishy odor will be noted by addition of KOH to the discharge.

Correct Answer C: *Treatment should be delayed for pregnant patients.* The patient has bacterial vaginosis. Treatment should not be delayed in symptomatic patients, regardless of pregnancy status, because of complications associated with preterm labor and PROM. Treatment includes metronidazole 500 mg bid orally for 7 days. In the first trimester of pregnancy, metronidazole 0.75%, one applicator intravaginally bid for 5 days may be given. The fishy odor is present when KOH is added to the discharge is known as a positive whiff (amine) test.

139. A 20-year-old female presents with pelvic pain. Exam reveals painful vesicles on an erythematous base in the vulvovaginal area. The patient has had no prior episodes. What is the best treatment for this patient?

    A. Valacyclovir 1 g bid for 7 to 10 days
    B. Metronidazole 500 mg bid for 7 days
    C. Fluconazole 150 mg po as a single dose
    D. Benzathine penicillin (PCN) G 2.4 million units intramuscular as a single dose

Correct Answer A: *Valacyclovir 1 g bid for 7 to 10 days.* Patient's presentation is consistent with herpes simplex. Primary infections present after an incubation period of 7 to 10 days, with painful vesicular lesions which progress to shallow-based ulcers. Metronidazole is used in treatment of bacterial vaginosis, which would have a frothy gray-white discharge. Fluconazole 150 mg as a single dose can be used in treatment of candida vaginitis, which would have a thick white discharge. Benzathine PCN G would be used to treat syphilis, which is characterized by a painless chancre or ulcer.

140. A 30-year-old lactating female, 4 weeks postpartum, presents with right breast pain. Her vitals are as follows: temp, 101°F; HR, 100; BP, 120/60; RR, 18; and O_2 sat 100% on RA. The upper outer quadrant of her breast is warm and erythematous. What is the appropriate treatment?

    A. Vancomycin
    B. Penicillin (PCN)
    C. Dicloxacillin
    D. Metronidazole

Correct Answer C: *Dicloxacillin.* The patient has postpartum mastitis, which is commonly caused by *Staphylococcus aureus*. Dicloxacillin would be the best choice because it is a penicillinase-resistant PCN. Vancomycin would be appropriate for methicillin-resistant staphylococcal infections. PCN would not provide appropriate coverage. Metronidazole would be helpful for infections caused by anaerobes.

141. The most commonly torn rotator cuff tendon in overuse injuries:

    A. Teres minor
    B. Teres major
    C. Infraspinatus
    D. Supraspinatus
    E. Subscapularis

Correct Answer D: *Supraspinatus.* The rotator cuff is made up of four muscles—supraspinatus, infraspinatus, teres minor, and subscapularis. The supraspinatus is located on the superior aspect of the joint responsible for shoulder abduction and passes through the subacromial space. With repetitive overhead activity, this can cause stress on this muscle tendon, increasing risk of injury.

142. A 35-year-old male with a history of diabetes and a recent right shoulder sprain that has kept his shoulder in a sling for 1 week now presents with limited and painful range of motion. Exam reveals no fever or erythema, but has restricted and painful external rotation. The most likely diagnosis is:

    A. Frozen shoulder
    B. Rotator cuff tear
    C. Septic arthritis
    D. Impingement syndrome

Correct Answer A: *Frozen shoulder.* Risk factors include prior injury and immobility, diabetes mellitus, connective tissue disorders. Most common finding is limited shoulder external rotation.

Treatment is conservative, including nonsteroidal anti-inflammatory drugs, rest, ice, compression, elevation, but may require manipulation under general anesthesia to break up adhesions. Presentation is not consistent with septic arthritis as no fever or redness, less likely impingement syndrome, or rotator cuff injury as he has worsening pain despite immobilization.

143. A 27-year-old runner presents with atraumatic left anterior knee pain. The patient denies swelling, redness, or paresthesias. Pain worsens when going up or down stairs and recalls it being very painful recently when standing after watching a 2-hour movie. X-ray is negative for acute bony abnormality. The clinical diagnosis is most consistent with:

    A. Osteosarcoma
    B. Patellofemoral syndrome
    C. Meniscal tear
    D. Anterior cruciate ligament tear
    E. Posterior cruciate ligament tear

Correct Answer B: *Patellofemoral syndrome.* This is the most common cause of anterior knee pain. "Theater sign" or pain worsening after prolonged sitting is often described. Meniscal tear typically presents with joint line tenderness. No trauma or instability makes anterior cruciate ligament or posterior cruciate ligament tear less likely. Osteosarcoma is a malignant bone neoplasm which may be seen on x-ray.

144. A 30-year-old female with history of intravenous drug use (IVDU) presents with red warm right knee and fever 101. Joint aspirate is concerning for septic arthritis. Which antibiotic is the most important to include in the initial empiric treatment?

    A. Ceftriaxone
    B. Vancomycin
    C. Azithromycin
    D. Augmentin
    E. Gentamycin

Correct Answer B: *Vancomycin.* Given the patient's history of IVDU, Methicillin-resistant *Staphylococcus aureus* (MRSA) must be suspected and vancomycin is the only listed option, which covers for MRSA. A second- or third-generation cephalosporin such as ceftriaxone should also be added for additional gram-negative coverage.

145. A positive Finkelstein test would be indicative of what condition?

    A. Carpal tunnel syndrome
    B. Tarsal tunnel syndrome
    C. De Quervain tenosynovitis
    D. Achilles tendon rupture
    E. Plantar fasciitis

Correct Answer C: *De Quervain tenosynovitis.* This is an inflammation of the extensor pollicis brevis and abductor pollicis longus tendon sheaths thought to be due to repetitive activity. Grasping the thumb, which is quickly ulnar deviated, performs the test. Sharp pain over the distal radius would indicate a positive test.

146. Which antibiotic is linked to atraumatic Achilles tendon rupture?

    A. Cephalexin
    B. Vancomycin
    C. Doxycycline
    D. Ciprofloxacin

Correct Answer D: *Ciprofloxacin.* Other fluoroquinolones are also linked and carry black-box warnings for tendonitis and tendon rupture. The exact mechanism is unclear, but may be due to interruption in joint blood supply or collagen formation.

147. What physical exam findings would be consistent with L3 to L4 lumbar disc radiculopathy?
     A. Decreased sensation lateral malleolus
     B. Weakness of great toe dorsiflexion
     C. Weakness of ankle dorsiflexion
     D. Weakness of ankle plantar flexion

Correct Answer D: *Weakness of ankle dorsiflexion.* It may also find decreased patellar reflex and sensation medial malleolus. L4 to L5 would reveal weakness of great toe dorsiflexion, and L5 to S1 would be consistent with weakness of ankle plantar flexion.

148. An 8-year-old male presents with mild right hip pain and a limp for 3 weeks. There is no known trauma or inciting event. On exam, afebrile with decreased internal rotation. X-rays show a mildly flattened femoral head. What is the most likely diagnosis?
     A. Transient synovitis
     B. Septic arthritis
     C. Legg–Calvé–Perthes syndrome
     D. Slipped capital femoral epiphysis

Correct Answer C: *Legg–Calvé–Perthes syndrome.* The pain and limp are due to avascular necrosis of the femoral head, sometimes not seen on x-ray and may require MRI for further evaluation. Although slipped capital femoral epiphysis can present similarly, x-rays show dissociation of the femoral epiphysis with the metaphysis that may result in avascular necrosis, and most cases require orthopedic surgical treatment. This presentation is not consistent with transient synovitis or septic arthritis as no history of fever or recent viral illness.

149. A patient presents to the emergency department complaining of hip pain. When asked further questions regarding this pain, the patient trails off telling unrelated stories about irrelevant topics, but eventually returns to the original subject at hand. What process is this person demonstrating?
     A. Circumstantiality
     B. Tangentially
     C. Flight of ideas
     D. Mania

Correct answer A: *Circumstantiality.* This implies that the original topic or question is returned to despite deviating from this topic along the way. Tangentially is incorrect because it means the person will go off on a tangent of topics, but does *not* return to the original topic of discussion. Flight of ideas implies that the person will discuss whatever topic enters his or her brain spontaneously, even if they are unrelated to each other. Mania is characterized by a state or period of intense elation, and often lack of sleep, grandiose gestures, and feeling invincible.

150. A patient presents to the emergency department complaining of foot pain. He is found to have multiple recent visits for various different complaints that have been worked up with negative results. The patient is convinced he has a medical disorder that is causing these unrelated issues and continued to have new complaints frequently. What is the most likely diagnosis?
     A. Obsessive compulsive disorder
     B. Hypochondriasis
     C. Panic disorder
     D. Schizophrenia

Correct answer B: *Hypochondriasis.* This is a condition in which individuals are convinced they have a variety of health concerns when there is often no diagnosis found. Obsessive compulsive disorder is often characterized by impulsive gestures that are irrational and the person recognizes as such. Panic disorder is when patients suffer from frequent panic attacks that can be triggered by a variety of scenarios. Disorganized thinking, delusions, and hallucinations characterize schizophrenia.

151. Which of the following medications can precipitate a manic event in an individual with suspected depression?
    A. Olanzapine
    B. Aripiprazole
    C. Sertraline
    D. Nortriptyline

Correct answer C: *Sertraline.* Patients with an underlying history (or family history) of bipolar disorder can be thrown into a manic event when given selective serotonin reuptake inhibitors (SSRIs) for treatment of depression. The mechanism by which this happens is directly related to the inhibition of serotonin reuptake in the synaptic space. Patients who have had a suspected manic episode in the past should not be started on SSRIs as initial management of depression. The remaining medications in this list act on different neurotransmitters (or less heavily on serotonin) and are therefore unlikely to propagate a manic episode.

152. A 38-year-old female is brought to the emergency department after she was missing for several days. She did not return back to her home after dropping her kids off from school one morning. She was found in the next town over from her home. When questioned about her disappearance, the woman provides you with a different name and profession, and is unable to identify her family members. What is the most likely diagnosis?
    A. Bipolar disorder
    B. Dissociative fugue
    C. Dementia
    D. Histrionic personality disorder

Correct answer B: *Dissociative fugue.* Dissociative fugue is when an individual removes himself/herself from his or her prior identity and lifestyle, and assumes a new identity. Bipolar disorder involves both episodes of depression and mania, but does not mean people change their names, profession, etc. Dementia is often age related and occurs gradually over time. Histrionic personality disorder is characterized by excessive attention-seeking behavior and attempted manipulation.

153. Which of the following trio of symptoms suggests a diagnosis of schizophrenia?
    A. Depression, anxiety, suicidal ideation
    B. Flight of ideas, word salad, tics
    C. Disorganized thinking, grandiose gestures, emotionally labile
    D. Auditory hallucinations, visual hallucinations, disorganized thinking

Correct answer D: *Auditory hallucinations, visual hallucinations, disorganized thinking.* Hallucinations (both auditory and visual) and disorganized thinking or behavior are characteristic traits of schizophrenia. Depression, anxiety, and suicidal ideation can be linked to major depressive or generalized anxiety disorder. Option B includes speech characteristics that collectively do not pertain to a specific diagnosis. Individually, tics often occur in individuals with Tourette syndrome. Grandiose gestures are often used to describe someone's activity when he or she is in a manic episode. Emotional lability describes incontrollable crying or laughing that often occurs after a brain injury.

154. A mother brings her 8-year-old daughter to the emergency department with the complaint that she has been having diarrhea. The child appears dehydrated and malnourished; so she

is admitted to the hospital for further workup. Upon further investigation, the child has been brought to her pediatrician multiple times for the same complaint, and has repeatedly given a diagnosis of acute gastroenteritis. While admitted to the hospital, the child has a single episode of nonbloody, watery diarrhea that quickly resolves after admission. On hospital day 2, she is able to tolerate food and liquids without any difficulty. Her hospital workup shows normal blood work and negative stool cultures. Immediately after returning home, the mother calls the pediatrician's office again complaining that the child's diarrhea has returned, is now associated with nonbilious nonbloody vomiting, and the hospital must not have done their job correctly. What is the most likely diagnosis?

    A. Ulcerative colitis
    B. Crohn disease
    C. Munchausen by proxy
    D. Foodborne illness

Correct answer C: *Munchausen by proxy syndrome*. This syndrome occurs when individuals create or fabricate health concerns for individuals they take care of. In this scenario, the mother is thought to be inducing diarrhea in her daughter, since her symptoms completely resolve once the child is under someone else's care. In addition, her negative workup suggests that this diarrhea would resolve on its own if it was not self-inflicted. Ulcerative colitis and Crohn's disease are often characterized by bloody diarrhea and are accompanied by abdominal pain, bloating, and elevated white blood cell count. Foodborne illness often occurs approximately 6 hours after ingesting the affected substance, and usually resolves after 24 hours. In addition, foodborne illness might have positive stool culture results in the case of *Salmonella*, *Campylobacter*, *Shigella*, etc.

155. Which of the following medications should be avoided in an individual with a known prolonged QT interval?

    A. Ondansetron
    B. Quetiapine
    C. Levofloxacin
    D. All of the above

Correct answer D: *All of the above*. All of the listed medications can potentially further elongate someone's QT interval, resulting in sudden arrhythmia and sometimes death.

156. A woman goes to her doctor's office and demands to be seen immediately by a practitioner, claiming she is the Queen of England and has a serious health issue. She is told that she must call to make an appointment due to the office's booked schedule, but she refuses to leave. She begins to cause a disturbance in the waiting room; so security is called to escort her out of the office. She continues to discuss her royal stature and attempts to flirt with the security guard in order to divert the trouble. After being escorted out of the office, the patient gets extremely agitated and begins weeping in the lobby of the building. What is the most likely diagnosis?

    A. Borderline personality disorder
    B. Histrionic personality disorder
    C. Conversion personality disorder
    D. Bipolar personality disorder

Correct answer B: *Histrionic personality disorder*. This is characterized by excessive attention-seeking behavior and attempted manipulation, as this patient exhibits by claiming to be the Queen of England. It is often accompanied by exaggerated and frequently changing emotions, as exemplified by her flirtation that quickly turned to agitation. Borderline personality disorder is often described by one's interpersonal relationships. Individuals with this diagnosis have difficulty maintaining friendships, have fear of abandonment, and have difficulty handling their emotions.

Conversion personality disorder often presents as a loss in sensory or motor function that is unexplained by a medical workup. Bipolar disorder is characterized by episodes of both depression and mania.

157. What is the recommended first-line therapy in someone with newly diagnosed generalized anxiety disorder (GAD)?

    A. Atypical antipsychotics
    B. Benzodiazepines
    C. Tricyclic antidepressants
    D. Low-dose selective serotonin reuptake inhibitors (SSRIs)

Correct answer D: *Low-dose selective serotonin reuptake inhibitors (SSRIs).* These have been found to be effective in treating GAD, and are recommended as the initial therapy. Benzodiazepines are often used in conjunction with SSRIs for breakthrough anxiety, but alone are not sufficient for treatment of GAD. In addition, benzodiazepines have several side effects that prevent them from being used on a regular basis (such as sedation, psychomotor impairment, and withdrawal symptoms). Tricyclic antidepressants are often used to treat major depressive disorder in patients who have failed SSRIs. Atypical antipsychotics are traditionally used to treat personality disorders and are not indicated as treatment for GAD.

158. A 55-year-old male is brought into the emergency department by emergency medical services after being found unresponsive on a park bench. Upon arrival to the emergency department, the patient appears disheveled, unkempt, and smells of alcohol. The patient responds to aggressive sternal rub, but otherwise appears somnolent. His blood alcohol level returns at 405. The patient has not been treated at this hospital before, and prior medical records are unable to be obtained. After several hours in the emergency room, one of the nurses comes out of his room and reports he appeared tremulous, diaphoretic, and agitated. What is the best next step in the care of this patient?

    A. Administer intravenous lorazepam immediately
    B. Administer intranasal Narcan
    C. Give a 1 L bolus of IV fluid
    D. Discharge the patient home

Correct answer A: *Administer intravenous lorazepam immediately.* The patient is exhibiting signs of alcohol withdrawal. The appropriate management for alcohol withdrawal in an acute setting is benzodiazepines, as they decrease the symptoms of withdrawal by enhancing γ-aminobutyric acid receptor activity. If the patient continued to withdraw from alcohol and no treatment was administered, he would be at risk for experiencing withdrawal seizures. Narcan is useful when it is suspected that someone has overdosed on opioids, and is ineffective at treating symptoms of alcohol withdrawal. Administering IV fluids in a patient who is intoxicated is helpful to achieve hydration, but will not have any effect on symptoms of alcohol withdrawal. Discharging the patient home is an inappropriate option given the patient could experience delirium tremens if not properly treated.

159. A 25-year-old male presents to the emergency department with "a black eye." He states last night he was in a fight with his roommate and was punched in the left eye. Today he woke up with blurry vision and pain. On exam you note ecchymosis and edema of the periorbital tissues, subconjunctival hemorrhage, and that the left eye remains fixed when the patient gazes upward. What condition are you concerned about?

    A. Entrapment of the inferior oblique muscle
    B. Blowout fracture with entrapment of the inferior rectus muscle
    C. Mandible fracture with inferior rectus and lateral rectus muscle rupture
    D. Blowout fracture with entrapment of the superior rectus muscle

Correct Answer B: *Blowout fracture with entrapment of the inferior rectus muscle.* This question tests the examinee's ability to correctly identify the disorder and its complications. Options A and D are incorrect as these muscles do not control upward gaze. Option C is incorrect as there is no indication in the history of a mandibular fracture.

160. The patient from question 1 has a CT scan showing fracture of the medial wall and orbital floor with air. What is the appropriate treatment course and discharge plan?

    A. Transport to the operating room for emergent surgical intervention
    B. Discharge home with referral to ENT
    C. Discharge home with sinus precautions, decongestants, Augmentin 875/125 bid ×
       7 days, and plan for surgery within 2 weeks
    D. Discharge home with nasal splint, oxycodone, and erythromycin ointment

Correct Answer C: *Discharge home with sinus precautions, decongestants, Augmentin 875/125 bid × 7 days, and plan for surgery within 2 weeks.* This question relies on the examinee's ability to correctly identify the injury and its treatment plan. Isolated blowout fractures are rarely operative and certainly not urgently. We do not splint these fractures, and although ENT referral is indicated, there are other instructions the patient needs.

161. A 35-year-old male is brought to the emergency department from a softball game with co-workers holding his face. He tells you that he walked behind a friend swinging a bat and was struck in the face with a metal bat. He "blacked out for a few seconds." He is holding a bloodstained shirt to his face and is complaining of severe facial pain, and has no other complaints. You obtain a maxillofacial CT scan and note a pyramidal fracture of the central maxilla and palate. What type of fracture is this?

    A. Nasal fracture
    B. LeFort I
    C. LeFort II
    D. LeFort III
    E. LeFort IV

Correct Answer C: *LeFort II. LeFort II fracture is pyramidal fracture of the central maxilla and palate.* A nasal fracture involves only the nasal bones. LeFort I is a transverse fracture that separates the maxilla from the lower portion of the pterygoid plate and nasal septum. LeFort III or craniofacial dissociation is a fracture line through the nasofrontal and frontomaxillary sutures, extending along the medial wall of the orbit through the ethmoid bones, along the floor of the orbit to the zygomatic arch. Facial tugging causes the entire face. LeFort IV fractures include the frontal bone and midface.

162. A 75-year-old male with a medical history of atrial fibrillation, hypertension, and non-insulin-dependent diabetes is brought in by ambulance after an unwitnessed fall. He states he was walking in his kitchen when he "fell out." The next thing he remembers is his wife standing over him shouting. Emergency medical services reports that his vital signs in the field are as follows: temp, 97.4°F; HR, 130; irregular BP, 100/60; RR, 20; and O_2 sat 95% on RA. Upon walking into the room you find the patient on a backboard with C-spine immobilization, awake, moaning in obvious distress with the right leg externally rotated and shortened. Your next step is:

    A. Obtain IV access and ECG and give fluid bolus
    B. Obtain vital signs, check pulses in all limbs, and complete the secondary survey
    C. Give 10 mg of oxycodone and Tylenol
    D. Place the right leg in traction

Correct Answer B: *Obtain vital signs, check pulses in all limbs, and complete the secondary survey.* This is the next step in the advanced trauma life support algorithm. The vital signs listed were pretransport. In addition, the examinee should recognize this patient has a potential hip fracture and/or dislocation, which could compromise the affected limb. Checking pulses is the first step in identifying vascular compromise. Getting IV access, EKG, putting leg in traction are all necessary actions, but not the next step in the algorithm. This patient should be kept NPO until further evaluation; so he should not receive oxycodone and Tylenol.

163. The family of the above patient is concerned that the C-spine collar is making the patient too uncomfortable and wants you to remove it. Do you need to image this patient's C-spine?

    A. Yes, because he has an altered level of consciousness
    B. Yes, because he has a distracting painful injury
    C. No, he is awake and alert and does not have any midline C-spine tenderness
    D. Both A and B

Correct Answer B: *Yes, because he has a distracting painful injury.* This question tests the examinee's knowledge of Nexus criteria for C-spine imaging, which states the C-spine of a trauma can be safely cleared without imaging if none of the following are present: Focal neurologic deficit, midline spine tenderness, altered level of consciousness, intoxication, distracting injury.

164. To provide optimal analgesia for the above patient and continue to adequately care for the patient, you:

    A. Give 100 µg fentanyl and 2 mg midazolam
    B. Subcutaneous morphine 2 mg every 1 hour up to three doses
    C. Ultrasound-guided femoral nerve block with 0.5% bupivacaine
    D. Intubate using rapid sequence intubation and sedate with propofol

Correct Answer C: *Ultrasound-guided femoral nerve block with 0.5% bupivacaine.* The block allows you to use safe, effective, and resource-conscious analgesia. It is minimally invasive, and provides excellent sustained analgesia without sedation or airway compromise. Fentanyl and midazolam serve as both an analgesic and sedative medication effectively inducing conscious sedation. This would require extra nursing staff to monitor the patient and puts the patient at risk for airway compromise. Although sedation may be necessary to reduce this patient's hip, adequate analgesia can be obtained prior to the reduction procedure without sedating the patient. Morphine 2 mg subcutaneous is incorrect as it is too low a dose to provide analgesia for this patient's injuries. This patient is protecting his airway with a normal mental status, and intubation should not be the first management strategy for this patient.

165. An 85-year-old female comes to the emergency department with chest wall pain after a fall forward hitting her right chest on the corner of her nightstand 3 days ago. She has taken Tylenol without any improvement. Her chest x-ray shows nondisplaced fractures of the right ribs 3, 4, and 5 and small right lower lobe patchy opacity concerning for atelectasis or early pneumonia. Your plan is:

    A. Place a Lidoderm patch to the area, advise the patient to take Tylenol 1,000 mg every 8 hours alternating with ibuprofen 800 mg every 8 hours, prescribe a azithromycin 5-day pack, and schedule follow-up in 1 week with her primary care physician (PCP).
    B. Prescribe oxycodone/acetaminophen 5/500 1 to 2 tabs every 6 hours, ibuprofen 800 mg every 8 hours, and azithromycin 5-day pack and schedule follow-up in 3 days with her PCP.
    C. Admit to the hospital for pain management and antibiotics and respiratory physical therapy.
    D. Either A or B

Correct Answer C: *Admit to the hospital for pain management and antibiotics and respiratory physical therapy.* This patient is at high risk for complications of her rib fractures and may already have a small pneumonia. As she is elderly, she is at risk for oversedation with opiate analgesics and should be admitted to the hospital for close monitoring, pain control, and antibiotics.

166. On your way home from work, you arrive at the scene of a high-speed motor vehicle crash. Paramedics are already on scene, and you offer your assistance. Upon evaluation of the unbelted driver of the vehicle, you find him lying on the ground, anxious, gasping for breath, a respiratory rate of 35, with tracheal deviation to the right and distended neck veins. You correctly identify the patient has a

    A. Tension pneumothorax
    B. Pulmonary contusion
    C. Fractured C-spine
    D. Cardiac contusion

Correct Answer A: *Tension pneumothorax.* This patient has clinical signs of a tension pneumothorax.

167. On the above patient, you immediately perform the following intervention improving his clinical status.

    A. Needle decompression of the right lung with 14-gauge IV catheter in the second intercostal space midclavicular line
    B. Apply C-spine immobilization
    C. Needle decompression of the left lung with 14-gauge IV catheter in the second intercostal space midclavicular line
    D. Tube thoracostomy

Correct Answer C: *Needle decompression of the left lung with 14-gauge IV catheter in the second intercostal space midclavicular line.* In tension pneumothorax, tracheal deviation points away from the lung under tension (the left in this case) and that needle decompression is the first choice when a tube thoracostomy cannot be placed immediately (as is the case in this scenario). C-spine immobilization may be necessary for this patient, but does not treat the immediate life-threat of tension pneumothorax. A tube thoracostomy cannot be accomplished in a safe, clean, and fast manner on this patient.

168. A 25-year-old female is brought in from the scene of a motor vehicle crash with chest pain. Paramedics tell you the patient was the belted driver of a sedan when she fell asleep and struck a telephone pole at 45 mph. Airbags did deploy. The patient has been having escalating chest pain during transport with minimal improvement after morphine 2 mg IV. Vital signs are as follows: temp, 97.8°F; HR, 140; BP, 90/50; RR, 22; and O_2 sat 95% on RA. She is awake, but pale. You order a screening portable chest x-ray that shows an abnormal mediastinum and a hemothorax increasing your suspicion for

    A. Aortic dissection
    B. Cardiac contusion
    C. Rib fracture
    D. None of the above

Correct Answer A: *Aortic dissection.* The most life-threatening injury that could result from rapid deceleration described in this scenario and the clinical symptoms and signs are of aortic dissection/rupture. A motor vehicle accident with chest wall trauma could cause cardiac contusion and rib fracture, but the chest x-ray findings of an "abnormal mediastinum" should clue the examinee to think of aortic dissection.

169. To confirm the injury in the questions above, you order which of the following:

    A. Thoracotomy

    B. CT-angiogram of the chest/abdomen/pelvis

    C. MRI of the chest/abdomen/pelvis

    D. Transesophageal echocardiogram

Correct Answer B: *CT-angiogram of the chest/abdomen/pelvis.* This test will give the most rapid and extensive evaluation of this patient's thorax. Thoracotomy is incorrect as it is too invasive for this semistable patient. MRI and echo require additional resources and technicians to perform and are therefore too time consuming for this patient scenario.

170. Emergency medical services arrives with a 40-year-old otherwise healthy male who fell off a 10-ft ladder landing on his feet. He has a Glasgow Coma Scale of 15 and stable vital signs. You confirm that he has bilateral calcaneal fractures. What other injury is most often associated with his injuries?

    A. Rib fracture

    B. Lumbar spine fracture

    C. Concussion

    D. Bladder rupture

Correct Answer B: *Lumbar spine fracture.* This is a dangerous mechanism and often has associated spinal fractures. It is important to think of other areas where the patient might have injuries when he has another painful injury. Although a rib fracture and concussion may be present, these are not the most common associated injuries. Bladder rupture is incorrect because the patient would be in more distress and have other notable physical exam findings.

171. A 32-year-old male patient presents after falling off his snowmobile at 15 mph. He was helmeted and did not lose consciousness. He is awake and alert with severe pain in his left leg and an open distal tibia-fibular fracture. Vital signs are as follows: temp, 97.8°F; HR, 120; BP, 100/70; RR, 24; and O_2 sat 96% on 2 L by nasal cannula. You perform a bedside _____, which identifies fluid between the liver and kidney and the spleen and kidney.

    A. Focused assessment with sonography for trauma (FAST)

    B. Plain film kidney, ureter, and bladder and upright chest

    C. CT-angiogram of the chest/abdomen/pelvis

    D. Diagnostic peritoneal lavage

Correct Answer A: *Focused assessment with sonography for trauma (FAST).* A FAST is a bedside procedure that is standard in the current evaluation of the trauma patient. Relevant findings of these tests are the only routine bedside procedure that specifically identifies fluid in these two locations.

172. While you are doing the focused assessment with sonography for trauma, the blood pressure drops to 90/65. Your next step is:

    A. Call the general surgeon and arrange for urgent exploratory laparotomy

    B. Call the orthopedic surgeon and arrange for urgent repair of his open fracture

    C. Give a bolus of normal saline IV fluids

    D. Given fentanyl 100 μg and reduce the ankle

Correct Answer C: *Give a bolus of normal saline IV fluids.* Giving IV fluids is the correct next step based on advanced trauma life support guidelines. You should be concerned that the patient is clinically deteriorating, likely has an intra-abdominal hemorrhage, and needs urgent intervention. Calling the surgeon for an ex-lap will most likely be necessary, but the clinician must first treat the patient, then coordinate disposition. Calling ortho and giving fentanyl are incorrect as the ankle fracture is not the priority injury at this time is unlikely the cause of the patient's hypotension.

173. You are caring for an elderly man with a recent fall from a small (3 step) stepladder. He is complaining of deep hip pain and an inability to walk. The nurses call your attention to bleeding at the urethral meatus. This finding confirms your suspicion for what two related injuries?

    A. Dementia and bladder infection
    B. Intra-abdominal bleeding and femur fracture
    C. Bladder rupture and hip fracture
    D. Urethral injury/tear and pelvic fracture

Correct Answer D: *Urethral injury/tear and pelvic fracture.* The patient has clinical signs of a urethral injury. Dementia and bladder infection are more likely to present in a more insidious manner and not the most acutely concerning illness. Options B and C include high-risk injuries that occur together with significant trauma, which is not the case with this scenario.

174. A 15-year-old boy is brought to your community emergency department (ED) after a particularly hard hit on the football field. He tells you he passed out after he was tackled and bystanders noted he was unresponsive for about 15 seconds. In the ED he is awake and alert, but cannot tell you his name, the date, or his home address; he has equal grip strength in both the upper and lower extremities and can hold both arms and legs off the stretcher for 4 seconds. This patient has a Glasgow Coma Scale of:

    A. 14
    B. 16
    C. 13
    D. 10

Correct Answer A: *14.* This question tests the ability to apply the standard scale used to indicate a patient's level of consciousness. The patient gets a 4 for eye response, 4 for verbal response, and 6 for motor response for a total of 14.

175. On the above patient, you decide to do a CT scan of the brain, which has no evidence of hemorrhage or skull fracture. You do which of the following?

    A. Transfer to a trauma center for neurology evaluation
    B. Discharge home with his parents and do urgent follow-up in the pediatric concussion clinic with clear return instructions and no sports until reevaluation
    C. Observe for 6 hours and repeat the head CT
    D. None of the above

Correct Answer B: *Discharge home with his parents and do urgent follow-up in the pediatric concussion clinic with clear return instructions and no sports until reevaluation.* As this patient does not have any evidence of intracranial hemorrhage, he does not need urgent neurosurgical or neurological intervention, although he does need close monitoring by a family or friend and clear return precautions. The examinee should also recognize the importance of subsequent head trauma and restrict this patient from high-risk sports, such as football.

176. You are examining one of the homeless men who frequently comes to your community emergency department intoxicated with alcohol. Typically, he is pleasant and cooperative despite his intoxication. Today, he is combative, has no odor of alcohol, and his gate is more unsteady than baseline. You are concerned and order a CT scan of the brain. What finding warrants acute neurosurgical evaluation?

    A. Large chronic subdural hematoma with acute bleeding and 3 mm of midline shift
    B. Large chronic subdural hematoma
    C. White matter changes and lacunar infarcts of undetermined age
    D. Large territorial ischemic stroke

Correct Answer A: *Large chronic subdural hematoma with acute bleeding and 3 mm of midline shift.* This is the only choice that necessitates urgent neurosurgical evaluation and evacuation of the hemorrhage. Large territorial ischemic stroke necessitates an urgent neurological evaluation.

177. Emergency medical services brings in a 50-year-old male with complaints of neck pain and paresthesias of both arms after a 30-lb barrel fell onto his head from a shelf. He has no other medical problems and takes no medications. His initial exam is notable for vital signs of the following: temp 98.7°F, HR 100, BP 130/80, RR 20, O_2 sat of 97% on RA, a Glasgow Coma Scale of 14, moderate confusion, tenderness of C3-4, and diminished sensation on bilateral upper extremities. What initial imaging studies do you obtain?

    A. Chest x-ray and pelvis x-ray
    B. MRI/MRA brain
    C. CT brain and CT C-spine
    D. All of the above

Correct Answer C: *CT brain and CT C-spine.* This patient has neurological injuries after an axial load to the skull that may have caused either intracerebral trauma or cervical spine injury. Option A does not address this patient's neurologic complaints, and option B does not include cervical imaging.

178. Imaging on the above patient reveals a Jefferson fracture (C1 burst fracture). Your next step is:

    A. Clinically clear the patient from C-spine immobilization and discharge with orthopedics follow-up in 3 days
    B. Consult a spine surgeon
    C. Give oral pain medicines, oxycodone, ibuprofen, and Tylenol until the patient's pain improves
    D. Obtain imaging of the remainder of the patient's spine
    E. Both B and D

Correct Answer E: *Both B and D.* This patient has potentially unstable spine fractures, and there may be additional injuries not noted on the first exam. A C1 fracture is potentially unstable and needs urgent evaluation by a spine surgeon so that immobilization should not be cleared. Oral pain medications are incorrect, as this patient should remain NPO until evaluation by a surgeon for operative planning.

179. A 32-year-old female, with a history of polycystic ovary syndrome, hypertension, hyperlipidemia, and a body mass index >40, presents to the emergency department with a severe headache and requires a lumbar puncture for concern of pseudotumor cerebri. What is the best method for performing a lumbar puncture on this patient?

    A. By assuming the fetal position with the spine parallel to the bed
    B. In the seated position facing away from the operator with spine perpendicular to the bed
    C. In the seated position bending over a bedside table to maximize lumbar flexion
    D. Place in the decubitus position after the spinal needle has been placed in the seated position over a bedside table tray

Correct Answer D: *Place in the decubitus position after the spinal needle has been placed in the seated position over a bedside table tray.* Positioning is a key aspect of performing a lumbar puncture. In obese patients, the best way to achieve maximal lumbar flexion is in the seated position bending over a bedside table. However, cerebrospinal fluid pressure, which is diagnostic of pseudotumor cerebri, is only properly assessed in the supine position. Therefore, once the needle has been inserted into the spinal canal, the patient can be carefully repositioned lie in the decubitus position to accurately measure pressure.

180. Roughly 5% to 40% of patients develop a postdural headache after a lumbar puncture (LP) is performed. What is the best way to prevent postdural puncture headache?

   A. Using the smallest gauge needle
   B. Place patient in seated position while performing LP
   C. Immediately lay patient supine after procedure for 1 hour
   D. Prophylactically fluid bolus the patient before the procedure

Correct Answer A: *Using the smallest gauge needle.* The incidence of postdural headache is directly correlated with needle gauge, thus using the smallest gauge needle can help minimize this occurrence. The patient's position during and immediately following LP does not appear to be associated with the development of prevention of a headache, nor does administration of a periprocedure fluid bolus.

181. Which of the following is not the standard of care in verifying the placement of a nasogastric tube (NG)?

   A. Chest x-ray
   B. Insufflation of air, resulting in borborygmi over the epigastrium
   C. Aspiration of contents
   D. Normal clear speech

Correct Answer A: *Chest x-ray.* Radiographic verification is the most sensitive test to detect proper placement of NG tube, but not the standard of care. The best methods of verifying placement are air bubbles heard within the stomach, aspiration of gastric contents, and in a conscious patient a normal speech without coughing.

182. A 35-year-old male is brought in by ambulance after a high-speed motor vehicle crash with direct head trauma against steering wheel. The patient is alert and oriented, with multiple midface fractures seen on CT. There is concern for a transdiaphragmatic hernia, and placement of a nasogastric tube (NGT) is warranted. Supplies are gathered at the bedside. What is the next best step in placement of this NGT?

   A. Estimation of tube length by measuring from patient's tip of the nose to earlobe, to the xiphoid process
   B. Assessing for patency of nares
   C. Anesthetizing the oropharynx with lidocaine 4%
   D. None of the above

Correct Answer D: *None of the above.* Placement of NGT in patients with cribriform plate or midface fractures is a contraindication given the susceptibility to intracranial placement of NGT. Therefore, the NGT should not be placed in this patient and alternative methods should be discussed. Typically, estimation of tube length is the first step in placement of an NGT.

183. During the insertion of a chest tube after the patient has been properly positioned, what are the appropriate steps?

   A. Sterilize the skin over insertion site on the anterior thorax and midaxillary line, drape the surrounding area, anesthetize, and make an incision over the superior aspect of the rib
   B. Sterilize the skin over insertion site on the lateral thorax and anterior axillary line, drape the surrounding area, anesthetize, and make an incision over the inferior aspect of the rib
   C. Sterilize the skin over insertion site on the anterior thorax and posterior axillary line, drape the surrounding area, anesthetize, and make an incision over the inferior aspect of the rib
   D. Sterilize the skin over insertion site on the lateral thorax and midaxillary line, drape the surrounding area, anesthetize, and make an incision over the superior aspect of the rib

Correct Answer B: *Sterilize the skin over insertion site on the lateral thorax and anterior axillary line, drape the surrounding area, anesthetize, and make an incision over the inferior aspect of the rib.* Chest tubes are inserted in the *lateral* thorax at the *anterior* axillary line, just lateral to the nipple at the level of 4th or 5th intercostal space, ensuring that it is above the diaphragm. Incisions must be made on the *inferior* aspect of the rib to avoid the neurovascular bundle that is located superior to the rib.

184. A 60-year-old male with a history of benign prostatic hyperplasia (BPH) was brought into the emergency department after mechanical slip and fall with obvious left hip deformity and an unstable pelvis. A Foley catheter is needed. What should you do in preparation for placing this Foley catheter?
   A. Grab a 14F coudé catheter
   B. Lubricate the urethra
   C. Perform a prostate exam
   D. Sterilize the glans and urethral meatus

Correct Answer C: *Perform a prostate exam.* A digital rectal exam must be performed before a catheter is inserted in a male patient with major blunt trauma. Specifically feel for free-floating prostate or gross blood escaping from the urethra, which signifies urethral rupture and is an absolute contraindication to Foley placement. Generally, patients with BPH require 20 to 22F coudé catheter. Lubricating and sterilizing the urethra are necessary steps in Foley catheter placement, which are typically performed after donning sterile gloves.

185. Which statement is false regarding arterial blood gas (ABG) sampling?
   A. Allen test must be performed before sampling.
   B. Can be performed in the same arm as arteriovenous (AV) fistula.
   C. Needle is held at a 45-degree angle aiming caudally, with wrist in extension.
   D. Air bubbles must be removed from the syringe for accurate analysis.

Correct Answer B: *Can be performed in the same arm as arteriovenous (AV) fistula.* The presence of AV fistulas and vascular grafts are a contraindication to ABG sampling of that same arm. Allen test must be performed to assess adequate collateral blood flow of the hand. Air bubbles that are left in the syringe can alter PO_2 and PCO_2 values and lead to false interpretation; therefore, these must be removed prior to analysis.

186. What are the appropriate steps in performing a central venous catheter?
   A. Use ultrasound to assess patency of internal jugular vein, insert needle into vein, place guide wire through lumen of the needle, using scalpel make small incision in the skin where the wire penetrates, advance dilator over the wire and into the lumen of the vein, advance the catheter over the guide wire, remove the guide wire
   B. Insert needle into vein, use ultrasound to assess patency of internal jugular vein, using scalpel make small incision in the skin where needle penetrates, advance guide wire through the lumen of the needle, use dilator over wire and into the lumen of the vein, advance the catheter over the guide wire, remove the guide wire
   C. Use ultrasound to assess patency of the vein, insert needle in internal jugular vein, place guide wire through the lumen of the needle, advance catheter over guide wire, using scalpel make small incision in the skin where the catheter penetrates, remove the guide wire
   D. Insert needle into vein, use ultrasound to assess patency of internal jugular vein, place guide wire through lumen of the needle, using scalpel make small incision in the skin where the wire penetrates, advance dilator over the wire and into the lumen of the vein, advance the catheter over the guide wire, remove the guide wire

Correct Answer A: *Use ultrasound to assess patency of internal jugular vein, insert needle into vein, place guide wire through lumen of the needle, using scalpel make small incision in the skin where the wire penetrates, advance dilator over the wire and into the lumen of the vein, advance the catheter over the guide wire, remove the guide wire.* Ultrasound must be performed first to assess patency of the vein as thrombus or stenosis of the vessel is contraindication to performing central venous access. Needle is inserted; guide wire is placed through the lumen of the needle, and needle is removed. A scalpel is used to make incision; a dilator is passed over the guide wire to create a tract for the pliable catheter to follow. The dilator is removed, the catheter is advanced over the wire and into the lumen of the vein, and the guide wire is removed. This method is referred to as the Seldinger technique.

187. Which of the following is true regarding wound care?
    A. Closed wounds are best treated with moist dressings
    B. Open wounds are best treated with dry dressings
    C. Petrolatum dressings (Xeroform) decrease the rate of epithelialization in partial-thickness wounds
    D. Immobilization of the wound may delay wound healing

Correct Answer C: *Petrolatum dressings (Xeroform) decrease the rate of epithelialization in partial-thickness wounds.* Partial-thickness wounds are better treated with ointment dressings (Bacitracin, Neosporin) or nonadherent occlusive dressings. Closed wounds are best treated with dry dressings, because moist dressings cause maceration of the skin and invite bacterial invasion. Open wounds are best treated with moist dressings to the open wound surface and dry dressings on top to achieve a capillary effect. Immobilization of the wound enhances resistance to infection and actually accelerates wound healing.

188. A 22-year-old male, otherwise healthy, presents to the emergency department after sustaining a laceration to his thumb using electric hedge clippers. What is the preferred method of wound irrigation?
    A. Hydrogen peroxide
    B. Normal saline
    C. Ionic soap/detergent
    D. 1% povidone-iodine

Correct Answer B: *Normal saline.* Washing the open wound with saline under pressure removes most of the surface bacteria. Hydrogen peroxide may be useful for removing debris and blood clots; however, there is a risk of cytotoxicity. Ionic soap and detergents are extremely irritating to tissues and increase the potential for infection if used directly on the wound. The use of concentrated iodine has been associated with a slightly decreased rate of wound infection but at risk of cytotoxicity. When diluted, there is no advantage to using this over normal saline.

189. Which of the following is contraindication to rapid sequence intubation (RSI)?
    A. Cardiac arrest
    B. Oral trauma
    C. Angioedema
    D. Recent mandibular open reduction internal fixation
    E. All of the above

Correct Answer E: *All of the above.* With cardiac arrest, there is no indication for muscle relaxation/paralysis. With oral trauma and mandibular fixation, there is a high likelihood of difficulty with bag valve mask ventilation if the RSI fails and there is no backup rescue ventilation option. With angioedema, first attempt should be made with an awake nasal intubation with plan for surgical airway as the backup.

190. A 90-year-old female presents to the emergency department (ED) with onset of palpitations, shortness of breath, and chest pressure that started 30 minutes prior. Emergency medical services found her with a heart rate of 160, BP of 110/74, respiratory rate of 26, and O_2 saturation of 96% on room air. On arrival to the ED she is diaphoretic, pulse is 170, and BP is 70/palp. EKG reveals an irregularly irregular narrow-complex tachycardia. The next treatment would be:

    A. Diltiazem 20 mg intravenous pyelogram (IVP)
    B. Metoprolol 5 mg IVP
    C. Adenosine 6 mg IVP
    D. Synchronized cardioversion at 100 J
    E. Unsynchronized cardioversion at 200 J

Correct Answer D: *Synchronized cardioversion at 100 J.* In a hemodynamically unstable patient, the treatment of choice is synchronized cardioversion. Unsynchronized cardioversion (option E) for atrial fibrillation can cause other arrhythmias. Medications (options A, B, and C) are not first-line treatment for new onset of hemodynamically unstable atrial fibrillation.

191. Which of the following patient is most appropriate for transcutaneous pacing?

    A. Asystolic cardiac arrest
    B. Hypothermic drowning victim with pulse 30 and BP 80/60
    C. Patient with second-degree Mobitz atrioventricular (AV) block and BP 70/40
    D. Patient with third-degree AV block and BP 120/80

Correct Answer C: *Patient with second-degree Mobitz atrioventricular (AV) block and BP 70/40.* The most appropriate patient is the patient with a high-degree AV block and unstable vital signs or clinical course. There has been no data to support benefit from pacing an asystolic cardiac arrest (option A). In hypothermia (option B), the heart is unable to respond to the electrical stimulus. In option D, the patient is hemodynamically stable and transcutaneous pacing is not the best first treatment choice.

192. Which of the following is not associated with a chest x-ray finding indicative of pulmonary embolus?

    A. Fleischner sign
    B. Hampton hump
    C. Hoover sign
    D. Westermark sign

Correct Answer C: *Hoover sign.* This sign indicates inward movement of the rib cage during inspiration and is associated with chronic obstructive pulmonary disease. Fleisher sign (indicative of an enlarged pulmonary artery), Hampton hump (peripheral wedge of airspace opacity due to pulmonary infarction), and Westermark sign (regional oligemia from vessel collapse distal to the pulmonary embolus) are all associated with pulmonary embolus.

193. Which patient would be the best candidate to receive succinylcholine as part of rapid sequence intubation?

    A. Patient brought in acutely with severe burns needing airway protection
    B. Patient with severe burns 36 hours ago
    C. Patient with a history of malignant hyperthermia
    D. Patient with penetrating ocular trauma
    E. Pediatric patient with unknown medical history
    F. Dialysis patient with last dialysis unknown

Correct Answer A: *Patient brought in acutely with severe burns needing airway protection.* This patient is the best candidate for succinylcholine. Option B is not indicated due to the increased risk of rhabdomyolysis and hyperkalemia in this patient. Succinylcholine can precipitate malignant hyperthermia (C) and also increases intraocular pressure (D). Option F is not the best choice due to the risk of hyperkalemia. There has been shown to be an increased risk of rhabdomyolysis/hyperkalemia/arrhythmia in pediatric patients with undiagnosed skeletal muscle disease; so it is avoided in pediatric populations.

194. Which of the following is a contraindication to cricothyroidotomy?
   A. Angioedema
   B. Oral trauma requiring airway protection
   C. History of laryngeal cancer with resection and radiation
   D. Pediatric trauma patient age 7 requiring airway protection
   E. Patient with recent mandibular open reduction internal fixation and needing airway protection

Correct Answer D: *Pediatric trauma patient age 7 requiring airway protection.* The pediatric patient is the only absolute contraindication to open cricothyroidotomy. There is controversy about the age, but generally in patients under 12, a needle cricothyrotomy is indicated given the small cricothyroid membrane in infant and pediatric patients along with their funnel-shaped larynx. The other patients will be difficult to intubate with rapid sequence intubation, and cricothyroidotomy would be the surgical airway of choice if necessary.

195. What is the most serious complication of the below injury:

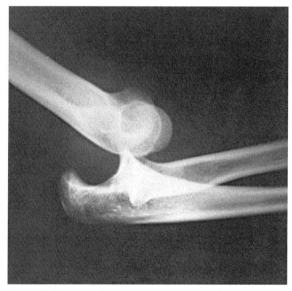

FIGURE 20.1. Radiograph reveals a complete posterolateral dislocation of the elbow.
(From Browner BD. *Skeletal Trauma.* 4th ed. Philadelphia, PA: W. B. Saunders; 2008. MD Consult.)

   A. Radial artery injury
   B. Ulnar artery injury
   C. Radial nerve injury
   D. Ulnar nerve injury
   E. Median nerve injury

Correct Answer A: *Radial artery injury.* This requires acute orthopedic consultation and intervention. The other injuries are seen in varying degrees with the same injury and would require orthopedics evaluation, but are not limb threatening.

196. A 34-year-old male, involved in high-speed motor vehicle crash, presents to the emergency department by emergency medical services (EMS). Vital signs on arrival via EMS are as follows: HR, 130; BP, 70/p; RR, 36. Ventilations are assisted by EMS via bag valve mask. Chest x-ray (CXR) on arrival is below. What is the next therapy indicated:

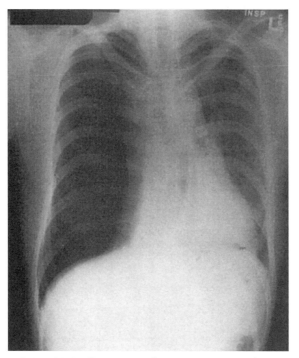

FIGURE 20.2. Chest x-ray of a tension pneumothorax with mediastinal shift to left.
(From Marx JA, Hockberger RS, Walls RM. *Rosen's Emergency Medicine—Concepts and Clinical Practice.* 8th ed. Philadelphia, PA: Mosby Elsevier. Figure 77-3 A. MD Consult.)

A. Intubate for airway protection
B. Repeat CXR in 1 hour
C. Consult trauma surgery for evaluation
D. Needle decompression
E. Insert chest tube

Correct Answer D: *Needle decompression.* The patient has a tension pneumothorax. Intubation (option A) would increase chest pressures via positive pressure ventilation and exacerbate the clinical picture. This is an emergent, life-threatening condition, and options B and C would not be indicated in this unstable patient until needle decompression is performed. Chest tube insertion (option E) would be performed after needle decompression.

197. A 3-year-old boy presents to the emergency department with his parents complaining of right elbow pain, and on exam he is guarding. Patient was walking; mom pulled on his outstretched arm to lift him up, and he had onset of pain. The treatment would be:

A. Splint and follow-up with orthopedics
B. Reduction with longitudinal traction
C. Reduction with supination of forearm and elbow flexion past 90 degrees with pressure over the radial head
D. X-rays of elbow

Correct Answer C: *Reduction with supination of forearm and elbow flexion past 90 degrees with pressure over the radial head.* The patient has a nursemaid's elbow or radial head subluxation. X-rays are not indicted if there is no other trauma. Reduction is performed by supinating the forearm and flexing the elbow past 90 degrees with pressure over the radial head. A pop is then often felt, and after a short period of observation, the patient will then resume normal activity and use of the elbow.

198. A 75-year-old female presents from home via emergency medical services. History via family is she had a headache then rapid onset of altered mental status and lethargy. After initial assessment in the emergency department (ED), head CT is obtained and shown below. Glasgow Coma Scale is now 5 in the ED. Then next steps would be:

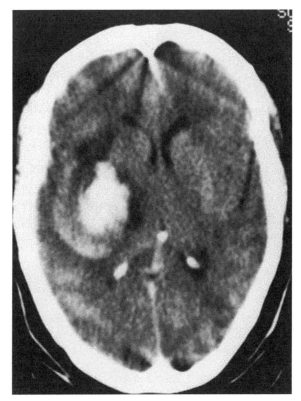

FIGURE 20.3. Right putaminal hemorrhage.
(From Daroff RB, Fenichel GM, Jankovic J, et al. *Bradley's Neurology in Clinical Practice.* 6th ed. Philadelphia, PA: Saunders Elsevier; 2012. Figure 51B.10. MD Consult.)

   A. Obtain MRI and admit
   B. Neurosurgery consultation and intubate via rapid sequence intubation (RSI)
   C. Administer aspirin and admit
   D. Neurology consultation and intubate not using RSI as patient is minimally responsive

Correct Answer B: *Neurosurgery consultation and intubate via rapid sequence intubation (RSI) for airway protection.* RSI will prevent any increase in BP and pulse from intubation in this patient with a very large intracerebral hemorrhage. MRI is not indicated. Intubating the patient without RSI even in a minimally responsive patient can still increase BP, which should be avoided in this case.

199. A 20-year-old male presents to the emergency department complaining of abdominal pain with nausea, vomiting, and diarrhea. He reports to you that he has felt ill recently and thought he had the flu. He has been taking multiple over-the-counter flu remedies every 2 hours for his cough and rhinorrhea, Tylenol 1,000 mg for fever every 4 hours and two tablets of Percocet, left over from when he had his wisdom teeth taken out last month every 3 hours for his myalgias. He has been consistent with this routine for 24 hours now. His vital signs are as follows: temp, 99.9°F; HR, 113; BP, 110/80; RR, 18; and O_2 sat 98% on RA. On exam, he is diaphoretic and irritable. He has normal cardiac, pulmonary, and abdominal exams. Your next step is:

A. Administer Narcan
B. Administer N-acetylcysteine
C. Send off laboratory studies and initiate treatment with intravenous fluids
D. Administer Flumazenil

Correct Answer B: *Administer N-acetylcysteine.* The patient presents with symptoms of Tylenol overdose and provides a history that is consistent with overuse of Tylenol. He inappropriately used multiple medications that all contain Tylenol. He more likely has ingested more than the recommended amount of daily Tylenol and is thus at risk for severe liver damage. The best course of action would be to initiate treatment with N-acetylcysteine immediately since this is the antidote for Tylenol overdose. Option A is not the correct answer since Narcan is the reversal agent for opiate overdose, and although this patient has taken narcotics, his history and examination are inconsistent with opiate overdose. While option C may place a role in the patient's overall care, it should not be your first step in his care. Option D is not the correct answer because flumazenil is the reversal agent for benzodiazepine overdose, not Tylenol overdose.

200. A 26-year-old female is brought into the emergency department for fever and hallucinations. She was found agitated by family on the floor of her bathroom with empty bottles of diphenhydramine, hydroxyzine, meclizine, and dextromethorphan surrounding her. On your exam, the patient is agitated and tells you that she sees spiders on the walls. She is febrile to 102°F, tachycardic to 125 bpm, and hypertensive to 180/90 mm Hg. Her pupils are dilated, cheeks are flushed, and mucous membranes are dry; she is tremulous and now becoming somnolent. You suspect the patient has overdosed, and you plan to treat her with the following medication:

A. Physostigmine salicylate
B. Flumazenil
C. Activated charcoal
D. N-Acetylcysteine

Correct Answer A: *Physostigmine salicylate.* This patient presents with the classic symptoms of anticholinergic overdose, and the symptoms can be recalled using the mnemonic blind as a bat (dilated pupils), red as a beet (vasodilation), hot as a hare (hyperthermia), dry as a bone (dry skin), and mad as a hatter (hallucinations/agitation). Physostigmine salicylate is the antidote for life-threatening anticholinergic overdoses. Flumazenil is not the correct choice as it is the antidote for benzodiazepine overdose, not anticholinergic overdose. Activated charcoal can be used for a variety of overdoses, but is not the treatment of choice for life-threatening anticholinergic overdoses. N-Acetylcysteine is the treatment for Tylenol overdose.

201. A 32-year-old male presents to the emergency department complaining of chest pain for the past 2 hours. He admits to using cocaine prior to the onset of chest pain. His vital signs are as follows: temp, 98.1°F; HR, 102; BP, 170/90; RR, 16; and O_2 sat 99% on RA. His EKG is nonischemic. Your workup includes complete blood count, chemistries, cardiac biomarkers, chest x-ray, and continuous cardiac monitoring. You plan to give all of the medications listed below *except*:

A. Nitroglycerin and aspirin
B. Benzodiazepines
C. Ca channel blocker
D. β-Blocker

Correct Answer D: β-Blocker. β-Blockers are contraindicated in the care of patients with cocaine-associated chest pain. β-Blockers are thought to exacerbate coronary vasoconstriction and increase blood pressure in patients with recent cocaine abuse and should therefore not be administered. Nitroglycerin and aspirin are standard of care in all patients who present with chest pain and should be given unless there are patient-specific contraindications. There is no contraindication to use these medications with cocaine-associated chest pain. Benzodiazepines help to relieve adrenergic stimulation that is caused by cocaine abuse and is effective in alleviating chest pain. Ca channel blockers decrease coronary vasoconstriction, thus helping to relieve chest pain that is caused by cocaine abuse.

202. The heavy metal responsible for interference with neurologic development, permanent learning disabilities, and behavior disorders in children is:

A. Mercury
B. Beryllium
C. Cadmium
D. Lead

Correct Answer D: Lead. Lead is still found in many old homes in paint and thus presents constant exposure to children in the form of ingested pain chips or ingested dust containing lead particles. Lead poisoning is known to cause abdominal pain, nausea, vomiting, decreased appetite, weight loss, decreased bone and muscle growth, anemia, and lethargy in addition to the symptoms listed above. Mercury poisoning typically results in sensory impairment, changes in sensation, and lack of coordination. Beryllium is identified as a carcinogen and would not cause these symptoms. Cadmium is a toxic metal found in industrial workplaces and not typically in the home or in places where children would be expected to readily have access.

203. The EKG finding that you would expect to see in a patient with known tricyclic antidepressant (TCA) overdose would be:

A. Peaked T waves
B. Widened QRS
C. Delta waves
D. Shortened PR interval

Correct Answer B: Widened QRS. TCAs are Na channel blockers that are cardiotoxic when ingested in large amounts. The most common and concerning EKG finding is widened QRS >100 ms caused by inhibition of the Na channels in the heart. Peaked T waves are found in hyperkalemia, not TCA overdose. Delta waves are indicative of Wolf–Parkinson–White syndrome. Shortened PR intervals are not seen in TCA overdose.

204. This drug when taken in excess or when combined with SSRIs or other drugs that increase serotonin levels in the body can lead to extreme diaphoresis, fever, tachycardia, hypertensive crisis, respiratory failure, coma, and possibly death.

A. Monoamine oxidase inhibitors (MAOIs)
B. Lithium
C. Cocaine
D. Heroin

Correct Answer A: *MAOIs*. Monoamine oxidase inhibitors (MAOIs) are older antidepressants that prevent the breakdown of neurotransmitters between neurons in the brain, thus leading to an increase in neurotransmitter concentrations. When MAOIs are combined with other medications that increase serotonin level, such as SSRIs, this can lead to serotonin syndrome, which presents as fever, tachycardia, hypertensive crisis, respiratory failure, and death. When combined with SSRIs, lithium does not lead to serotonin syndrome. The combination of cocaine and SSRIs do not lead to serotonin syndrome. Heroin and SSRIs in combination do not lead to serotonin syndrome.

205. A 20-year-old male with recent diagnosis of schizophrenia, who was started on Thorazine 6 days ago, presents with fever and altered mental status. On arrival, he is febrile to 101.7°F, and has a HR of 116 bpm with respiratory rate of 16 breaths per minute and O_2 saturation of 97% 2 L by nasal cannula. His blood pressures are fluctuating anywhere from 90/62 to 167/85 mm Hg. On exam, he is confused and profusely diaphoretic and his muscles seem rigid. Laboratory analysis reveals a white blood cell (WBC) of 16 and creatine kinase (CK) of 1526 IU/L. What are you most concerned for in this case?
    A. Serotonin syndrome
    B. Neuroleptic malignant syndrome (NMS)
    C. Meningitis
    D. Anticholinergic overdose

Correct Answer B: *Neuroleptic malignant syndrome (NMS)*. NMS is a life-threatening neurologic complication of antipsychotic use. This patient recently started Thorazine, which is known to cause NMS. Patients who recently start or have an increase in antipsychotics are most at risk for NMS. NMS presents as fever, tachycardia, bradykinesia, muscle rigidity, and autonomic instability. The diagnosis can be further confirmed with laboratory testing revealing an elevated WBC and CK. NMS is a true emergency, and rapid identification of this syndrome is crucial in order to initiate proper treatment. Serotonin syndrome does present with fever, tachycardia, and hypertension, but does not typically have fluctuating blood pressures, muscle rigidity, and elevated WBC or CK. Meningitis should be on the differential for any patient presenting with altered mental status, but in this case, with the patient presenting with a history of starting a new antipsychotic medication and having autonomic instability, meningitis is less likely the cause of this patient's symptoms. Anticholinergic overdose does not present with autonomic instability and does not have an elevated WBC or CK on laboratory analysis. Anticholinergic overdose symptoms can be recalled using the mnemonic blind as a bat (dilated pupils), red as a beet (vasodilation), hot as a hare (hyperthermia), dry as a bone (dry skin), and mad as a hatter (hallucinations/agitation).

206. A 42-year-old female with a history of bipolar disorder, on lithium, comes in to the emergency department with complaints of dizziness, muscle twitching, hand tremors, and diarrhea for 3 days. She states she has generally felt well until these symptoms started and notes that she had a recent visit to her primary care physician's office, where she was diagnosed with hypertension and started on hydrochlorothiazide. You suspect the patient has lithium toxicity. Your next step is:
    A. Activated charcoal
    B. Benzodiazepines
    C. Supportive therapy
    D. Meclizine

Correct Answer C: *Supportive therapy*. Supportive therapy that includes intravenous fluids and cardiac monitoring is the treatment of lithium toxicity. In this case, the patient was already on lithium when she was started on hydrochlorothiazide. Thiazide diuretics impair lithium excretion and can lead to increased serum levels of lithium. This patient has mild symptoms of lithium toxicity, and supportive care is appropriate. With more severe symptoms such as seizures, coma, and renal failure, hemodialysis may be used. Lithium is a monovalent cation and cannot bind to charcoal; so activated charcoal has no use in facilitating the excretion of lithium from the body. Benzodiazepines are not the treatment for lithium overdose. They may be used as an adjunctive therapy only if a patient experiences seizures. Meclizine is used to treat vertigo, not lithium toxicity.

207. Flumazenil is the antidote of choice for which of the following overdoses?

A. Heroin
B. Lithium
C. Benzodiazepine
D. Tylenol

Correct Answer C: *Benzodiazepine. Flumazenil is the reversal agent for benzodiazepine overdose.* It works by competing with benzodiazepines for the $GABA_A$ receptor in the brain and thus preventing benzodiazepines from taking effect on the body. Narcan is the antidote for heroin (option A) overdose. Lithium does not have a reversal agent. N-Acetylcysteine is the antidote for Tylenol (option D) overdose.

208. A 46-year–old female is brought to the emergency department with fever, nausea, vomiting, and tinnitus. The patient admits to an intentional overdose at home, but does not tell you with what medication. On exam, her vital signs are as follows: temp, 100.4°F; HR, 101; BP, 140/60; RR, 32; and O_2 sat 96% on RA. The patient is alert and oriented, and she is hyperactive. Other than being tachycardic, her entire exam is normal. You send off laboratory studies, including a toxicology screen. So far results reveal a metabolic acidosis and additional laboratory studies are still pending. In the meantime, the patient becomes confused and lethargic, and her respiratory rate has slowed to 10 breaths per minute. What medication do you suspect the patient has ingested?

A. Vicodin
B. Aspirin
C. Tylenol
D. Benadryl

Correct Answer B: *Aspirin.* Early acute symptoms of overdose of this medication include nausea, vomiting, and tinnitus. Later symptoms of this medication overdose include fever, hyperactivity that rapidly gives way to lethargy, hyperventilation that quickly progresses to hypoventilation, and finally respiratory arrest. Laboratory findings consistent with aspirin overdose include a respiratory alkalosis in the acute phase of ingestion followed by a compensatory metabolic acidosis. Hyponatremia and hypokalemia may also exist. Vicodin is combination pain medication consisting of hydrocodone and Tylenol. An overdose of Vicodin would lead to respiratory failure, but would not initially present with fever, tinnitus, and hyperactivity. Although Tylenol overdose can present with nausea and vomiting, it is not associated with tinnitus, hyperactivity, and hypoventilation. Benadryl is an antihistamine, and overdose of this medication would result in anticholinergic effects.

209. Which of the following clinical features is more common in hyperosmolar hyperglycemic state (HHS) than diabetic ketoacidosis (DKA)?

A. Mental obtundation and coma
B. Tachypnea and tachycardia
C. Abdominal pain and vomiting
D. Cheyne–Stokes respirations

Correct Answer A: *Mental obtundation and coma.* Neurologic deterioration is more common in HHS due to the greater degree of hyperosmolality. Patients with HHS may also exhibit focal neurologic signs and/or seizures. Mental obtundation may be seen in patients with DKA when severe acidosis exists. Other choices may be seen in both HHS and DKA.

210. A 39-year-old male, with insulin-dependent diabetes mellitus, presents to the emergency department with complaints of nausea, vomiting, and abdominal pain. Vital signs are as follows: temp, 97.2°F; HR, 110; BP, 110/68; RR, 22; and O_2 sat 98% on RA. Finger stick blood sugar is 410; labs are pending. Which of the following should be administered first?

    A. Insulin
    B. K
    C. IV fluids
    D. Bicarbonate

Correct Answer C: *IV fluids.* IV fluids (specifically isotonic saline) should be administered first to expand extracellular volume and stabilize cardiovascular status. Nearly all patients have significant total body K deficit despite often normal serum K levels. K repletion should follow and is based on serum K levels. Next, insulin should be administered but should be delayed until repletion of K has begun because insulin can worsen hypokalemia by driving K into cells, triggering cardiac arrhythmias. Finally, sodium bicarbonate may be given if pH is below 7.0.

211. Which of the following medication classes is least likely to cause hypoglycemia?

    A. Sulfonylureas
    B. Thiazolidinediones
    C. Meglitinides
    D. Both A and B

Correct Answer B: *Thiazolidinediones.* Thiazolidinediones are unlikely to cause hypoglycemia, although the mechanism is not well understood, whereas sulfonylureas and meglitinides increase insulin release from the pancreas, often leading to hypoglycemia.

212. All of the following are correct regarding hyperosmolar hyperglycemic state (HHS) compared to diabetic ketoacidosis (DKA) except?

    A. Patients with DKA generally have higher blood sugars (BS) than those with HHS.
    B. Both are treated with insulin.
    C. Blood pH is more likely to be low in patients with DKA.
    D. HHS most commonly occurs in patients with noninsulin-dependent diabetes mellitus (NIDDM).

Correct Answer A: *Patients with DKA generally have higher blood sugars (BS) than those with HHS.* Patients with DKA generally have serum glucose between 350 and 500 and generally below 800, whereas patients with HHS often have BS exceeding 1,000. Option B is correct as both DKA and HHS are treated with insulin. Option C is correct as blood pH is more likely to be low in patients with DKA as metabolic acidosis is often the major finding, and finally option D is correct as HHS is predominantly in patients with NIDDM, with illness being the major predisposing factor.

213. A 35-year-old female with history of "unknown thyroid problems," who has been off medication for many months due to insurance issues, is brought in by emergency medical services with nausea, vomiting, and abdominal pain. Her vital signs are as follows: temp, 103°F; HR, 140; BP, 103/55; RR, 18; and O_2 sat 98% on RA. Exam is notable for agitation, goiter, and exophthalmos. All of the following are potential treatments for this patient's condition except?

    A. β-Blocker
    B. Glucocorticoids
    C. Thionamide
    D. All of the above

Correct Answer D: *All of the above.* This clinical picture is most consistent with thyroid storm due to medication noncompliance. β-Blockers are used to control signs and symptoms of increased adrenergic tone, thionamides are used to block new hormone synthesis, and steroids are used to reduce T4 to T3 conversion, promote vasomotor stability, and possibly treat associated relative adrenal insufficiency. Other treatment options not listed here include iodine solution to block release of thyroid hormone and iodinated contrast agent to inhibit peripheral conversion of T4 to T3.

214. All of the following are true of myxedema coma except:
    A. It is more common in females than in males.
    B. You would expect low serum thyroid-stimulating hormone (TSH) and high free T4 values.
    C. The hallmark findings are decreased mental status and hypothermia.
    D. Hyponatremia is found in approximately half of patients.

Correct Answer B: *You would expect low serum thyroid-stimulating hormone (TSH) and high free T4 values.* Option B is incorrect as most cases are due to primary hypothyroidism and you would expect high serum TSH and low free T4. Option A is correct as females are more commonly affected. Patients often present with lesser degrees of altered mental status, but will progress to coma if untreated, and hypothermia is due to the decrease in thermogenesis that accompanies decreased metabolism. Hyponatremia is common due to impaired free water excretion secondary to inappropriate excess vasopressin secretion or impaired renal function.

215. Which of the following is an appropriate treatment for myxedema coma?
    A. Thyroid hormone therapy
    B. Stress dose steroids
    C. Supportive care
    D. All of the above

Correct Answer D: *All of the above.* There is debate regarding the preferred method of thyroid hormone therapy, but ultimately it is recommended. Stress dose steroids are imperative until the possibility of concomitant adrenal insufficiency has been excluded. Finally supportive care measures may include fluid resuscitation, electrolyte repletion, mechanical ventilation, correction of hypothermia, and treatment of possible predisposing infection.

216. All of the following are true about cerebral edema except:
    A. Treatment includes reducing fluid administration and administering mannitol or hypertonic saline.
    B. Cerebral edema is more common in children with newly diagnosed insulin-dependent diabetes mellitus.
    C. Patients with cerebral edema will have tachycardia.
    D. Abnormalities on head CT occur late in the development of cerebral edema.

Correct Answer C: *Patients with cerebral edema will have tachycardia.* Sustained heart rate deceleration is actually one of the major diagnostic criteria. Option A is the correct treatment regimen. Option B is a true statement as risk factors include younger children and those with newly diagnosed type I diabetes. Option D is a true statement, and therefore, decision to treat should be based on clinical exam and not CT.

217. 82-year-old female, with history of hypertension, noninsulin-dependent diabetes mellitus, and chronic kidney disease, currently being treated for a urinary tract infection presents to the emergency room with hypoglycemia in the 40s. Which of the following medications could be contributing to her hypoglycemia?
    A. Ciprofloxacin
    B. Atenolol

C. Lisinopril

D. All of the above

Correct Answer D: *All of the above.* Drug-induced hypoglycemia occurs more frequently in elderly patients, particularly those with underlying renal or hepatic dysfunction and in those taking insulin-lowering medications such as insulin or sulfonylureas. Fluoroquinolones, β-blockers, and angiotensin-converting enzyme inhibitors have all been associated with hypoglycemia.

218. Myxedema coma is associated with which of the following findings:

   A. Tachycardia

   B. Hyperthermia

   C. Hyperglycemia

   D. Hyponatremia

Correct Answer D: *Hyponatremia.* Hyponatremia is the result of the fluid retention in the body. The other answers are incorrect as bradycardia, hypothermia, and hypoglycemia are all results of severe hypothyroidism, which leads to the slowing of most organ systems.

219. A 62-year-old male presents to the emergency department slurring his words and smelling of alcohol. He is disheveled, but is able to give you a history of vomiting four to five times of bright red blood. He then vomits about 150 mL of bright red blood. Per hospital records he had known ETOH abuse. On physical exam vital signs are as follows: temp, 97.6°F; HR, 123; BP, 84/40; RR, 26; and O_2 sat 97% on RA. He is jaundice appearing with scleral icterus and mild diffuse abdominal tenderness with ascites. What should be the next emergency department intervention to be started?

   A. Omeprazole

   B. Metronidazole

   C. Octreotide

   D. Propranolol

Correct Answer C: *Octreotide.* It is a medication used to help reduce hemorrhage in patients with upper gastrointestinal bleed caused by esophageal varices. This diagnosis is likely due to the patient's known alcohol abuse and liver disease consistent with scleral icterus, jaundice, and ascites. Omeprazole is an oral proton pump inhibitor and since the patient is vomiting he would not tolerate it. Metronidazole is used for abdominal infections and would not play a role in treating the vomiting. Propranolol is a β-blocker that can be used for prophylaxis or varices, but not for acute hemorrhage.

220. A 40-year-old male presents to the emergency department with mild lower abdominal pain for 3 days. No other associated symptoms. He denies alleviating or aggravating symptoms. He is otherwise healthy, and he denies any daily medication use. Vital signs are within normal limits, he is well appearing, in no acute distress with a soft, nondistended abdomen with mild left lower quadrant abdominal tenderness to palpation without rebound or guarding. You suspect diverticulitis as your leading diagnosis. What is the next most appropriate management for this patient?

   A. Broad-spectrum IV antibiotics

   B. Oral metronidazole and ciprofloxacin

   C. General surgery consultation

   D. Abdominal and pelvic CT scan

Correct Answer B: *Oral metronidazole and ciprofloxacin.* The next more appropriate treatment for uncomplicated diverticulitis is oral antibiotics, antiemetics, liquid diet for 2 to 3 days, and close follow-up. Due to the patient being otherwise healthy and afebrile without associated symptoms, there is not surgical intervention or need for broad-spectrum IV antibiotics. The infection can be treated with oral antibiotics. A CT of the abdomen and pelvis could be considered to confirm the diagnosis, but if the patient's symptoms improve with the initial treatment, he should not be exposed to unnecessary radiation.

221. A mother brings her otherwise healthy 18-month-old daughter to be evaluated for a dark red blood in her diaper. This has never happened before. The patient has otherwise been acting appropriately, eating and drinking well, and not complaining of pain or crying with bowel movements. On exam vital signs are within normal limits, well appearing, and playful child. Exam is unremarkable except for dark red blood in the diaper with a nontender rectum. You decide to send the patient for a nuclear medicine scan. Based on this information what is the most likely diagnosis?
    A. Meckel's diverticulum
    B. Intussusception
    C. Internal hemorrhoid
    D. Volvulus

Correct Answer A: *Meckel's diverticulum.* This diagnosis usually starts with a large amount of rectal bleeding without any other associated signs or symptoms. The diagnostic study of choice is a Meckel scan. Intussusception is a telescoping of one part of the intestine into the other, which causes intense pain and cramping. Without patient having associated symptoms, this diagnosis is very unlikely. Volvulus or intestinal malrotation is rare, causes vascular comprise to the intestine, and can lead to necrosis. The patient would have other associated symptoms such as fever, pain or vomiting. An internal hemorrhoid would be palpable on rectal exam and likely cause painful bowel movements.

222. A 32-year-old female with a history of 1 week of abdominal pain, fevers, vomiting, and diarrhea presents with worsening symptoms and now bloody diarrhea. She denies any known medical history, but had an appendectomy as a child. On exam, her vital signs are significant for a temp 100.7°F, HR 109, and BP 106/78. She appears uncomfortable with dry mucous membranes, diffuse abdominal tenderness with voluntary guarding, and guaiac positive stool. What is the next step in management for this patient?
    A. Abdominal and pelvic CT scan
    B. Broad-spectrum antibiotic
    C. General surgery consultation
    D. Oral antibiotics

Correct Answer A: *Abdominal and pelvic CT scan.* Patient's symptoms could represent many intra-abdominal pathologies, including toxic megacolon, infectious bowel disease, and inflammatory bowel disease. The next step in being able to appropriately manage this patient is to send her for an abdominal and pelvic CT scan. Due to the patient's history, broad-spectrum antibiotics should be initiated rather than oral as well as surgical consultation, but this is all pending the results of the abdominal and pelvic CT scan.

223. An elderly patient with a medical history of coronary artery disease, hypertension, hyperlipidemia, diabetes, and rate controlled atrial fibrillation is at risk for developing which of the following intra-abdominal emergencies?
    A. Aortic dissection
    B. Mesenteric ischemia
    C. Volvulus
    D. Diverticulitis

Correct Answer B: *Mesenteric ischemia.* Atrial fibrillation can be a common contributor in the development of mesenteric ischemia because atrial fibrillation can cause an arterial embolism of the abdominal vasculature that originates from the heart. Atrial fibrillation plays no role in developing diverticulitis, which starts with diverticulosis of the bowel that becomes infected. Volvulus is malrotation of the intestines, which leads to vascular compromise of the bowel, but is not caused by an embolism. With an aortic dissection, the cause is due to a tear in the aortic intima not initiated by an embolism.

224. A 28-year-old male, with no medical history, presents with right lower abdominal pain since yesterday morning. Pain is worse with walking and extension of his right hip. He also reports decreased appetite, but denies fevers, chills, nausea, vomiting, or diarrhea. Vital signs are as follows: temp, 100.2°F; HR, 98; BP, 117/68; RR, 18; O_2 sat 98% on RA. He appears mild uncomfortable lying on his left side, heart is regular, clear lungs to auscultation bilaterally, abdominal exam reveals normal active bowel sounds, nondistended, with mild right lower quadrant tenderness. You send the patient for an abdominal and pelvic CT scan, which shows an enlarged appendix with streaking and free fluid around the surrounding bowel. What is the next step in the management of this patient?

   A. Laparoscopic appendectomy
   B. Parental antibiotics
   C. Parental steroids
   D. Endoscopic retrograde cholangiopancreatography (ERCP)

Correct Answer B: *Parental antibiotics.* Prior to the patient needing an urgent appendectomy for a likely ruptured appendix, the patient with need to be started on broad-spectrum antibiotics to help reduce the risk of becoming septic with two large-bore IVs giving fluids. ERCP has no treatment benefits for appendicitis; it is used for the treatment of retained or obstructing gall stones in the common bile duct. Steroids are not the treatment of choice for an acute appendicitis as it does not aid in the healing process.

225. First-line treatment for *Helicobacter pylori* includes all of the following except?

   A. Amoxicillin
   B. Clarithromycin
   C. Pantoprazole
   D. Oral vancomycin

Correct Answer D: *Oral vancomycin.* Triple therapy should be initiated for first-line treatment of *H. pylori*, including a proton pump inhibitor, amoxicillin, and clarithromycin for 7 to 14 days. There is no data on the effects of oral vancomycin for treatment of this bacterium. It is most commonly used for treatment of *Clostridium difficile.*

226. 54-year-old male presents with his wife to the emergency department for altered mental status. The wife reports the patient was in his usual state of health until 3 days ago when he started complaining of nausea and abdominal pain. He has never had similar symptoms in the past, and there is no vomiting or diarrhea. On exam he is ill appearing, alert, and oriented. Labs show a white blood cell of 21, elevated alkaline phosphate, and bilirubin. You and your attending do a bedside ultrasound (US) that shows significant narrowing of the common bile duct. Which of the following diagnostic tests would be most appropriate?

   A. Official right upper quadrant (RUQ) US
   B. Abdominal and pelvic CT scan
   C. Barium swallow
   D. Emergent laparotomy
   E. ERCP: endoscopic retrograde cholangiopancreatography

Correct Answer E: *ERCP: endoscopic retrograde cholangiopancreatography.* The patient likely had cholangitis obstructing the common bile duct and will need an ERCP to decompress the dilation and obstructing stone. With a bedside RUQ US showing narrowing of the common bile duct, an official US would not show any further information as well as an abdominal CT. Emergency laparotomy is not indicated at this time because the management of obstructing cholangitis needs internal decompression with the ERCP. If there were intra-abdominal complications warranting an ex-lap, then surgery would be consulted and intervened at that time.

227. What is the most common side effect of an endoscopic retrograde cholangiopancreatography (ERCP)?
    A. Cholangitis
    B. Small bowel obstruction
    C. Adhesion
    D. Pancreatitis

Correct Answer D: *Pancreatitis.* Inflammation of the pancreas is the most common complication after a patient undergoes an ERCP. If it does occur, most cases are mild with epigastric abdominal pain and nausea. This usually resolves within a few days with hospitalization for fluids and anti-emetics. Although the other three options could be side effects based on research, the percentage is extremely low.

228. Less than one-third of patients preset with the classic Charcot triad, but in the event, you see a patient with these symptoms. Which of the following is the correct combination?
    A. Fever, leukocytosis, and right upper quadrant pain
    B. Fever, right upper quadrant pain, and jaundice
    C. Right upper quadrant pain, jaundice, and leukocytosis
    D. Right upper quadrant pain, leukocytosis, and elevated lipase

Correct Answer B: *Fever, right upper quadrant pain, and jaundice.* These three signs and symptoms represent the classic triad. Leukocytosis, elevated alkaline phosphate and bilirubin levels can help guide the diagnosis.

229. A 39-year-old male presents with painful rectal bleeding for the past 6 days. It is worse with bearing down while trying to have a bowel movement. He reports blood streaks in his stool as well as with wiping. On physical examination, you appreciate an anal fissure. What is not the next step in management for this patient?
    A. Abdominal and pelvic CT scan and blood work
    B. Stool softeners
    C. Sits baths
    D. High-fiber diet and stool softener

Correct Answer A: *Abdominal and pelvic CT scan and blood work.* Answers B, C, and D are all conservative treatment for uncomplicated anal fissures.

230. A 28-year-old, G1P0, 30 weeks gestation, presents to the emergency department for a painful bowel movements with bright red blood on toilet paper. On exam she is well appearing with normal vital signs, abdomen is soft, consistent with uterus above the umbilicus, and non-tender. Rectal exam shows a thrombosed internal hemorrhoid, which you are unsuccessful at reducing. Your next step should be which of the following?
    A. Elliptical excision
    B. Topical anesthetics

C. Surgical consultation

D. Topical nitroglycerine

Correct Answer C: *Surgical consultation.* Internal hemorrhoids that become thrombosed and irreducible are very likely to become necrotic and need emergency surgical consultation for further management. Topical anesthetics and nitroglycerine are conservative treatment for nonthrombosed external hemorrhoids. Elliptical excision is an option for an external hemorrhoid that is not already thrombosed and needs to be drained.

231. You are covering the microbiology reports for the emergency department today, and you come across a patient's hepatitis panel, which shows the following results; anti-HBs positive, anti-HBC negative, and HBcAg negative. What is the correct representation of the viral panel?

A. Acute exposure to hepatitis B

B. Chronic exposure to hepatitis B

C. Vaccination to hepatitis B

D. Acute exposure to hepatitis C

E. Chronic exposure to hepatitis C

Correct Answer C: *Vaccination to hepatitis B.* If patients are vaccinated against hepatitis B, the core antigen will be negative (HBcAg). Patients who are exposed to hepatitis B will develop antibodies to the surface showing positive anti-HBs.

232. What is the most common way hepatitis B is transmitted?

A. Oral route

B. Blood

C. Fecal route

D. Respiratory droplets

Correct Answer B: *Blood.* Both hepatitis B and C are transmitted by body fluids and blood. Hepatitis A and E are transmitted by the oral–fecal route.

233. Abdominal pain that is felt in the midline and bilaterally around the midline and epigastrium is known as what type of abdominal pain?

A. Parietal abdominal pain

B. Somatic abdominal pain

C. Diffuse abdominal pain

D. Visceral abdominal pain

Correct Answer D: *Visceral abdominal pain.* This is pain in the midline and bilaterally around the midline because it follows the blood supply. Parietal abdominal pain occurs when there is irritation to the peritoneal lining, making the pain more severe and easier to localize. Diffuse abdominal pain is as it sounds, usually all over without ability to localize a more tender area than the other. Somatic pain is well localized. It is usually located asymmetrically and becomes worse with deep inspiration or pressure on the abdominal wall.

234. A 29-year-old female presents with nausea, nonbloody, nonbilious vomiting, and diffuse abdominal pain for 3 days. Patient states her symptoms have progressively worsened over the past 24 hours and has had no relief with home prescriptions of Ondansetron and metoclopramide. She has a known medical history for cyclic vomiting syndrome and has had multiple emergency department visits for similar symptoms. On exam patient is uncomfortable appearing, but nontoxic, vital signs are notable only for a heart rate of 114 and an abdominal exam with positive normal active bowel sounds, nondistended abdomen with diffuse

tenderness to palpation without rebound or guarding. You start IV fluids and IV antiemetics. What should be your next step in managing this patient?

A. Gastrointestinal consultation
B. Abdominal ultrasound (US)
C. Abdominal and pelvic CT scan
D. Laboratory studies including complete blood count, comprehensive metabolic panel, urinalysis, and urine pregnancy
E. Nothing, continue IV fluids and antiemetics as needed

Correct Answer D: *Laboratory studies.* Although patient has had many similar presentations, she still needs laboratory studies obtained for further management. Many patients will have hypokalemia or hyponatremia that needs to be repleted. She should also have a urinalysis. The patient should be medically managed prior to any imaging unless her physical exam is concerning. There may be an intra-abdominal pathology causing her symptoms and not the cyclical vomiting.

235. A 27-year-old female presents from her family lake house on a hot summer day with sudden onset of nausea, vomiting, and cramping abdominal pain 3 hours ago. She was in her usual state of health prior the onset of symptoms, is otherwise healthy, and denies daily medications. Patient reports eating hot dogs, potato salad, salad, and corn on the cob. Her sister has had three episodes of diarrhea as well. What should be the next step in this patient's emergency department treatment course?

A. Oral metronidazole
B. Oral ciprofloxacin
C. Abdominal and pelvic CT scan
D. Symptomatic treatment including IV fluids and antiemetics

Correct Answer D: *Symptomatic treatment.* In an otherwise healthy female who was in her usual state of health just prior to eating food on a hot summer day likely has an infectious gastrointestinal pathogen, most commonly *E. coli.* Conservative treatment including IV fluids and antinausea medications should be more than appropriate for this patient as the infection will run its course usually lasting between 12 and 48 hours. If the patient's symptoms persist and do not improve with IV fluids, CT scan of the abdomen and pelvis should be considered then pending results adding antibiotics.

236. A 25-year-old male presents to the emergency department with right lower quadrant abdominal pain, nausea, and nonbloody diarrhea for the past 2 to 3 days. He has had symptoms like this before. Vital signs are within normal limits; he is ill appearing with dry mucous membranes and nondistended abdominal with moderate tenderness to the right lower and mid-abdomen with voluntary guarding. Negative psoas and obturator signs. Laboratory results are revealing for leukocytosis, an elevated lactate, a normal lipase, liver panel, and urinalysis. CT of abdomen and pelvis shows an inflammatory mass in the right lower quadrant associated with wall thickening and narrowing of the lumen of the terminal ileum. This is most consistent with which of the following diagnoses?

A. Crohn's disease
B. Ulcerative colitis
C. Diverticulitis
D. Mesenteric ischemia

Correct Answer A: *Crohn disease.* It is an inflammatory response extending through intestinal wall from mucosa to serosa, and can involve any part of the intestine (distal small bowel most common). Common symptoms are abdominal pain, nausea, and nonbloody diarrhea. CT findings of wall thickening in the distal ileum are consistent with Crohn's. Ulcerative colitis is a disease of the colon with ulcers and typically causes bloody diarrhea. Diverticulitis is when the diverticula form within the wall of the colon and then becomes inflamed by bacteria. Mesenteric ischemia is vascular compromise of the bowel usually from emboli that can lead to necrosis of the bowel.

237. For the patient above in question #18, what is the next most appropriate intervention for ultimate diagnosis?

   A. Endoscopy and colonoscopy
   B. Endoscopic retrograde cholangiopancreatography (ERCP)
   C. Hepatobiliary iminodiacetic acid scan
   D. Abdominal ultrasound

Correct Answer A: *Endoscopy and colonoscopy.* The patient will need a gastrointestinal consultation and further workup includes endoscopy and colonoscopy to directly visualize where the disease lies as well as how invasive. Abdominal ultrasound and ERCP have no importance in providing further information about the characteristics of the bowel.

238. A 40-year-old obese female presents with almost 2 months of daily epigastric pain, nausea, reflux, and few episodes of vomiting. Patient reports she has been seen by her Primary Care Provider twice for the same symptoms and started on an H2 blocker and then a protein pump inhibitor (PPI) both with some improvement, but it has not completely resolved. Her symptoms usually are better during the day and worse at night. You get a test that confirms *H. pylori*. What should be initiated next to the patient's treatment plan?

   A. Ibuprofen to decrease inflammation
   B. Ondansetron to control nausea
   C. Antibiotics
   D. Endoscopy

Correct Answer C: *Antibiotics.* She needs an antibiotic for triple therapy treatment to eradicate the infection. If her symptoms still persist after this, then she may need an endoscopy for further workup.

239. What are the most common signs and symptoms in a patient whom you suspect sclerosing cholangitis?

   A. Leukocytosis and elevated alkaline phosphate
   B. Elevated lipase and amylase
   C. Jaundice and conjugated hyperbilirubinemia
   D. Jaundice and elevated transaminitis

Correct Answer C: *Jaundice and conjugated hyperbilirubinemia.* The hyperbilirubinemia is caused by biliary duct obstruction, and jaundice is usually clinically seen with bilirubin levels around 3 mg per dL and associated with intense itching.

240. What is the most common hereditary cause of elevated bilirubin?

   A. Sickle cell disease
   B. Autoimmune hemolytic anemia
   C. Cholangitis
   D. Gilbert syndrome

Correct Answer D: *Gilbert syndrome.* This syndrome is hereditary causing the enzyme that breaks down bilirubin to inefficiently break down bilirubin, which then causes the rise in the blood levels.

Sickle cell disease and autoimmune hemolytic anemia are defects in the blood hemoglobin and antibodies. Cholangitis is not a hereditary disease and is caused by an infection of the common bile duct.

241. A 70-year-old female, who is healthy and active for her age, reports some mild epigastric pain over the past few days and then had two separate episodes of hematemesis with clots. During your detailed history, the patient starts to appear more ill, diaphoretic, and then vomits a large amount of bright red blood into the emesis basin. Her BP has dropped to 80/56 with a heart rate increased to 118. You appreciate moderate epigastric tenderness. Further history reveals daily nonsteroidal anti-inflammatory drug (NSAID) use for arthritis and bloody stools. The patient vomits a second time with a similar amount of bright red blood. What is the definitive step in managing the patient's hematemesis?

    A. EGD (esophagogastroduodenoscopy)
    B. Octreotide
    C. IV pantoprazole
    D. Nasogastric tube

Correct Answer A: *EGD (esophagogastroduodenoscopy).* The patient needs an emergency EGD to help stop the bleeding from the upper gastrointestinal bleed likely from peptic ulcer disease caused by the daily NSAID usage. Although she will likely receive IV pantoprazole as well as an nasogastric tube, this will not visualize the bleed to assess how the bleeding should be controlled. Octreotide is first line in acute gastroesophageal varices.

242. Dad brings in his 2-year-old daughter because she has been "fussy" for the past 24 hours with decreased appetite and pointing to her abdomen that it hurts. Dad reports his daughter is otherwise healthy and suddenly he noticed her lying on the couch crying in the fetal position. After a few moments she felt better but has had multiple episodes. On exam she is well appearing with normal vital signs. Her abdomen is soft, but she is nervous for you to fully palpate her abdomen. No masses are found. During further history talking with dad, the patient begins to cry and draw her knees to her chest. What is the next most appropriate step to managing this patient?

    A. Air enema
    B. Abdominal ultrasound (US)
    C. Abdominal and pelvic CT scan
    D. Nothing, supportive care with fluids

Correct Answer A: *Air enema.* This study of choice is diagnostic as well as therapeutic for intussusception. The classic signs of abdominal pain and drawing the knees to the chest are most consistent with intussusception as well. CT scans are not advised in young children, as there are other options such as kidney, ureter, and bladder (KUB) x-ray to assess the anatomy of the bowel. Abdominal US may give some information if intussusception is present, but it is not therapeutic.

243. An 83-year-old male is brought in by his family, who is concerned about intermittent altered mental status over the past few days. Patient has a past medical history for hypertension, hyperlipidemia, hepatic encephalopathy, and diabetes mellitus. Per patient he has felt well but does report having a few moments of confusion. He also reports not being fully compliant with his daily medications, which include metoprolol, omeprazole, simvastatin, and lactulose. Vital signs are stable. He is well appearing, alert, and oriented to person, place, and time, and abdominal exam is unremarkable. Laboratory workup reveals an elevated ammonia (NH_3). What is the next step in management for this patient?

    A. Abdominal and pelvic CT scan
    B. Endoscopic retrograde cholangiopancreatography
    C. IV fluids and antiemetics
    D. Initiate oral lactulose

Correct Answer D: *Initiate oral lactulose.* With a known history of hepatic encephalopathy, mild altered mental status, elevated NH_3, and noncompliance with home medications, the patient needs to start lactulose to titrate to 3 to 4 bowel movements per day to help reduce NH_3 level. This is the treatment of choice in patients with mild signs and symptoms of hepatic encephalopathy. IV fluids and antiemetics can be added but are more for symptoms control not treatment.

244. What is the most common cause of a small bowel obstruction?
    A. Infection
    B. Adhesions
    C. Mass
    D. Hernia

Correct Answer B: *Adhesions.* Adhesions from previous abdominal surgeries are fibrous bands between the tissues and organs that can act as an internal scar connecting tissues that are not normally connected, leading to an obstruction of the bowel. Infection, masses, and hernia are all causes of small bowel obstruction, but adhesions are still the most common cause.

245. Which of the following is the most common type of hernia?
    A. Inguinal
    B. Umbilical
    C. Femoral
    D. Incisional

Correct Answer A: *Inguinal.* Inguinal hernias account for almost 30% of all hernias. There are two different types of inguinal hernias, direct and indirect. Femoral hernias are the most common type of hernia in women but not over all. Umbilical hernias are usually present at birth and resolve with time or are chronic.

246. A 33-year-old male presents with the emergency department for left groin pain since yesterday. He is otherwise healthy and well appearing. Vital signs are within normal limits, and physical exam is positive for a palpable mass at the left inguinal area and some fullness to the left scrotum. This likely represents which type of hernia?
    A. Direct inguinal hernia
    B. Indirect inguinal hernia
    C. Ventral hernia
    D. Incisional hernia

Correct Answer B: *Indirect inguinal hernia.* Most common and congenital, it is described as a passage of the intestines through the inguinal ring down the inguinal canal, thus making this diagnosis most consistent with fullness in the scrotum. Incision hernias are in the area of a previous incision. Direct hernia is a hernia through a weak point in the fascia of the abdominal wall and does not follow the inguinal canal into the scrotum. Ventral hernia is a bulging of the abdominal wall usually in the midline.

247. A 19-year-old male is brought to the emergency department by his friends, because they noticed blood in the patient's vomit. He is intoxicated, disheveled, and smells of alcohol. The patient's friends report he drank a pint of vodka and then vomited five times with small amount of blood in the last episode of emesis that made them concerned. Vital signs are stable, and physical exam is unremarkable. You start IV fluids and antiemetics, and observe the patient for any change in his condition. What was the most likely cause of the hematemesis?
    A. Esophageal varices
    B. Peptic ulcer disease
    C. Small tear in the gastroesophageal junction
    D. *Helicobacter pylori*

Correct Answer C: *Small tear in the gastroesophageal junction.* Patient's symptoms and history of forceful vomiting are most consistent with a Mallory–Weiss tear, which is a tear in the esophagus generally at the gastroesophageal junction. Most resolve on their own without treatment. Peptic ulcer disease would cause more epigastric discomfort with signs of reflux and possibly lead to melena. *H. pylori* is a bacterial infection in the stomach, which is not associated with acute hematemesis but reflux, epigastric fullness and pain.

248. A 16-year-old male with a history of poorly controlled diabetes mellitus (DM) arrives to urgent care with a fever of 102.4, heart rate of 110, respiratory rate of 22, O_2 saturation of 97% on room air, and blood pressure of 110/63. He and his mother relate to you that he has had a sore throat and left ear pressure for 2 weeks. Mom reports that yesterday morning he developed a high fever and shaking chills. Physical exam reveals a febrile but otherwise mildly ill appearing young man. He has TMs that are bilaterally occluded by wax. He has mild blanching erythema of the left posterior auricular area. Pharynx is clear. Positive left-sided neck and submandibular lymphadenopathy. Rate is tachycardic but regular. Lungs are clear to auscultation. Abdomen is soft and nontender. Your likely diagnosis given the information above is:

    A. Otitis media
    B. Viral pharyngitis
    C. Ludwig's angina
    D. Acute mastoiditis

Correct Answer D: *Acute mastoiditis.* **This is more frequently seen in patients with DM, and usually presents with fever, and posterior ear swelling and erythema.** Otitis generally does not cause posterior ear pain and erythema. Viral pharyngitis is also seen with upper respiratory symptoms and generally does not present with posterior ear pain and erythema. Ludwig's angina generally also presents with submandibular pain, lower facial pain, and is associated with underlying dental caries.

249. A 4-year-old girl arrives with her mother to the emergency department (ED) for evaluation of slow onset of drooling and cough. Her father reports 2 to 3 days of sore throat and hoarse cough. She is leaning forward, drooling, breathing 24 times a minute with loud inspiratory sounds. You obtain chest x-ray to evaluate for pneumonia and neck x-ray to evaluate for possible obstructing foreign body. Chest x-ray shows no infiltrate; neck x-ray shows no visible foreign body but does show a thumb print sign. Your next step in management is.

    A. Immediate intubation and airway support
    B. Arrange for emergent anesthesia evaluation, and transport of the child to the operating room (OR) with ENT for possible surgical airway while maintaining supportive airway management in the ED
    C. Give racemic epinephrine and admit for observation
    D. Preform blind finger sweep for foreign body

Correct Answer B: *Arrange for emergent anesthesia evaluation, and transport of the child to the operating room (OR) with ENT for possible surgical airway while maintaining supportive airway management in the ED.* You would want to ensure that you have specialized airway assistance available if needed as any manipulation of the airway in these patients can lead to sudden worsening of her clinical condition and may require surgical airway, which is always better obtained in a controlled setting with specialty care. Intubation is appropriate, but anticipation of a difficult airway is more appropriate, and you would normally like to ensure that you have anesthesia and OR available for possible surgical airway if needed. Racemic epinephrine is not the appropriate treatment for this scenario; this patient needs emergent ENT evaluation and backup for airway intervention if needed. Blind finger sweep is incorrect because this procedure is not indicated in this patient and may in fact worsen her condition.

250. A 26-year-old male with no medical history presents to urgent care for evaluation of 3 days of watery rhinorrhea, sneezing, nonproductive cough, malaise, and sore throat. His vital signs reveal temp 98.6°F, HR 82, BP 123/64, RR 16, and O_2 sat 98% on RA. This patient's most likely diagnosis is.

   A. Influenza
   B. *Streptococcus pharyngitis*
   C. Viral upper respiratory infection
   D. Respiratory syncytial virus (RSV)

Correct Answer C: *Viral upper respiratory infection.* Most upper respiratory infections are caused by rhinoviruses and are generally self-limiting. Influenza would generally present with high fever. *S. pharyngitis* would generally be marked with unilateral exudate and fever, which was not described in this case. RSV would be uncommon in a patient of this age.

251. A 49-year-old male presents with 3 days left tooth pain and left-sided upper facial swelling. Exam reveals tooth 13 periodontal swelling and fluctuance. His likely diagnosis and treatment are:

   A. Pulpitis, treat with doxycycline and discharge patient home with close dental clinic follow-up
   B. Dental caries, treat with NSAIDs, and discharge patient home with close dental clinic follow-up
   C. Dental abscess, attempt incision and drainage, and treat with clindamycin. Discharge patient home with dental clinic follow-up in the next 1 to 2 days
   D. Deep space infection, initiate broad-spectrum antibiotics, and transfer for emergent ENT evaluation

Correct Answer C: *Dental abscess, attempt incision and drainage, and treat with clindamycin. Discharge patient home with dental clinic follow-up in the next 1 to 2 days.* There is clinical evidence of dental abscess. The exam is not consistent with dental caries. There is no evidence of deep space infection, and there is no role in the case for IV antibiotics.

252. A 92-year-old male with history of hypertension, coronary artery disease, chronic obstructive pulmonary disease, nasal polyps, aortic valve replacement on Coumadin arrives to the emergency department with 3 hours of epistaxis. His vital signs are stable. His exam reveals profuse bleeding from the left nare without visualized focal area of bleeding; there is no visualized posterior nasal bleeding. Laboratory evaluation reveals white blood cell of 9.2, hematocrit of 39, platelets of 170, partial thromboplastin time of 33.4, and international normalized ratio (INR) of 2.6. Your initial treatment option would be.

   A. Attempt anterior nasal packing and initiate Coumadin reversal with vitamin K IV
   B. Hold manual anterior nasal pressure for 20 minutes and reevaluate
   C. Electrocautery of source of bleeding
   D. Reverse INR with vitamin K and transfer for emergent ENT evaluation

Correct Answer B: *Hold manual anterior nasal pressure for 20 minutes and reevaluate.* In this case, the most appropriate first intervention would be to hold manual pressure in attempt to stop the bleeding. Reversal of anticoagulation in artificial valve should be carefully considered, and in this case, there is no evidence of posterior bleeding, thus symptomatic treatment should be attempted first. There is no clear source of bleeding identified in this case; therefore, pressure control should be attempted first.

253. A tall 29-year-old male with a 7 pack-year history presents to the emergency department complaining of right-sided chest pain and increased shortness of breath on exertion. The patient states yesterday he sneezed and felt a sudden, sharp pain in the right side of

his chest. The pain is worse with deep inspiration, but otherwise nonradiating. He feels he is becoming more short of breath even going up two flights of stairs. No significant medical history. Vital signs: BP, 110/90; HR, 90; RR, 17; and O_2 sat 96% on RA, but will drop to 94% when the patient is explaining his symptoms. This presentation is most consistent with what diagnosis?

A. Aortic dissection
B. Pulmonary embolism (PE)
C. Tension pneumothorax
D. Spontaneous pneumothorax

Correct Answer D: *Spontaneous pneumothorax.* The patient's history and vitals are most consistent with a spontaneous pneumothorax. The patient is a tall male with a history of smoking. It is thought that taller individuals are at increased risk of spontaneous pneumothoraces due to the increase in negative pressure generated at the lung apices. Smoking also increases an individuals' risk up to 20× that of a nonsmoker. The patient's BP and HR are within normal limits, and consequently, no tension physiology is being seen at this time. Without a known history of connective tissue disease (i.e., Marfan, Ehlers–Danlos), and without radiating pain to the back, aortic dissection in an otherwise healthy 29-year-old male becomes very unlikely. PE could be considered with this patient's constellation of symptoms; however, with the sudden onset of symptoms after a sneeze in the context of the rest of the history without known risk factors, PE also becomes less likely.

254. An otherwise healthy 43-year-old female presents after sustaining a mechanical trip and fall, at which time she hit the right side of her chest against the side of her table. She noted immediate pain in the right ribs, worse with inspiration. Over the past 30 minutes, she has become increasingly short of breath, slightly dyspneic and decides to dial 911. On arrival she is in moderate respiratory distress, vitals are as follows: HR 126, BP 84/58, RR 25, and O_2 sat of 88% on RA. On exam her trachea appears slightly deviated from midline, absent breath sounds on the right, and there is slight jugular venous distention. She tells you "Help me! I can't breathe, I feel like I'm going to pass out!" What is the first thing you should do for this patient?

A. Place her on high-flow O_2
B. Start an IV and begin intravenous fluids resuscitation
C. Obtain a chest x-ray
D. Needle decompression

Correct Answer D: *Needle decompression.* The patient's history and physical exam should immediately make you concerned for a tension pneumothorax. The patient reports mild trauma to the ribs with progressive worsening shortness of breath and dyspnea. She presents hypotensive, tachycardiac, and hypoxic with the feeling she cannot breathe. Exam demonstrates absent breath sounds and a slightly shifted trachea. In this setting, there is no need for chest x-ray to confirm diagnosis prior to needle decompression. This time lapse may cause the patient to further deteriorate. All of the other potential answers should be done; however, they are not the first things that need to be done in a patient with a tension pneumothorax. Once it is decompressed, further stabilization of the patient should be performed and, possibly, tube thoracotomy.

255. A 20-year-old male with no significant medical history presents with spontaneous right-sided, pleuritic chest pain. Chest x-ray demonstrates a small pneumothorax. Repeating x-ray 6 hours later demonstrates the pneumothorax is stable. Prior to discharging the patient, he

tells you he is scheduled to fly in 2 days and wants to know if it is safe for him to fly. You explain to him that:

A. It is *safe* to fly as long as the flight is <12 hours long.

B. It is *unsafe* to fly because, in accordance with Boyle law, the pneumothorax will increase in size and, potentially, convert into a tension pneumothorax.

C. It is *safe* to fly as long as the flight is <6 hours long.

D. It is *safe* to fly because, in accordance to Boyle law, the pneumothorax will actually shrink, making it completely safe to fly.

Correct Answer B: *It is unsafe to fly because, in accordance with Boyle law, the pneumothorax will increase in size and, potentially, convert into a tension pneumothorax. An active pneumothorax is a contraindication to flight.* The reason for this is explained via Boyle law, which states that pressure and volume are inversely proportional to a gas at a stable temperature. Consequently, at elevation, the pressure within the cabin is decreased (in comparison to ground level), which allows for an increase in gas volume (the pneumothorax). This could possibly lead to an inflight emergency if a previously simple, small pneumothorax converted into a tension pneumothorax or resulted in significant hypoxia and dyspnea due to its increase in size. In patients with underlying pulmonary or cardiac disease, such as chronic obstructive pulmonary disease or coronary artery disease, the decreased O_2 level due to an increase in size puts them at even a greater risk as such things as worsening hypoxia, ischemia, or potentially myocardial infarction.

256. A 28-year-old female on the oral contraceptive pill presents complaining of left-sided chest pain for 24 hours. The patient states the previous day she was walking when she developed a sudden onset of sharp left-sided chest pain. The pain radiates slightly into the left side of her back, is worse with deep inspiration, and has otherwise been associated with exertional dyspnea and a transient episode of lightheadedness when her symptoms first began. Medical history is otherwise significant for a recent partial tear of her gastrocnemius muscle, which she reports has minimized her physical activity as of late. There is no significant family history. Vitals: HR, 110; BP, 108/80; RR, 17; and O_2 sat 95% on RA. The classic EKG findings that would be most consistent with this patient's diagnosis is:

A. Delta waves

B. Diffuse ST elevations and PR depression

C. Electrical alternans and diffuse low voltage

D. Prominent S wave in I with Q waves and inverted T waves in III

Correct Answer D: *Prominent S wave in I with Q waves and inverted T waves in III.* The patient described above is presenting with a pulmonary embolism (PE). She has a number of risk factors, including the oral contraceptive pill, recent immobility, and recent trauma to the lower extremity. Other risk factors for PE include pregnancy, surgery within the past 4 weeks, long flights, immobilization, personal history of deep venous thrombosis/PE, and known hypercoagulopathy. The EKG findings that have been reported to be "classic" for PE include the S1Q3T3 findings. EKG findings in PE, however, are both nonsensitive and nonspecific and can also include sinus tachycardia alone, right axis deviation, a new right bundle branch block, or T-wave inversions in V1 to V4. Diffuse ST elevations with PR depression are classically found in pericarditis. Electrical alternans and diffuse low voltage are findings seen in patients with pericardial effusions. Delta waves are found in Wolf–Parkinson–White syndrome.

257. A 67-year-old male with a history of chronic obstructive pulmonary disease (COPD), hypertension, and high cholesterol with notably decreased physical activity due to his exertional dyspnea presents to the emergency department (ED) complaining of increased shortness of breath and chest tightness. The patient reports that 2 days ago he developed a fairly sudden onset of increased shortness of breath and left-sided chest tightness. The chest tightness was worse with inspiration and radiated toward his left upper back. He has not noticed an increase in his baseline cough but did notice some blood-tinged sputum, which was new. He denies fevers/chills, diaphoresis, weakness, nausea/vomiting. Vitals demonstrate temp 99.1°F, HR 110, BP 110/82 in bilateral arms, RR 18, and O_2 sat of 92% on RA. On exam there is no jugular venous distention or peripheral edema. Chest x-ray (CXR) shows findings consistent with COPD, but no acute cardiopulmonary disease. EKG shows sinus tachycardia with nonspecific ST-T wave changes. He receives two Duoneb treatments, but notices no change. What is the most likely diagnosis?

A. Pulmonary embolism (PE)
B. Congestive heart failure (CHF)
C. COPD exacerbation
D. Atypical pneumonia

Correct Answer A: *Pulmonary embolism (PE).* Patients with a history of COPD presenting to the ED with shortness of breath and chest tightness can often be labeled as COPD exacerbations, as up to 30% of exacerbations may not have a clear etiology. These patients, however, who tend to have other comorbidities, increased inflammation, and immobility, can be at increased risk for PE. Studies have shown that in patients presenting with severe COPD exacerbations requiring hospitalization or exacerbations with unclear etiology, PE was the cause in up to 25% of the cases. This patient has no findings consistent with CHF. He is afebrile with a normal CXR and had a fairly sudden onset of symptoms, which makes an atypical pneumonia an unlikely diagnosis.

258. A 38-year-old male who was born in Africa presents to the emergency department (ED) complaining of fevers, night sweats, and cough. The patient reports he has been in the United States over the past few years but has not received any medical attention. His medical history is significant for intravenous drug use (IVDU), but otherwise denies smoking. He states he was seen for these same symptoms approximately 3 weeks ago and treated for a presumed pneumonia; however, his symptoms never improved and continued to persist. He denies any unexplained weight loss. Vitals demonstrate temp 100.1°F, HR 87, BP 130/82, and O_2 sat of 97% on RA. Physical exam is unremarkable, and no murmur, rash, or lymphadenopathy are present. A chest film obtained in the ED demonstrates a single cavitary lesion in the right upper lobe (RUL) with right hilar lymphadenopathy; no other lesions or left hilar lymphadenopathy is noted. What is the most likely diagnosis?

A. Tuberculosis (TB)
B. Infective endocarditis (IE)
C. Lymphoma
D. Sarcoidosis

Correct Answer A: *Tuberculosis (TB).* The patient is currently suffering from reactivated TB. Reactivated TB most often occurs in patients who develop weakened immune systems, such as patients on immunocompromising medications or HIV patients. Other risk factors for TB infection include age (infants and elderly), close contact with a person with known TB, residing in a nursing home, and travelling to areas with high rates of TB. The patient mentioned above has at least one major risk factor, as Africa is known to have a high prevalence of TB. He also has a history of IVDU, which puts him at risk for HIV and becoming immunocompromised, which could then lead to active TB infection. The patient's physical exam demonstrates no rash consistent with Osler nodes or Janeway lesions and has no heart murmur, both of which would be more consistent with IE. Pulmonary findings in sarcoidosis classically include bilateral hilar lymphadenopathy and interstitial lung disease. Although night sweats and fevers may at first make one concerned for lymphoma, the chest x-ray findings, and lack of weight loss, lymphadenopathy on exam makes the diagnosis of TB most likely.

259. A 35 year-old female now 2 weeks postpartum from an uncomplicated pregnancy and vaginal delivery presents to the emergency department minimally responsive after a witnessed syncopal event. The husband is able to report that the patient had been complaining of mild chest discomfort earlier in the day and felt she was more short of breath. They were walking prior to arrival when she suddenly gripped her chest and collapsed to the ground. On arrival she is receiving respiratory support via a bag valve mask, her BP is 82/50 in bilateral arms, radial pulses are faint but appear equal, femoral pulses are palpable and equal bilaterally, HR is 140s, and O_2 saturation is 80%. On rapid assessment her lungs are clear; there is no peripheral edema. Bedside ultrasound demonstrates significant right ventricular (RV) strain, but otherwise unremarkable. The most likely cause of this patient's syncopal event is:

A. Postpartum dilated cardiomyopathy
B. Pulmonary embolism (PE)
C. Aortic dissection
D. Vasovagal

Correct Answer B: *Pulmonary embolism (PE).* The most likely cause of her syncope is a large pulmonary embolism. Pregnancy is a well-known risk factor for deep venous thrombosis/PE, and the risk for thromboembolic events can be present up to 6 weeks after delivery. The history of chest pain and shortness of breath prior to the syncope, as well as RV strain noted on cardiac ultrasound, makes PE the most likely diagnosis. Postpartum dilated cardiomyopathy would have more findings consistent with congestive heart failure, and bedside ultrasound would demonstrate cardiomegaly and decreased ventricular function. Dissection is less likely given there were no ultrasound findings consistent with dissection and bilateral arm blood pressures as well as pulses were equal.

260. A 23-year-old male with a history of intravenous drug use presents to the emergency department via emergency medical services (EMS) after a friend called 911 after the patient became increasingly difficult to arouse and appeared to be breathing very slowly. EMS reports his initial vital signs were as follows: HR, 122; BP, 98/60; RR, 6; and O_2 sat 82% on RA. When you see the patient, he is nodding off continually, is peripherally cyanotic with slight perioral cyanosis, and has clear lungs on exam. His vitals continue to demonstrate hypoxia, and an end-tidal CO_2 demonstrates hypercapnia. Blood gas demonstrates $PaCO_2$ of 60 and PaO_2 of 50. This would be defined as what time of respiratory failure?

A. Type I respiratory failure
B. Type II respiratory failure
C. Cardiogenic
D. None of the above

Correct Answer B: *Type II respiratory failure.* Type II respiratory failure is defined by inadequate gas exchange that results in hypercapnia with a $PaCO_2$ >50. This is often accompanied by hypoxemia. Type II respiratory failure is caused by inadequate alveolar minute ventilation. This can be a result of both acute and chronic problems such as increased airway resistance (chronic obstructive pulmonary disease, asthma), reduced breathing effort (drug/alcohol induced, brainstem lesions), decreased volume for airway exchange, or neuromuscular disease.

261. A patient presents via emergency medical services (EMS) shortly after receiving Narcan. The patient is awake and alert coming into the emergency department. EMS reports that despite being wide awake during the ride in, the patient continued to be hypoxic with an O_2 sat of

72% on room air. Despite supplemental O_2, the patient continues to have an O_2 sat of 82%. Chest x-ray demonstrates diffuse pulmonary edema. Blood gas demonstrates PaO_2 of 50, and $PaCO_2$ is normal. The patient is currently in what type of respiratory failure?

A. Type I respiratory failure
B. Type II respiratory failure
C. The patient is not in respiratory failure.
D. None of the above

Correct Answer A: *Type I respiratory failure.* Type I respiratory failure is defined by hypoxemia without hypercapnia, with a PaO_2 of <60. This is often caused by V/Q mismatch. Common causes of type I failure include pulmonary embolism, acute respiratory distress syndrome, pneumonia, right-to-left shunts, or early acute alveolar hypoventilation.

262. A 70-year-old with a history of congestive heart failure (CHF) presents with increased short-ness of breath, dyspnea, and peripheral edema. She reports over the past few days she was on vacation and was not following her usual diet and thinks she may have missed a dose or two of her Lasix. She denies any fevers/chills, chest pain, cough, and hemoptysis. Her vitals shows BP 160/98, HR 95, and O_2 sat of 84% on RA. She appears to be in moderate respira-tory distress. Arterial blood gas (ABG) demonstrates PaO_2 of 55, and $PaCO_2$ is normal. Chest x-ray shows pulmonary edema consistent with failure. Her O_2 sat increases to 89% on high-flow O_2. What type of respiratory failure is this, and what type of ventilatory support should be attempted at this point?

A. Type I, continuous positive airway pressure (CPAP)
B. Type II, CPAP
C. Type I, intubation
D. Type II, intubation

Correct Answer A: *Type I, CPAP.* This patient is presenting with a CHF exacerbation. Her vital signs and ABG are consistent with a type I respiratory failure, with a low PaO_2 and nor-mal $PaCO_2$. The patient's O_2 saturation improved to 89% on high-flow O_2. The next best type of ventilatory support for this patient would be CPAP. Constant positive airway pressure will help both recruit/maintain opened alveoli and increase the intra-alveolar pressure, which will begin to help with the pulmonary edema by pushing fluid back into the vascular system. Research has shown that patients with CHF exacerbation requiring intubation have a signifi-cantly higher mortality rate than those able to be managed via CPAP and other typical CHF treatment.

263. A 56-year-old male, is brought to the emergency department by ambulance after house fire, where he sustained burn injuries to the face, anterior torso, and bilateral anterior arms. What percentage of his body surface area is involved?

A. 31.5
B. 36
C. 40.5
D. 45

Correct Answer A: *31.5.* Percentage of body surface is calculated using the rule of 9s. The head is estimated at 9% (face 4.5%), each arm 9% (4.5% anterior, 4.5% posterior), anterior torso 18%, posterior torso 18%, each leg 18% (anterior 9%, posterior 9%), genital 1%. Smaller burn areas can use the back of the hand to estimate burn size, with the back of the hand representing 1% body surface area. In this example, the patient sustained burns to the face (4.5%), bilateral anterior arms (4.5% each arm), and anterior torso (18%).

264. A 54-year-old female, without any medical history, is brought in by ambulance after house fire. The patient was intoxicated and fell asleep with a lit cigarette. On exam, her vitals are as follows: temp, 99°F; HR, 112; BP, 110/74; RR, 20; and O_2 sat 91% on RA. She has a partial-thickness facial burn, soot in the upper airway, cough, use of accessory respiratory muscles, and diffuse wheezing. After starting O_2, what is the next step in the patient's care?

   A. Albuterol via nebulizer
   B. Chest x-ray
   C. Labs including blood gas, lactate, and toxicology screen
   D. Intubation

Correct Answer D: *Intubation.* The patient has an inhalation injury. Intubation is indicated, as deterioration may be precipitous. Risks for inhalation injury include decreased cognition and closed-space fires. Carbon monoxide poisoning should be suspected. Initial chest x-ray may be normal, though opacities are indicative of poor prognosis. Labs should be sent, but are not the immediate concern. Inhaled β-adrenergic agonists are not sufficient management.

265. A 34-year-old male, diver with no medical history, comes to emergency department complaining of bilateral ear pain and fullness after returning from a dive trip 1 day ago. He denies fever, nasal congestion, sinus pain, or discharge from the ears. On exam, his vital signs are as follows: temp, 98.6°F; HR, 74; BP, 118/78; and RR, 16. Bilateral external auditory canals are without erythema or edema, and TMs are intact, with bilateral hemotympanum noted. What is the likely etiology of his symptoms?

   A. Otitis media
   B. Otitis externa
   C. Descent barotrauma
   D. Sinusitis

Correct Answer C: *Descent barotrauma.* Barotrauma results from pressure differences that exceed the body's ability to equalize. Rapid descent causing descent barotraumas is the likely etiology. Otitis media can present with ear pain and pressure, but would cause tympanic membrane erythema, bulging, fever. Otitis externa is associated with inflammation and discharge in the external canal. Sinus squeeze can also result from barotraumas, but typically associated with sinus pain and epistaxis.

266. A 3-year-old boy presents with vomiting and decreased mental status after he and his mother attempted to stay warm in their running car during power outage from winter storm. Patient is lethargic, and vital signs are as follows: temp, 96.8°F; HR, 150; BP, 76/48; RR, 30; and O_2 sat 99% on RA. Mother is complaining of a headache and nausea. What is the most important aspect of treatment?

   A. O_2 via nasal cannula at 2 L
   B. IV fluids
   C. 100% O_2 via facemask with reservoir
   D. Nasal swab for influenza

Correct Answer C: *100% O_2 via facemask with reservoir.* Initiate treatment with highest concentration of supplemental oxygen available. Beware false reassurance from the standard pulse oximetry, as it cannot differentiate between carboxyhemoglobin and oxyhemoglobin. The most reliable test to diagnose carbon monoxide poisoning is a blood sample for co-oximetry. After initial treatment with 100% supplemental oxygen, determine whether hyperbaric therapy is indicated. Patient's symptoms are not related to severe dehydration; so IV fluids are not mainstay of treatment.

267. A 32-year-old marathon runner presents with confusion, agitation, ataxia, and vomiting after mile 22 on an unseasonably warm day. Her temp 105°F, HR 164, BP 90/46, RR 50, and O_2 sat 91% on RA. Initial treatment includes:

   A. Evaporative cooling and/or ice water immersion if available
   B. High-flow O_2
   C. IV crystalloids with mean arterial pressure above 80 to 90
   D. All of the above

Correct Answer D: *All of the above.* The patient has exertional heat stroke. This has a high mortality rate, which is increased when cooling is delayed. Resuscitation including evaluation of airway, breathing, circulation (ABCs) and treatment with O_2 and crystalloids is essential, though volume requirements may be modest.

268. In January, a homeless male, with unknown medical history, appearing approximately 50 years old is brought into emergency department. On exam, he is stuporous, smelling of alcohol, temp 87.8°F (31°C), HR 46, BP 90/48, RR 10. Finger stick glucose is 180. What is true about his diagnosis?

   A. Ethanol is an uncommon contributing factor in the urban setting.
   B. Passive external rewarming via removing wet clothing and covering with blankets is sufficient.
   C. Both passive and active rewarming are recommended.
   D. Most hypothermic patients are tachycardic.

Correct Answer C: *Both passive and active rewarming are recommended.* This patient has moderate hypothermia. Given the likely involvement of alcohol and unknown medical history, the patient is unlikely to have sufficient metabolic reserve to generate endogenous rewarming. Examples of active external and internal rewarming include warmed humidified oxygen and forced air warming systems. For mild hypothermia (core temp 35 to 33°C [95 to 91.4°F]), passive external rewarming is the treatment of choice. Severe hypothermia is core temperature below 28°C (82.4°F). Ethanol is a major contributing cause of hypothermia. Progressive bradycardia develops after initial tachycardia, and if tachycardia persists despite lower core temperatures, contributing factors such as hypoglycemia, hypovolemia, or drug ingestion should be sought.

269. A 65-year-old right-hand-dominant female with medical history of asthma, depression, and anxiety presents with puncture wound on left hand from cat bite. The cat and patient both are up-to-date on immunizations. What is the first-line antibiotic?

   A. Amoxicillin-clavulanate 875/125 mg bid × 10–14 days
   B. Amoxicillin 500 mg tid × 7 days
   C. Doxycycline 100 mg bid × 7 days
   D. Cephalexin 500 mg qid × 3 days

Correct Answer A: *Amoxicillin-clavulanate 875/125 mg bid × 10–14 days.* Amoxicillin-clavulanate 875/125 mg bid × 10–14 days is the first-line oral antibiotic for prophylaxis with cat bites, in order to cover *Pasteurella* species. Infection develops rapidly as early as 12 hours following injury. Alternative regimens include doxycycline or trimethoprim-sulfamethoxazole, which have coverage against *Pasteurella multocida* plus clindamycin or metronidazole for anaerobic coverage. Cephalexin has poor activity against *P. multocida* and should be avoided.

270. A 37-year-old hiker, nonsmoker, with no medical history, is brought in by friends after the third night of a hiking trip with dry cough and impaired exercise capacity. They had been heavily exerting themselves attempting a rapid ascent. His vitals are as follows: temp, 98.8°F; HR, 114; BP, 144/90; RR, 22; and O_2 sat 88% on RA. Lungs exam reveals generalized rales. Chest x-ray shows interstitial infiltrates. What is the likely diagnosis?

A. Congestive heart failure
B. Pulmonary embolism
C. High altitude pulmonary edema
D. Myocardial infarction

Correct Answer C: *High altitude pulmonary edema.* The key to making the diagnosis of high altitude pulmonary edema is suspicion in the appropriate clinical context. Here, the history of a rapid ascent should prompt early consideration. Pulmonary embolism, congestive heart failure, and myocardial infarction are also in the differential with patient's symptoms and exam findings, but less likely given clinical context and lack of risk factors.

271. A 19-year-old female college student presents with excruciating pain after being stung by stingray on her left ankle while on spring break. She has a 3 cm linear laceration to the left ankle. What treatment neutralizes the venom?

A. Apply acetic acid (vinegar)
B. Apply ice packs
C. Give antivenom
D. Submerge in hot water

Correct Answer D: *Submerge in hot water.* The correct answer is submerge in hot, nonscalding water for up to 90 minutes or until pain improves. Other treatment includes aggressive cleaning, antibiotics, analgesia, tetanus immunization, and x-ray to find and remove stingers. Vinegar is applied to injuries sustained by nematocysts (jellyfish, corals, Portuguese man-of-war, anemones). Antivenom is also treatment for certain nematocysts (box jellyfish).

272. A 22-year-old male presents with two fang marks on lower right leg, with associated pain, but no erythema or edema after a bite by copperhead while hiking 3 hours before presenting. He denies nausea, vomiting, weakness, or paresthesias. IV access is established, pain is managed, and labs including complete blood count, coagulation panel, and blood typing are sent. Local wound care is provided, and tetanus immunization is updated. What is the appropriate emergency department course?

A. Immediately administer Polyvalent Crotalidae Fab (FabAV) 4 to 6 vials, and plan to admit to ICU
B. Monitor for progression of symptoms for 8 hours, if no evidence of envenomation, discharge to home with strict return precautions
C. Do skin testing for Polyvalent Crotalidae Fab (FabAV) prior to administering according to package insert
D. Apply tourniquet to extremity

Correct Answer B: *Monitor for progression of symptoms for 8 hours, if no evidence of envenomation, discharge to home with strict return precautions.* The patient sustained snakebite from copperhead, which is a pit viper. Only 25% of pit viper bites result in envenomation. Any erythema should be marked, and extremity measured above and below the bite. Signs of envenomation include erythema, ecchymosis, and progressive edema. Systemic symptoms include nausea, vomiting, weakness, or more severely tachycardia, tachypnea, and mental status change. Coagulopathies may develop. If no signs or symptoms of envenomation occur in 8 hours, then a dry bite can be assumed. Unlike with older antivenoms, skin testing is not necessary prior to administering Polyvalent Crotalidae Fab (FabAV), and the usual initial dose is four to six vials. Constricting bands should only be placed within 30 minutes of bites to gently constrict venous flow until antivenom can be obtained (if indicated).

273. A 26-year-old male is brought to your small community hospital with full-thickness burns to hands, arms, and chest sustained while lighting fireworks 30 minutes prior to arrival. The most appropriate first step is to:
    A. Arrange for immediate transfer to the nearest burn center
    B. Assess the airway
    C. Start wound debridement
    D. Start aggressive fluid resuscitation
    E. Administer IV narcotics for pain management

Correct Answer B: *Assess the airway.* The principles of management of the traumatic patient are well defined by the American College of Surgeons. Here, the initial steps are assessment of the airway with airway maintenance with cervical spine protection, followed by assessment and management of breathing and ventilation, followed by assessment of circulation and hemorrhage control as needed, neurologic exam, complete exposure of the patient, and environmental control. These initial steps are included in the primary survey and should take precedence over wound debridement, fluid resuscitation, pain management, and transfer to the nearest burn center.

274. Which of the following statements is true with regards to applying the rule of nines to infants?
    A. The head accounts for 18% of total body surface area (TBSA).
    B. The posterior thorax accounts for 9% of TBSA.
    C. Each leg accounts for 18% of TBSA.
    D. The percentage of body surface area assigned to each section of an infant is the same for a child and an adult.
    E. All of the above

Correct Answer A: *The head accounts for 18% of total body surface area (TBSA).* The rule of nines is a guide meant for quick estimation of TBSA affected by a burn. These estimates are adjusted in the infant to account for the differences in infant anatomy when compared to that of an adult. For instance, the head of an infant is proportionately larger to that of an adult and, therefore, accounts for a larger total body surface area. The head of an adult accounts for 9% of TBSA, whereas the head of an infant accounts for 18%.

275. Emergency medical services arrives to your facility with a 46-year-old previously healthy female who sustained a fall from a balcony. She opens her eyes briefly and moans incomprehensively to sternal rub. She withdraws her right upper extremity after pressure is applied to her nail bed of her left middle finger. You calculate her Glasgow Coma Scales (GCS) as:
    A. 4
    B. 6
    C. 8
    D. 9
    E. 12

Correct Answer C: *8.* The GCS is a tool used for the quick assessment of brain function and is particularly useful when assessing the traumatic patient. Here, eye opening, verbal response, and motor response are evaluated, and a score is calculated. The lowest possible score is 3, while the highest possible score is 15. The patient in this question receives a score of 2 out of 4 for opening her eyes to painful stimuli, a score of 2 out of 5 for incomprehensible moans, and 4 out of possible 6 for withdrawing her hand to pain.

276. A 25-year-old male was brought into the emergency department after being stabbed once in the mid-abdomen. The patient is confused and lethargic. On exam you find an actively bleeding 4 cm linear laceration just superior to the umbilicus and fluid in Morrison pouch on focused assessment with sonography for trauma exam. The patient appears to weigh approximately 70 kg and his vital signs are as follows: temp 98.0; HR, 142; BP, 82/50; RR, 36; and O_2 sat 99% on RA. Based on the patient's exam, the patient's estimated blood loss is:

   A. Zero
   B. Up to 15% blood volume
   C. 15% to 30% blood volume
   D. 30% to 40% blood volume
   E. >40% blood volume

Correct Answer E: >40% blood. The American College of Surgeons classifies traumatic hemorrhage based on a patient's initial presentation into Classes I to IV. Here, an uncomplicated hemorrhage in a trauma victim who has lost <15% of blood volume would be classified as Class I, and a trauma victim with significant, near-terminal bleeding of >40% blood volume (>2,000 mL in the average 70 kg person) would be classified as Class IV. This classification system uses pulse rate, systolic pressure, respiratory rate, urine output, and mental status help, estimates blood loss in terms of volume, both milliliters and percentage of total body volume, and guides initial fluid replacement with crystalloid or a combination of both crystalloid and blood. A trauma victim with loss of >40% blood volume would be expected to have a rapid heart rate, decreased systolic pressure, decreased pulse pressure, rapid respiratory rate, and negligible urine output, and appear confused and lethargic on initial presentation. Patients with Class IV traumatic hemorrhage are frequently managed with rapid blood transfusion and surgical intervention.

277. You are seeing a trauma patient with hemorrhage of approximately 10% of blood volume. Your patient is an otherwise healthy adult who weighs 70 kg and has no other associated injury. His estimated blood loss is most commonly associated with:

   A. Heart rate >130
   B. Heart rate <100
   C. Hypotension
   D. Tachypnea
   E. Lethargy

Correct Answer B: Heart rate <100. The American College of Surgeons uses a four tier classification system for estimated blood loss based on a trauma victim's initial presentation. The above-mentioned patient with uncomplicated hemorrhage of approximately 10% of blood volume is not expected to cause significant increase in heart rate, tachypnea, hypotension, or lethargy. If significant vital sign abnormality or mental status change is found in a patient with estimated blood loss of <10% blood volume, care should be taken to find another source of injury.

278. Emergency medical services arrives to your department with a 35-year-old female who was extracted from a house fire. Which of findings below is consistent with a suspected inhalation injury?

   A. Singed nasal hairs
   B. Carbonaceous sputum
   C. Normal chest x-ray
   D. Answers A and B
   E. Answers A, B, and C

Correct Answer E: Answers A, B, and C. Inhalation injury, as a consequence of heat exposure to the airway, can be determined through history or physical exam. Some clinical indications of inhalation injury include face and/or neck burns, singeing of facial hair, including eyebrows and nasal hairs, carbonaceous sputum or carbon deposits in the oropharynx or nose, acute inflammation in the oropharynx, hoarse voice, history of mental status change or confinement in a smoke or fire-filled space, explosion, or elevated carboxyhemoglobin level in a patient exposed to a fire- or smoke-filled environment. Plain radiographs of the chest may appear normal early after inhalation injury and should not mislead the clinician in the seriousness of the injury.

279. Which patient in the following scenarios is candidate for emergent, resuscitated open thoracotomy in the emergency department (ED)?

   A. A 30-year-old patient in PEA (pulseless electrical activity) cardiac arrest after a single gunshot wound to the chest in a regional trauma center
   B. A 36-year-old patient with severe chest pain and hypotension after high-speed motor vehicle accident
   C. An 18-year-old patient in cardiac arrest with multiple stab wounds of the chest, abdomen, and neck in a small community hospital without surgical capabilities
   D. 70-year-old patient with atraumatic chest pain radiating to the back and asymmetric blood pressure readings in the upper extremities
   E. All of the above

Correct Answer A: *A 30-year-old patient in PEA (pulseless electrical activity) cardiac arrest after a single gunshot wound to the chest in a regional trauma center*. The best candidates for emergent resuscitative open thoracotomy in the ED are those with penetrating thoracic injury who arrive to a trauma facility pulseless, but with electrical myocardial activity (PEA cardiac arrest). The goals of resuscitative thoracotomy are to evacuate any pericardial blood causing tamponade, provide access for direct control of hemorrhage, open cardiac massage, and cross clamping of the descending aorta to increase blood delivery to the brain and heart while minimizing ongoing hemorrhage when there is injury below the diaphragm. Emphasis should be placed on the surgical capabilities of the facility since definitive surgical management of the injury will be necessary.

280. Emergency medical services brings a middle-aged female to your emergency department who was an unhelmeted cyclist who struck a tree. Her vitals are as follows: HR, 100; BP, 110/64; RR, 16; and O_2 sat, 99% on 2 L by nasal cannula. She does not respond to commands, but responds to vigorous sternal rub with a brief moan and opening of her eyes. She withdraws her right upper extremity to painful stimuli. Which of the following is the best first step in management of this patient?

   A. Plain films of the pelvis
   B. Endotracheal intubation while maintaining in-line stabilization of the cervical spine
   C. Fluid resuscitation with 2 L of crystalloid
   D. Head CT scan
   E. Portable chest x-ray

Correct Answer B: *Endotracheal intubation while maintaining in-line stabilization of the cervical spine*. This patient fits into the category of severe brain injury based on a Glasgow Coma Scale score of 8. Her impaired consciousness makes her at risk for airway compromise and aspiration if she begins to vomit. In addition to this, hypoxia and apnea associated with severe brain injury can cause secondary brain injury. For these reasons, early intubation in patients with brain injury and impaired consciousness should be performed while paying special attention to cervical spine in-line stabilization due to potential concomitant cervical spine injury. Once the airway has been secured, the remainder of the primary and secondary survey, along with other resuscitative efforts, can be performed.

281. A patient presents with loss of motor strength in bilateral upper extremities disproportionate to the loss of motor strength to the bilateral lower extremities after a fall forward from

standing. This patient also sustained facial injuries from this fall. He complains of severe weakness in bilateral upper extremities, moderate weakness in lower extremities, bladder dysfunction, and variable degrees of sensory loss of bilateral upper extremities, trunk, and lower extremities. This presentation is most consistent with:

A. Cauda Equina syndrome
B. Complete cord transection
C. Anterior cord syndrome
D. Central cord syndrome
E. Brown-Séquard syndrome

Correct Answer D: *Central cord syndrome.* Central cord syndrome can be caused by a slow-growing central spinal cord lesion or by hyperextension injury in an individual with preexisting cervical spondylosis. Central cord syndromes caused by trauma often manifests as disproportionate motor loss in bilateral upper extremities when compared to bilateral lower extremities, bladder dysfunction, and variable degrees of sensory loss. Cauda equina syndrome is a loss of function of any two of the nerve roots of the Cauda equina and may manifest as asymmetric radicular pain, loss of plantar flexion strength, sensory loss of the affected nerve root, and loss of bowel and bladder function. A complete cord transection will manifest as a complete loss of sensation and motor function below the level of injury. Anterior cord syndrome manifests as weakness along with loss of pain and temperature sensation; however, position, deep pressure sensation, and vibration sense tend to be preserved. Brown-Séquard syndrome is usually caused by penetrating trauma, causing hemisection of the cord. Brown-Séquard syndrome manifests as loss of ipsilateral motor function and position sense that is associated with a contralateral loss of pain and temperature sensation below the level of injury.

282. A patient arrives to your burn facility with full-thickness burns of approximately 40% of total body surface area (TBSA). The patient's wife reports that prior to this injury the patient was otherwise healthy and weighs approximately 200 lb. Using the Parkland formula to guide your initial approach to fluid resuscitation, you can estimate that the patient should receive:

A. 7 units of cross matched packed red blood cells over 8 hours
B. 7.2 L of crystalloid over the first 8 hours based on the time of injury
C. 7.2 L of colloid fluids over the first 24 hours based on the time of injury
D. Continuous infusion at 2 L an hour for 24 hours
E. 1 L of crystalloid solution for every 1 L of urine output

Correct Answer B: *7.2 L of crystalloid over the first 8 hours based on the time of injury.* In general, fluid resuscitation in adults can be monitored by physiologic response such as heart rate, blood pressure, and urine output, with a goal urine output for adults being 0.5 mL/kg/hour. Patients with severe burns and adequate fluid resuscitation with minimal or inadequate urine output generally have poor prognosis. The Parkland formula is a commonly utilized tool for estimating initial fluid requirements in a severely burned patient. Superficial burns are excluded from this formula. The Parkland formula dictates that 4 mL per kg of body weight multiplied by the TBSA burned be given in the first 24 hours, with the first half of given over the first 8 hours based on the time of injury and the remaining half given over the subsequent 18 hours.

Applying the Parkland formula to the patient mentioned above:

4 mL × 90 kg × 40% TBSA = approximately 14,500 mL over the first 24 hours. 7,250 mL crystalloid should be given in the first 8 hours based on time of injury (at a rate of approximately 905 mL per hour), and the remaining 7,250 mL crystalloid should be given over the subsequent 16 hours (at a rate of approximately 450 mL per hour).

Colloids and blood are not recommended as standard treatment for severe burns without evidence of other trauma.

283. A 35-year-old healthy male presents with complaint of right-sided flank pain worsening over the past 3 days. He reports subjective fevers and nausea/vomiting today. Vitals signs are notable for temp of 101.2 and HR of 120. He appears uncomfortable, but nontoxic. On exam, there is marked right costovertebral angle tenderness and mild right lower quadrant pain on deep palpation without rebound or guarding. Labs reveal white blood count 16, blood urea nitrogen/Cr within normal limits. Urinalysis reveals urinary tract infection. CT abdomen/pelvis is obtained and shows an 8 mm obstructing right proximal ureteral calculus. What is the most likely disposition for this patient?

 A. Home after 2 L intravenous fluids (IVF) with prescriptions for antibiotics, α-blockers, and symptom control with primary care physician follow-up in 2 to 3 days
 B. Admission to general medicine for IVF, IV antibiotics, and monitor
 C. Admission to urosurgical service for emergent surgical decompression of infected stone
 D. Home after single dose of IV antibiotics with prescription for oral antibiotics, symptom control, and encourage oral fluid hydration with urology follow-up in 1 week

Correct Answer C: *Admission to urosurgical service for emergent surgical decompression of infected stone.* The management of obstructing urinary calculus in the presence of infection requires emergent urologic intervention. It is appropriate to begin IV antibiotics, antipyretics, and symptom control; however, these are not definitive treatments for this patient's condition.

284. Pelvic inflammatory disease (PID) is most commonly caused by which of the following sexually transmitted organisms?

 A. *Neisseria gonorrhoeae*
 B. *Chlamydia trachomatis*
 C. *Haemophilus influenzae*
 D. *Gardnerella vaginalis*

Correct Answer B: *Chlamydia trachomatis.* In the United States, *C. trachomatis* is the primary sexually transmitted organism that causes PID. *N. gonorrhoeae* is the second most common sexually transmitted disease; it is also commonly associated with PID, but with less frequency than Chlamydia. *H. influenzae* and *Gardnerella* are also associated with PID, but with much lower incidences.

285. In a patient presenting with symptoms concerning for urinary tract obstruction, which imaging test is the most sensitive and specific for confirming this diagnosis?

 A. Renal ultrasound
 B. CT scan
 C. Kidney, ureter, and bladder (KUB) x-ray
 D. Urinalysis

Correct Answer A: *Renal ultrasound.* Renal ultrasound is the initial and most sensitive and specific test for identifying hydronephrosis and can be done quickly at the bedside. CT scan is helpful in identifying the cause of an obstruction and is very helpful as secondary imaging. KUB may reveal stones but will not confirm obstruction. Urinalysis cannot confirm obstruction.

286. A 17-year-old male presents with complaint of acute onset of right testicular pain 2 hours ago while playing basketball with friends. While being interviewed, the patient becomes nauseated and vomits. Exam is notable for a tender swollen scrotum with a negative Prehn sign. The right testis appears high riding compared to the left. Examiner is unable to elicit a cremasteric reflex on the right. What is the treatment for this condition?

 A. Bedside ultrasound and reevaluate in 2 to 3 hours for improvement
 B. Emergent surgical intervention

C. Symptom control and antibiotics

D. Surgical intervention if symptoms do not improve within 6 hours of onset

Correct Answer B: *Emergent surgical intervention.* Testicular torsion is a surgical emergency. Delaying surgery beyond 6 hours after symptom onset is a risk for testicular infarction, and ultimately the testicle may not be salvageable. A bedside ultrasound is an important tool in helping diagnose testicular torsion for epididymitis, but it is nontherapeutic. Antibiotics and pain control are an appropriate treatment approach for epididymitis, which this patient does not have given the sudden onset of his symptoms.

287. In the setting of renal failure, which of the following is *not* considered an absolute indication for emergent dialysis?

A. Intractable metabolic acidosis

B. Hypertensive emergency refractory to antihypertensive agents

C. Persistent hyperkalemia

D. Elevated creatinine

Correct Answer D: *Elevated creatinine.* Elevated creatinine level is not an absolute indication for emergent dialysis. The indications for emergent dialysis include severe metabolic acidosis, severe persistent electrolyte disturbances such as hyperkalemia and hypermagnesemia, life-threatening fluid overload such as pulmonary edema and hypertensive emergency that are refractory to other treatments, drug toxicity, and severe uremia.

288. In a patient with acute renal failure, the presence of which of the following casts on urinalysis is pathognomonic for acute tubular necrosis (ATN)?

A. Hyaline casts

B. Red blood cell (RBC) casts

C. Muddy brown casts

D. Fatty casts

Correct Answer C: *Muddy brown casts.* ATN is a renal cause of acute renal failure, which is diagnosed by the presence of muddy casts on urinalysis and a FENa >3%. Hyaline casts are seen in prerenal failure, RBC casts indicate glomerular disease, and fatty casts indicate nephrotic syndrome.

289. A 30-year-old healthy nonpregnant female is diagnosed with pyelonephritis. Which of the following is an appropriate outpatient antibiotic regimen for this diagnosis?

A. Trimethoprim/sulfamethoxazole (TMP/SMX) (double strength) 1 tablet po two times daily for 3 day

B. Fosfomycin 3 g po daily for 3 days

C. Nitrofurantoin 100 mg po two times daily for 5 days

D. Ciprofloxacin 500 mg po daily for 10 days

Correct Answer D: *Ciprofloxacin 500 mg po daily for 10 days.* This is an acceptable outpatient treatment for pyelonephritis. TMP/SMX is an acceptable treatment for pyelonephritis; however, the treatment course should be at least 7 to 10 days. Nitrofurantoin and fosfomycin should not be used in the treatment of pyelonephritis, as they do not achieve adequate renal tissue penetration

290. A 21-year-old male presents with complaint of left testicular pain and dysuria worsening over the past 2 days. History reveals multiple sexual partners with intermittent barrier contraception use. Vital signs are stable. On exam the left testis is exquisitely tender with scrotal redness and edema. There is a small amount of purulent discharge at the penile meatus.

Prehn sign is positive. Doppler ultrasonography reveals increased blood flow to the left epididymis. What is the most likely diagnosis?

A. Testicular torsion
B. Epididymitis
C. Ureterolithiasis
D. Inguinal hernia

Correct Answer B: *Epididymitis.* The patient's exam is consistent with epididymitis. Epididymitis is most common in sexually active adolescent males; it is most often infectious in etiology with the most common organisms being *Chlamydia trachomatis and Neisseria gonorrhoeae*. In acute cases of infectious epididymitis, exam is often notable for extreme tenderness and swelling over the involved epididymis. Patients with testicular torsion usually present with acute onset of symptoms within the past few hours; bedside Doppler would reveal decreased blood flow to the affected testis. Inguinal hernia would more likely present as pain in the groin or abdomen. Ureterolithiasis is more likely to cause flank and abdominal pain than testicular pain.

291. You are working in a pediatric emergency department when a mother and father present with their 8-day-old son, appearing very concerned. History reveals a normal vaginal delivery without complications. The mother explains that a visiting relative was changing their son's diaper and was very concerned that his foreskin could not be retracted and suggested they be seen right away as this could be dangerous for the baby. Vital signs are stable. Inspection reveals a calm sleeping infant. Foreskin is intact and pliant with an unscarred preputial orifice covering the glans penis. There is no redness or swelling. The diaper is wet with yellow urine. What is the most appropriate plan?

A. Urgent urologic consultation for paraphimosis
B. Obtain urine to rule out urinary tract infection (UTI) as uncircumcised infants are at a high risk for urinary infections
C. Assure the parents that phimosis is normal for infants and can be followed by the pediatrician
D. Attempt to gently retract foreskin at bedside using topical anesthetic, if unsuccessful then urologic consult will be required for evaluation of pathologic phimosis

Correct Answer C: *Assure the parents that phimosis is normal for infants and can be followed by the pediatrician.* The patient has physiologic phimosis which is a normal exam finding in almost all uncircumcised males. Manual retraction at the bedside is not indicated as physiologic phimosis resolves spontaneously; attempting to retract a physiologic phimosis can put the infant at risk for developing a paraphimosis. The patient has no evidence of pathologic phimosis, which would be evident by a nonpliant foreskin that appears scarred down around the preputial orifice. The patient does not have paraphimosis as this is characterized by a retracted foreskin that cannot be returned to normal position. There is no indication to rule out UTI as the infant is afebrile and producing adequate urine and otherwise well.

292. Which of the following is a common complication of acute kidney injury (AKI)?

A. Metabolic acidosis
B. Metabolic alkalosis
C. Hypovolemia
D. Hypokalemia

Correct Answer A: *Metabolic acidosis.* In AKI, the reduced glomerular filtration rate impairs the kidney's ability to excrete acid, K, Na, and H_2O as well the ability to uptake bicarbonate. Decreased acid excretion and bicarbonate uptake leads to metabolic acidosis. Decreased excretion of K and

Na leads to hyperkalemia and hypervolemia, respectively. Metabolic alkalosis, hypovolemia, and hypokalemia are not common complications of AKI for the above reasons.

293. A 32-year-old pregnant female sustained a laceration. She is not up-to-date on her tetanus immunization. She also asks if it is safe for her to get the varicella vaccine. You respond with:

    A. It is safe for both.
    B. It is not safe for either.
    C. The tetanus is safe but the varicella is not.
    D. The tetanus is not safe but the varicella is.

Correct Answer C: *The tetanus is safe but the varicella is not.* According to the latest Centers for Disease Control and Prevention recommendations, it is safe for pregnant women to get the tetanus vaccine, but not the varicella vaccine.

Suggested Readings

....

CHAPTER 1—ABDOMINAL AND GASTROINTESTINAL DISORDERS

Adams JG, Barton ED, Collings J, et al, eds. *Emergency Medicine: Clinical Essentials*. 2nd ed. Philadelphia, PA: Elsevier; 2013.

Afdhal NH. Acute cholangitis. In: Basow DS, ed. *UpToDate*. Waltham, MA: UpToDate; 2013.

Hodin RA. Small bowel obstruction: clinical manifestations and diagnosis. In: Basow DS, ed. *UpToDate*. Waltham, MA: UpToDate; 2013.

Kitagawa S. Intussusception in children. In: Basow DS, ed. *UpToDate*. Waltham, MA: UpToDate; 2013.

Martin RJ. Acute appendicitis in adults: clinical manifestations & diagnosis. In: Basow DS, ed. *UpToDate*. Waltham, MA: UpToDate; 2013.

Zakko SF. Pathogenesis, clinical features, and diagnosis of acute cholecystitis. In: Basow DS, ed. *UpToDate*. Waltham, MA: UpToDate; 2013.

Zakko SF. Uncomplicated gallstone disease in adults. In: Basow DS, ed. *UpToDate*. Waltham, MA: UpToDate; 2013.

CHAPTER 2—CARDIOVASCULAR DISORDERS

Bakris GL. Management of severe asymptomatic hypertension (hypertensive urgencies). In: Basow DS, ed. *UpToDate*. Waltham, MA: UpToDate; 2013.

Brusche JL. Infective endocarditis. *Medscape Reference*. April 09, 2013. WebMD LLC. Accessed July 20, 2013.

Burns E. Junctional escape rhythm. *Life in the Fast Lane*. The Frontier Group and Global Medical Education Project. http://lifeinthefastlane.com/ecg-library/junctional escape-rhythm/. Accessed July 10, 2013.

Dallman R, Mell M. Management of asymptomatic abdominal aortic aneurysm. In: Basow DS, ed. *UpToDate*. Waltham, MA: UpToDate; 2013.

de Jong JSSG, Postema PG. AV conduction. *ECGpedia*. http://en.ecgpedia.org/wiki/AV_Conduction. Published March 3, 2009. Accessed July 10, 2013.

Jim J, Thompson RW. Clinical features and diagnosis of abdominal aortic aneurysm. In: Basow DS, ed. *UpToDate*. Waltham, MA: UpToDate; 2013.

Jim J, Thompson RW. Management of symptomatic (non-ruptured) and ruptured abdominal aortic aneurysm. In: Basow DS, ed. *UpToDate*. Waltham, MA: UpToDate; 2013.

Kaplan N. Drug treatment of hypertensive emergencies. In: Basow DS, ed. *UpToDate*. Waltham, MA: UpToDate; 2013.

Longo DL, Fauci AS, Kasper DL, et al, eds. *Harrison's Principles of Internal Medicine*. 18th ed. New York, NY: McGraw Hill Companies, Inc; 2012.

Martindale JL, Brown DF, eds. *Rapid Interpretation of ECGs in Emergency Medicine. A Visual Guide*. Philadelphia, PA: Lippincott Williams & Wilkins; 2012.

Mayersak RJ. Facial trauma in adults. In: Basow DS, ed. *UpToDate*. Waltham, MA: UpToDate; 2013.

Mick N, Peters JR, Egan D, et al, eds. *Emergency Medicine*. Malden, MA: Blackwell Publishing; 2006.

Patel K. Deep venous thrombosis. *Medscape Reference*. July 08, 2013. WebMD LLC. Accessed July 20, 2013.

Sabatine MS, ed. *Aortic Aneurysm. Pocket Medicine*. 4th ed. Philadelphia, PA: Lippincott Williams & Wilkins; 2011.

Sabatine MS, ed. *Hypertension. Pocket Medicine*. 4th ed. Philadelphia, PA: Lippincott Williams & Wilkins; 2011.

Sovari AA. Cardiogenic pulmonary edema treatment and management. *Medscape Reference*. February 03, 2012. WebMD LLC. Accessed July 20, 2013.

Sprangler S. Acute pericarditis. *Medscape Reference*. June 03, 2013. WebMD LLC, Accessed July 20, 2013.

Tang WHW. Myocarditis. *Medscape Reference*. April 15, 2013. WebMD LLC. Accessed July 20, 2013.

Types of Aneurysms. National Institutes of Health. U.S. Department of Health and Human Services. April 01, 2011. http://www.nhlbi.nih.gov/health/health topics/topics/arm/types.html. Accessed July 10, 2013.

Withers K, Carolan-Rees G, Dale M. Pipeline™ embolization device for the treatment of complex intracranial aneurysms. *Appl Health Econ Health Policy*. 2013;11(1):5–13.

CHAPTER 3—DERMATOLOGIC DISORDERS

Davidovici B, Wolf R. Emergencies in dermatology: diagnosis, classification and therapy. *Expert Rev Dermatol*. 2007;2(5):549–562. http://Medscape.com/viewarticle/565823. Accessed August 17, 2013.

Sandy N, Usantine R. Dermatologic emergencies. *Am Fam Physician*. 2010;82(7):773–780.

Stern R. Exanthemous drug eruptions. *N Engl J Med*. 2012;366:2492–2501.

Swanson D, Vetter R. Bites of brown recluse spiders and suspected necrotic archnisdism. *N Engl J Med*. 2005;352:700–707.

CHAPTER 4—ENDOCRINE, METABOLIC, AND NUTRITIONAL DISORDERS

Adams JG, Barton E, Collings J, et al, eds. *Emergency Medicine*. Philadelphia, PA: Saunders; 2008.

Auth PC, Kerstein MD, eds. *Physician Assistant Review*. 4th ed. Philadelphia, PA: Lippincott Williams and Wilkins; 2013.

Kitabchi AE, Umpierrez GE, Miles JM, et al. Hyperglycemic crises in adult patients with diabetes. *Diabetes Care*. 2009;32:1335.

Shoback D. Hypoparathyroidism. *N Eng J Med*. 2008;359:391.

Tintinalli JE, Stapczynski JS, Cline DM, et al, ed. *Tintinalli's Emergency Medicine Manual*. 7th ed. NewYork, NY: McGraw Hill; 2012.

CHAPTER 5—ENVIRONMENTAL DISORDERS

Ayala C, Spellberg B, eds. *Boards and Wards*. 2nd ed. Malden, MA: Blackwell; 2003.

Clardy P, Scott M, Holly P. Carbon monoxide poisoning. In: Basow DS, ed. *UpToDate*. Waltham, MA: UpToDate; 2013.

Danzl DF. Accidental hypotermia. In: Marx JA, Hockberger RS, Walls RM, et al, eds. *Rosen's Emergency Medicine*. 7th ed. Philadelphia, PA: Mosby Elsevier; 2010:1868–1881.

Danzl DF. Frostbite. In: Marx JA, Hockberger RS, Walls RM, et al, eds. *Rosen's Emergency Medicine*. 7th ed. Philadelphia, PA: Mosby Elsevier; 2010:1861–1867.

McPhee S, Papadakis M. Tierney LM, eds. *Current Medical Diagnosis and Treatment*. 46th ed. New York, NY: McGraw-Hill Medical Publishing Division; 2007.

Mechem CC. Severe hyperthermia (heat stroke) in adults. In: Basow DS, ed. *UpToDate*. Waltham, MA: UpToDate; 2013.

O'Connor FG, Casa DJ. Exertional heat illness in adolescents and adults: management and prevention. In: Basow DS, ed. *UpToDate*. Waltham, MA: UpToDate; 2013.

O'Connor FG, Casa DJ. Exertional heat illness in adolescents and adults: epidemiology, thermoregulation, risk factors and diagnosis. In: Basow DS, ed. *UpToDate*. Waltham, MA: UpToDate; 2013.

Platt M, Vicario S. Heat illness. In: Marx JA, Hockberger RS, Walls RM, et al, eds. *Rosen's Emergency Medicine*. 7th ed. Philadelphia, PA: Mosby Elsevier; 2010:1882–1892.

Tintinalli JE, Kelen GD, Stapczynski JS, eds. *A Comprehensive Study Guide*. 6th ed. New York, NY: McGraw-Hill Medical Publishing Division; 2004.

Tintinalli JE, Kelen GD, Stapczynski JS, eds. *Emergency Medicine: A Comprehensive Study Guide*. 5th ed. New York, NY: McGraw-Hill; 2000.

Velissariou I, Cottrell S, Berry K, et al. Management of adrenaline (epinephrine) induced digital ischaemia in children after accidental injection from an EpiPen. *Emerg Med J*. 2004;21(3):387–388.

Wolfson AB Hendey GW, Ling LJ, et al, eds. *Hardwood-Nuss' Clinical Practice of Emergency Medicine*. 5th ed. Baltimore, MD: Lippincott Williams & Wilkins; 2010.

CHAPTER 6—HEAD, EAR, EYE, NOSE AND THROAT DISORDERS

Bosemani T, Izbudak I. Head and neck emergencies. In: Stead LG, Stead SM, Kaufman MS, eds. *First Aid for the Emergency Medicine Clerkship*. New York, NY: McGraw-Hill Medical Publishing Division; 2006:117+.

Estrada CM, Givens TG. In: Wolfson AB, Cloutier RL, Hendey GW, et al, eds. *Harwood-Nuss' Clinical Practice of Emergency Medicine*. 5th ed. Philadelphia, PA: Lippincott Williams & Wilkens; 2010.

Gappy C, Archer SM, Barza M. Orbital cellulitis and preseptal cellulitis. In: Post TW, ed. *UpToDate*. Waltham, MA: UpToDate; 2013.

Hedges TR III. Central and branch retinal artery occlusion. In: Basow DS, ed. *UpToDate*. Waltham, MA: UpToDate; 2013

Hendey GW, Cloutire RL, Ling LJ, et al, eds. *Harwood-Nuss' Clinical Practice of EmergencyMedicine*. Philadelphia, PA: Wolters Kluwer; 2013.

Manno M. Pediatric respiratory emergencies: upper airway obstruction and infections. In: Marx JA, Hockberger RS, Walls RM, et al, eds. *Rosen's Emergency Medicine*. 7th ed. Philadelphia, PA: Mosby Elsevier; 2010:2108–2112.

Rosen P, Barkin RM, Schaider J. Acute sinusitis. In: Rosen P, Barkin RM, Hayden SR, et al, eds. *5-Minute Emergency Medicine Consult*. Philadelphia, PA: Lippincott Williams & Wilkins; 2007:1020–1021.

Rosen P, Barkin RM, Schaider J. Cavernous sinus thrombosis. In: Rosen P, Barkin RM, Hayden SR, et al, eds. *5-Minute Emergency Medicine Consult*. Philadelphia, PA: Lippincott Williams & Wilkins; 2007:204–205.

Rosen P, Barkin RM, Schaider J. Hyperthyroidism. In: Rosen P, Barkin RM, Hayden SR, et al, eds. *5-Minute Emergency Medicine Consult*. Philadelphia, PA: Lippincott Williams & Wilkins; 2007:584–585.

Rosen P, Barkin RM, Schaider J. Hyperthyroidism. In: Rosen P, Barkin RM, Hayden SR, et al, eds. *5-Minute Emergency Medicine Consult*. Philadelphia, PA: Lippincott Williams & Wilkins; 2007:562–563.

Rosen P, Barkin RM, Schaider J. Ludwig angina. In: Rosen P, Barkin RM, Hayden SR, et al, eds. *5-Minute Emergency Medicine Consult*. Philadelphia, PA: Lippincott Williams & Wilkins; 2007:646–647.

Rosen P, Barkin RM, Schaider J. Mastoiditis. In: Rosen P, Barkin RM, Hayden SR, et al, eds. *5-Minute Emergency Medicine Consult*. Philadelphia, PA: Lippincott Williams & Wilkins; 2007:672–673.

Rosen P, Barkin RM, Schaider J. Otitis externa. In: Rosen P, Barkin RM, Hayden SR, et al, eds. *5-Minute Emergency Medicine Consult*. Philadelphia, PA: Lippincott Williams & Wilkins; 2007:778–779.

Rosen P, Barkin RM, Schaider J. Otitis media. In: Rosen P, Barkin RM, Hayden SR, et al, eds. *5-Minute Emergency Medicine Consult*. Philadelphia, PA: Lippincott Williams & Wilkins; 2007:780–781.

Rosen P, Barkin RM, Schaider J. Peritonsillar abscess. In: Rosen P, Barkin RM, Hayden SR, et al, eds. *5-Minute Emergency Medicine Consult*. Philadelphia, PA: Lippincott Williams & Wilkins; 2007:838–839.

Rosen P, Barkin RM, Schaider J. Retropharyngeal abscess. In: Rosen P, Barkin RM, Hayden SR, et al, eds. *5-Minute Emergency Medicine Consult*. Philadelphia, PA: Lippincott Williams & Wilkins; 2007:966–967.

Weber PC. Etiology of hearing loss in adults. In: Deschler DG, ed. *UpToDate*. Waltham MA: UpToDate; 2013.

Weizer JS. Angle-closure glaucoma. In: Basow DS, ed. UpToDate. Waltham, MA: UpToDate; 2013.

Woods CR. Clinical features, evaluation and diagnosis of croup. In: Basow DS, ed. *UpToDate*. Waltham, MA: UpToDate; 2013.

CHAPTER 7—HEMATOLOGIC DISORDERS

2010 American Heart Association Guidelines for Cardiopulmonary Resuscitation and Emergency Cardiovascular Care. *Circulation*. 2010;122(suppl 3):S640–S656.

Arya R, Wander G, Gupta P. Blood component therapy: which, when and how much. *J Anaesthesiolo Clin Pharmacol*. 27(2):278–284.

Craig SA, Zich DK. Gastroenteritis. In: Marx JA, Hockberger RS, Walls RM, et al, eds. *Rosen's Emergency Medicine*. 7th ed. Philadelphia, PA: Mosby Elsevier; 2010:1206–1207.

Field J, DeBraun M. Acute chest syndrome in adults with sickle cell disease. *UpToDate*. December 12, 2012.

Field J, Vichinsky E, DeBaun M. Overview of the management of sickle cell disease. *UpToDate*. July 15, 2013.

Kaur P, Basu S, Kaur G, et al. Transfusion protocol in trauma. *J Emerg Trauma Shock*. 2011;4(1):103–108.

Niaudet P. Clinical manifestations and diagnosis of Shiga toxin associated (typical) hemolytic uremic syndrome in children. In: Basow DS, ed. *UpToDate*. Waltham, MA: UpToDate; 2013.

Niaudet P. Treatment and prognosis of Shiga toxin associated (typical) hemolytic uremic syndrome in children. In: Basow DS, ed. *UpToDate*. Waltham, MA: UpToDate; 2013.

Rick ME, Leung LL, Tirnauer JS. *Clinical Presentation and Diagnosis of vWD*. Waltham, MA: UpToDate; 2013.

Rodeghiero F, Castaman G, Tosetto A. How I treat vonWillebrand disease. *Blood*. 2009;114(6):1158–1165.

Rodgers G. Specific therapies for sickle cell disease. *UpToDate*. October 23, 2012.

Tan AJ. Hemolytic uremic syndrome in emergency medicine. In: Dronen SC, ed. *Medscape*. New York, NY: Medscape Reference; 2013.

Vichinsky E. *Overview of Cinical Manifestations of Sickle Cell Disease*. Waltham, MA: UpToDate. November 16, 2012.

CHAPTER 8—IMMUNE SYSTEM DISORDERS

Agrawal P, LeMaster C, Narayan K, et al. *Pocket Emergency Medicine*. 2nd ed. Philadelphia, PA: Wolters Kluwer; 2011.

Stead L, Stead S, Kaufman M. *First Aid for the Emergency Medicine Clerkship*. 2nd ed. New York, NY: The McGraw-Hill Companies; 2006.

CHAPTER 9—MUSCULOSKELETAL DISORDERS

Becker M. Clinical manifestations and diagnosis of gout. *UpToDate*. June 15, 2012.

Becker M. Treatment of acute gout. *UpToDate*. June 11, 2013.

Goldenberg D, Sexton D. Disseminated gonoccocal infections. *UpToDate*. November 16, 2012.

Goldenberg D, Sexton D. Septic arthritis in adults. *UpToDate*. April 22, 2013.

Hochman M. Approach to imaging modalities in the setting of suspected osteomyelitis. *UpToDate*. August 23, 2012.

Hu L. Clinical manifestations of lyme disease. *UpToDate*. February 15, 2013.

Levin K. Lumbar spinal stenosis treatment and prognosis. *UpToDate*. August 1, 2012.

Levin K. Lumbar spinal stenosis: pathophysiology, clinical features and diagnosis. *UpToDate*. May 11, 2012.

Linden H. Diagnosis of lyme disease. *UpToDate*. November 20, 2012.

Linden H. Treatment of lyme disease. *UpToDate*. October 10, 2012.

Schiff D. Clinical features and diagnosis of neoplastic spinal cord compression. *UpToDate*. July 30, 2013.

Schiff D, Brown P, Shaffrey M. Treatment and prognosis of neoplastic spinal cord compression. *UpToDate*. April 11, 2013.

Sexton D, McDonald M. Vertebral osteomyelitis and discitis. *UpToDate*. May 21, 2013.

Sexton D. Epidural abscess. *UpToDate*. September 7, 2012.

Tahaniyat L. Overview of osteomyelitis in adults. *UpToDate*. August 14, 2012.

CHAPTER 10—NERVOUS SYSTEM DISORDERS

Barton ED, Adams JG, Collings J, et al, eds. *Emergency Medicine*. Philadelphia, PA: Saunders; 2008.

Bird SJ. Clinical manifestations of myasthenia gravis. In: Shefner JM, ed. *UpToDate*. Waltham, MA: UpToDate; 2013.

Cline DM, Tintinalli JE, Stapczynski JS, et al, eds. *Tintinalli's Emergency Medicine Manual*. 7th ed. New York, NY: McGraw Hill; 2012.

Eisen A. Anatomy and localization of spinal cord disorders. In: Basow DS, ed. *UpToDate*. Waltham, MA: UpToDate; 2013.

Francis J, Young GB. Diagnosis of delirium and confusional states. In: Basow DS, ed. *UpToDate*. Waltham, MA: UpToDate; 2013.

Furman JM, Barton JJS. Approach to the patient with vertigo. In: Basow DS, ed. *UpToDate*. Waltham, MA: UpToDate; 2013.

Furman JM. Pathophysiology, etiology, and differential diagnosis of vertigo. In: Basow DS, ed. *UpToDate*. Waltham, MA: UpToDate; 2013.

Kattah JC, Talkad AV, Wang DZ, et al. HINTS to diagnose stroke in the acute vestibular syndrome: three-step bedside oculomotor examination more sensitive than early MRI diffusion-weighted imaging. *Stroke*. 2009;40:3504–3510. doi: 10.1161/STROKEAHA.109.551234.

Lowenstein DH. Seizures and epilepsy. In: Fauci AS, Kasper DL, Longo DL, et al, eds. *Harrison's Principles of Internal Medicine*. 17th ed. New York, NY: McGraw-Hill; 2008.

Mahadevan SV, Garmel GM. *An Introduction to Clinical Emergency Medicine*. 2nd ed. New York, NY: Cambridge University Press; 2012.

McPhee S, Tierney L, Papadakis M, eds. *Current Medical Diagnosis and Treatment*. New York, NY: McGraw Hill; 2010.

O'Connell CB, Zarbock SF, eds. *A Comprehensive Review for the Certification and Recertification Examinations for Physician Assistants*. 4th ed. Baltimore, MD: Lippincott Williams & Wilkins; 2010.

Press D, Alexander M. Treatment of dementia. In: Basow DS, ed. *UpToDate*. Waltham, MA: UpToDate; 2013.

Shadlen M. Evaluation of cognitive impairment and dementia. In: Basow DS, ed. *UpToDate*. Waltham, MA: UpToDate; 2013.

Stecker M. Status epilepticus in adults. In: Pedley PA, ed. Waltham, MA: UpToDate; 2013.

Vriesendorp FJ. Clinical features and diagnosis of Guillain-Barre syndrome in adults: In: Shefner FM, ed. *UpToDate*. Waltham, MA: UpToDate; 2013.

CHAPTER 11—OBSTETRICS AND GYNECOLOGY

Ananth CV, Kinzler WL. Placental abruption: clinical features and diagnosis. In: Basow DS, ed. *UpToDate*. Waltham, MA: UpToDate; 2013.

August P, Sibai BM. Preeclampsia: clinical features and diagnosis. In: Basow DS, ed. *UpToDate*. Waltham, MA: UpToDate; 2013.

Birnbaumer DM, Anderegg C. Sexually transmitted diseases. In: Marx JA, Hockberger RS, Walls RM, et al, eds. *Rosen's Emergency Medicine: Concepts and Clinical Practice*. 7th ed. Philadelphia, PA: Mosby Elsevier; 2010:1282–1296.

Chen KT. Endometritis unrelated to pregnancy. In: Basow DS, ed. *UpToDate*. Waltham, MA: UpToDate; 2013.

Chen KT. Postpartum endometritis. In: Basow DS, ed. *UpToDate*. Waltham, MA: UpToDate; 2013.

Dixon JM. Lactational mastitis. In: Basow DS, ed. *UpToDate*. Waltham, MA: UpToDate; 2013.

Dixon JM. Mastitis and other skin disorders of the breast. In: Basow DS, ed. *UpToDate*. Waltham, MA: UpToDate; 2013.

Fuller SS. Emergencies during pregnancy and the postpartum period. In: Ma OJ, Cline D, Tintinalli J, et al, eds. *Emergency Medicine Manual*. 6th. New York, NY: McGraw-Hill; 2004:294–298.

Growdon WB, Laufer MR. Ovarian and fallopian tube torsion. In: Basow DS, ed. *UpToDate*. Waltham, MA: UpToDate; 2013.

Houry DE, Salhi BA. Acute complications of pregnancy. In: Marx JA, Hockberger RS, Walls RM, et al, eds. *Rosen's Emergency Medicine: Concepts and Clinical Practice*. Philadelphia, PA: Mosby Elsevier; 2010:2279–2297.

Lockwood CJ, Russo-Stieglitz K. Clinical features, diagnosis and course of placenta previa. In: Basow DS, ed. *UpToDate*. Waltham, MA: UpToDate; 2013.

Marrazzo J. Acute cervicitis. In: Basow DS, ed. *UpToDate*. Waltham, MA: UpToDate; 2013.

Muto MG. Approach to the patient with an adnexal mass. In: Basow DS, ed. *UpToDate*. Waltham, MA: UpToDate; 2013.

Norwitz ER, Repke JT, Preeclampsia: management and prognosis. In: Basow DS, ed. *UpToDate*. Waltham, MA: UpToDate; 2013.

Oyelese Y, Ananth CV. Placental abruption: management. In: Basow DS, ed. *UpToDate*. Waltham, MA: UpToDate; 2013.

Sibai BM. HELLP syndrome. In: Basow DS, ed. *UpToDate*. Waltham, MA: UpToDate; 2013.

Tibbles CD. Selected gynecologic disorders. In: Marx JA, Hockberger RS, Walls RM, et al, eds. *Rosen's Emergency Medicine: Concepts and Clinical Practice*. 7th ed. Philadelphia, PA: Mosby Elsevier; 2010:1325–1332.

Wiesenfeld HC. Treatment of pelvic inflammatory disease. In: Basow DS, ed. *UpToDate*. Waltham, MA: UpToDate; 2013.

CHAPTER 12—PSYCHOBEHAVIORAL DISORDERS

Augustyn M. Diagnosis of austism spectrum disorder. *UpToDate*. February 14, 2014.

Bechtle K, Bennett BL. Evaluation of sexual abuse in children and adolescents. *UpToDate*. February 14, 2014.

Bernstein DA, Penner LA, Clark-Stewart A, et al. *Psychology*. 7th ed. Boston, MA: Houghton Mifflin Company; 2006.

Block S. Grief and bereavement. *UpToDate*. February 14, 2014.

Dyer CB, Halphen JM. Elder mistreatment: abuse, neglect and financial exploitation. *UpToDate*. February 14, 2014.

Fauci AS, Braunwald E, Kasper DL, et al. *Harrison's Manual of Medicine*. 17th ed. New York, NY: McGraw-Hill; 2009.

O'Connell CB, Zarbock SF. *A Comprehensive Review for the Certification and Recertification Examinations for Physician Assistants*. 4th ed. Philadelphia, PA: Lippincott Williams & Wilkins.

Searight HR, Burke JM. Adult attention deficit hyperactivity disorder. *UpToDate*. February 14, 2014.

Silk KR. Personality disorders. *UpToDate*. February 14, 2014.

Weil A. Intimate partner violence: intervention and patient management. *UpToDate*. February 14, 2014.

CHAPTER 13—PULMONARY DISORDERS

Auth P, Kerstein M, eds. *Physician Assistant Review*. 4th ed. Philadelphia, PA: Lippincott Williams and Wilkins; 2013.

Bartlett JG, Sethi S. Management of infection in acute exacerbations of chronic obstructive pulmonary disease. In: Sexton DJ ed. *UpToDate*. Waltham, MA: UpToDate; 2013.

King TE. Approach to the adult with interstitial lung disease: clinical evaluation. In: Flaherty KR, Hollingsworth H, eds. *UpToDate*. Waltham, MA: UpToDate; 2013.

Kleinschmidt P. Chronic obstructive pulmonary disease and emphysema in emergency medicine. In: Brenner BE, ed. *Medscape Reference*. Updated September 17, 2012.

Komanapalli CB, Sukumar MS. Thoracoscopic decortication. *The Cardiothoracic Surgery Network*. December 13, 2011. Accessed July 11, 2013.

Light R. Primary spontaneous pneumothorax in adults. In: Basow DS, ed. *UpToDate*. Waltham, MA: UpToDate; 2013.

Light R. Secondary spontaneous pneumothorax in adults. In: Basow DS, ed. *UpToDate*. Waltham, MA: UpToDate; 2013.

National Heart, Lung, and Blood Institute. "What is Sleep Apnea?" *Department of Health and Human Services*. Updated July 10, 2012. Accessed July 15, 2013.

Oulette DR. Pulmonay embolism. *Medscape Reference*. July 19, 2013. WebMD LLC. Accessed July 20, 2013.

Strohl KP. Overview of obstructive sleep apnea in adults. In: Basow DS, ed. *UpToDate*. Waltham, MA: UpToDate; 2013.

Tintinalli JE, Stapczynski J, Ma O, et al, eds. *Tintinalli's Emergency Medicine Manual*. 7th ed. New York, NY: McGraw Hill; 2011.

Wells AU, Hirani N. Interstitial lung disease guideline: the British Thoracic Society in collaboration with the Thoracic Society of Australia and New Zealand and the Irish Thoracic Society. *Thorax*. 2008, 63:v1.

CHAPTER 14—RENAL AND UROGENITAL DISORDERS

Curhan G, Aronson M, Preminger G. Diagnosis and Acute Management of Suspected Nephrolithiasis in Adults. *UpToDate*. July 1, 2013.

Hooton T. Acute complicated cystitis and pyelonephritis. *UpToDate*. In: Woods W, Young J, Just S, eds. *Emergency Medicine Recall* Baltimore, MD: Lippincott Williams & Wilkins; 2000.. October 5, 2012.

Meyrier A. Renal and perinephric abscess. *UpToDate*. November 19, 2012.

Preminger G. Management of ureteral calculi. *UpToDate*. March 19, 2013.

Sena A, Cohen M, Swygard H. Epididymitis, Treatment of uncomplicated gonococcal infections, Treatment of uncomplicated Chlamydia trachomatis infections. In: Baslow DS, ed. *UpToDate*. Waltham, MA: UpToDate; 2013.

Tintinalli J, Kelen G, Stapczymski J, eds. *Emergency Medicine A Comprehensive Study Guide*. New York, NY: McGraw-Hill; 2004.

CHAPTER 15—SYSTEMIC INFECTIOUS DISORDERS

Advisory Committee on Immunization Practices. Use of a reduced (4-dose) vaccine schedule for post-exposure prophylaxis to prevent human rabies. *MMWR*. 2010;59(RR-2):1–9. July 11, 2013.

Advisory Committee on Immunization Practices. Updated recommendations for use of tetanus tpxoid, reduced diptheria toxoid, and acellular pertussis vaccine (Tdap) in pregnant women—Advisory Committee on Immunization Practices (ACIP), 2012. *MMWR*. 2013;62(7):131–5.

Ahmed S. Schistosomiasis. *Medscape Reference*. http://emedicine.medscape.com/article/228392-overview. March 1, 2013.

Al-Nassir W. Brucellosis. *Medscape Reference*. http://emedicine.medscape.com/article/213430-overview. February 28, 2013.

Arnold L. Trichinellosis/trichinosis. *Medscape Reference*. http://emedicine.medscape.com/article/787591-overview. September 19, 2012.

Bennett N. HIV disease. *Medscape Reference*. http://emedicine.medscape.com/article/211316-overview. July 15, 2013.

Chandrasekar P. Strongyloidiasis. *Medscape Reference*. http://emedicine.medscape.com/article/229312-overview. March 8, 2013.

Cleveland K. Tularemia. *Medscape Reference*. http://emedicine.medscape.com/article/230923-overview. June 13, 2013.

Cunha B. Bacterial sepsis. *Medscape Reference*. http://emedicine.medscape.com/article/234587-overview. July 13, 2012.

Cunha B. Ehrlichiosis. *Medscape Reference*. http://emedicine.medscape.com/article/235839-overview. February 15, 2013.

Cunha B. Rocky Mountain Spotted Fever. *Medscape Reference*. http://emedicine.medscape.com/article/228042-overview. January 31, 2013.

Cunha B. West Nile Encephalitis. *Medscape Reference*. http://emedicine.medscape.com/article/234009-overview. February 6, 2013.

Cunha B. Babesiosis. *Medscape Reference*. http://emedicine.medscape.com/article/212605-overview. April 30, 2012.

Fernandez-Frackelton M. Bacteria. In: Marx JA, Hockberger RS, Walls RM, et al, eds. *Rosen's Emergency Medicine*. 7th ed. Philadelphia, PA: Mosby Elsevier; 2010:1681–6.

Godwin J. Neutropenia. *Medscape Reference*. http://emedicine.medscape.com/article/204821-overview. July 3, 2013.

Gompf S. Rabies. *Medscape Reference*. http://emedicine.medscape.com/article/220967-overview. May 16, 2013.

Haburchak D. Ascariasis. *Medscape Reference*. http://emedicine.medscape.com/article/212510-overview. November 21, 2011

Huh S. Pinworm. *Medscape Reference*. http://emedicine.medscape.com/article/225652-overview. October 26, 2012.

Lacasse A. Amebiasis. *Medscape Reference*. http://emedicine.medscape.com/article/212029-overview. May 1, 2013.

Meyerhoff J. Lyme disease. *Medscape Reference*. http://emedicine.medscape.com/article/330178-overview. May 16, 2013.

Nadel ES, ed. *Blueprints Emergency Medicine*. 2nd ed. Baltimore, MD: Lippincott Williams & Wilkens; 2006:90–92.

Nandalur M. Eastern equine encephalitis. *Medscape Reference*. http://emedicine.medscape.com/article/233442-overview. July 19, 2013.

Nazer H. Giardiasis. *Medscape Reference*. http://emedicine.medscape.com/article/176718-overview. January 3, 2013.

Schwartz R. Cutaneous Manifestations of HIV. *Medscape Reference*. http://emedicine.medscape.com/article/1133746-overview. March 21, 2013.

Sexton D. Immune Reconstitution Inflammatory Syndrome. *UpToDate*. http://www.uptodate.com/contents/immune-reconstitution-inflammatory-syndrome. March 22, 2013.

Tam A. Hookworm in emergency medicine. *Medscape Reference*. http://emedicine.medscape.com/article/788488-overview. September 27, 2012.

Thaker V. Cholera. *Medscape Reference*. http://emedicine.medscape.com/article/962643-overview. July 19, 2011.

Tolan R. Taenia Infection. *Medscape Reference*. http://emedicine.medscape.com/article/999727-overview. April 12, 2013.

Tolan R. Trypanosomiasis. *Medscape Reference*. http://emedicine.medscape.com/article/1000389-overview. April 12, 2013.

Tolan R. Whipworm. *Medscape Reference*. http://emedicine.medscape.com/article/1000631-overview. April 12, 2013.

Weber EJ, Ramanujam P. Rabies. In: Marx JA, Hockberger RS, Walls RM, et al, eds. *Rosen's Emergency Medicine*. 7th ed. Philadelphia, PA: Mosby Elsevier; 2010:1723–31.

CHAPTER 16—TOXICOLOGY DISORDERS

Ayala C, Brad S. *Boards and Wards*. 2nd ed. Malden, MA: Blackwell; 2003.

The Faculty, Staff and Associates of the California Poison Control System. *Poisoning & Drug Overdose*. 5th ed. New York, NY: Lange Medical Books/McGraw-Hill; 2007.

CHAPTER 17—TRAUMATIC DISORDERS

Andreoli CM, Gardiner MF. Traumatic hyphema: clinical features and management. In: Basow DS, ed. *UpToDate*. Waltham, MA: UpToDate; 2013.

Bloom J. Metacarpal neck fractures. In: Basow DS, ed. *UpToDate*. Waltham, MA: UpToDate; 2013.

Bulger EM. Inpatient management of traumatic rib fractures. In: Basow DS, ed. *UpToDate*. Waltham, MA: UpToDate; 2013.

deWeber K. Scaphoid fractures. In: Basow DS, ed. *UpToDate*. Waltham, MA: UpToDate; 2013.

Fiechtl J. Pelvic trauma: initial evaluation and management. In: Basow DS, ed. *UpToDate*. Waltham, MA: UpToDate; 2013.

Hammerberg E, Stracciolini A. Acute compartment syndrome of the extremities. In: Basow DS, ed. *UpToDate*. Waltham, MA: UpToDate; 2013.

Harrison A. Approach to the adult with epistaxis. In: Basow DS, ed. *UpToDate*. Waltham, MA: UpToDate; 2013.

Heegaard W, Biros M. Skull fractures in adults. In: Basow DS, ed. *UpToDate*. Waltham, MA: UpToDate; 2013.

Karlson KA. Initial evaluation and management of rib fracture. In: Basow DS, ed. *UpToDate*. Waltham, MA: UpToDate; 2013.

Light R. Primary spontaneous pneumothorax in adults. In: Basow DS, ed. *UpToDate*. Waltham, MA: UpToDate; 2013.

Light R. Secondary spontaneous pneumothorax in adults. In: Basow DS, ed. *UpToDate*. Waltham, MA: UpToDate; 2013.

Mayersak RJ. Facial trauma in adults. In: Basow DS, ed. *UpToDate*. Waltham, MA: UpToDate; 2013.

Petron D. Distal radius fractures in adults. In: Basow DS, ed. *UpToDate*. Waltham, MA: UpToDate; 2013.

Schaider J, Sherman S. Shoulder dislocation and reduction. In: Basow DS, ed. *UpToDate*. Waltham, MA: UpToDate; 2013.

Schmitt S. Treatment and prevention of osteomyelitis following trauma. In: Basow DS, ed. *UpToDate*. Waltham, MA: UpToDate; 2013.

Slabaugh M. Radial head and neck fractures in adults. In: Basow DS, ed. *UpToDate*. Waltham, MA: UpToDate; 2013.

CHAPTER 18—PROCEDURES AND SKILLS

Adams JG, Barton ED, Collings J, et al, eds. *Emergency Medicine: Clinical Essentials*. 2nd ed. Philadelphia, PA: Elsevier; 2008.

Doeken P. Placement and management of thoracostomy tubes. In: Basow DS, ed. *UpToDate*. Waltham, MA: UpToDate; 2013.

CHAPTER 19—OTHER COMPONENTS

Agrawal P, LeMaster C, Narayan K, et al. *Pocket Emergency Medicine*. 2nd ed. Philadelphia, PA: Wolters Kluwer; 2011.

Stead L, Stead S, Kaufman M. *First Aid for the Emergency Medicine Clerkship*. 2nd ed. New York, NY: The McGraw-Hill Companies, Inc; 2006.

Index